Your Body, Your Diet

Your Body, Your Diet

A Complete Program for Losing Weight, Boosting Energy, and Being Your Best Self

Elizabeth Dane, Ph.D.

BALLANTINE BOOKS • NEW YORK

A Ballantine Book
Published by The Ballantine Publishing Group
Copyright © 2001 by Elizabeth Dane, Ph.D.
Foreword copyright © 2001 by Ann Reinking

www.randomhouse.com/BB/

Library of Congress Cataloging-in-Publication Data
Dane, Elizabeth.
Your body, your diet : a complete program for losing weight, boosting energy, and being your best self /
Elizabeth Dane.— 1st ed.
       p.   cm.
   1. Nutrition.   2. Reducing diets.   3. Health.   4. Weight loss.   I. Title.
RA784 .D36 2001
613.7—dc21   2001018414

ISBN 0-345-43322-X

Manufactured in the United States of America

First Edition: July 2001

10 9 8 7 6 5 4 3 2 1

Book design by H. Roberts Design

To my three sons,
Randall, David, and Thomas

Contents

Acknowledgments

Individuals never accomplish the completion of endeavors, projects, or books by themselves. It takes a wide range of experiences and people to cull the lessons to be learned for one's self and to help others. We all are mirrors of each other. When we can see ourselves through the eyes and events of others, we have truly been given the gift of knowledge and self-exploration guiding us further along our path of evolution.

In this way, I have been greatly blessed, and it's now my turn to thank all those who have lighted my way in the creation of this book. First and foremost, to all of my clients in the United States, Great Britain, Europe, and India, I give you my deepest honor and gratitude; without you, this book would never exist. David: without all your encouragement, love, patience, and support, I would certainly have faltered along this journey.

To my wonderful agent, Barbara Lowenstein, I owe a debt of gratitude for spotting me in a magazine article, believing I had a book in me, and diligently working with me to hone the book's first concept. To a *great* editor: Leona Nevler who patiently guided me step-by-step until the finished product was realized. Heartfelt thanks to Carolyn Fireside who helped formulate the book's first concept, and to Sherri Crute for bringing life, form, and color to the pages. To Joy Cook: my profound thanks for her brilliant expertise and dedication in finalizing the writing of this book. My deep appreciation also goes to a fantastic copy editor, Sue Cohan, who really tied up all the "loose ends" and made it flow.

A very special thanks and acknowledgment goes to computer whiz David Muravez, whose magical skills with computers and computer art brought my thoughts into form—at all times of the day and night—and weekends! Particular gratitude is given to Frank Abdale, a gifted genius of foods and food preparation, who helped formulate and execute the *delicious* menus and recipes. Also many thanks go to Runcie Tatnall for the yogic and exercise illustrations.

Last, but not least, special thanks goes to Claire Ferraro, Jerry Croghan, Sandy Goldsmith, Helen Bransford, Carol Caldwell, Lester Hoffman, Laurie Weitzner, Christine Mirante, Janet Higgins, and many other friends and colleagues, too numerous to mention, who have helped and inspired me along the way.

Foreword

I was fortunate enough to discover Dr. Elizabeth Dane through my good friend and costar in the Broadway musical *Chicago*, Bebe Neuwirth. Now as anybody can see, Bebe Neuwirth does not need to lose weight, and at that time neither did I. My problem was that I had a virus that I just could not kick, and it was sapping absolutely all of my energy. Since I'm a dancer and an actress, that was the last thing I needed.

My name is Ann Reinking, and when Elizabeth Dane came to my rescue, I was working hard to get ready to open in *Chicago* while struggling with my health. Elizabeth helped me to get over the virus and get my energy back—and I was feeling just wonderful, for a while.

After the great success of *Chicago* on Broadway, however, it was time to take the show on the road. After a few weeks of airplane food, hotel food, crazy travel schedules, and jet lag, I was eating the wrong foods— giving in to my passion for high-fat snacks—and putting on weight. I looked great in street clothes (especially for a forty-eight-year-old mom), but carrying around an extra twenty pounds, when I had to wear revealing dancer's costumes every night, was definitely a problem.

I went back to Dr. Dane for help. On her diet plan I lost the first ten pounds very quickly, then the next ten began to come off. But it wasn't just the weight: I was sleeping better, I had more energy, and I had a much easier time recovering from jet lag. My skin got better. Even my eyes sparkled. The results were dramatic!

I also found the plan easy to follow because I was never hungry. The diet is so balanced, I always had plenty of good food to eat. I never even craved a giant hamburger, dripping with cheese (one of my former personal favorites). After a while I started saying to myself, "Well, wouldn't a bowl of asparagus be nice." I even learned to find healthy food in hotels.

These days I cheat on my plan a little bit—but not much. Because I find that when I do eat the wrong foods, I just don't feel very good afterward. Since my success on the plan, I've recommended a dear friend, my publicist, and my choreographer to Elizabeth. They all lost weight and ended up looking and feeling great. And as for me, the rigors of the road aside, I intend to stick with the plan and my healthy new lifestyle.

Ann Reinking

Part one

It's All about Your Metabolic Type

As an Alternative Health Care practitioner, I've learned that no one system, Eastern or Western, has all the answers to weight loss and health. Used together, however, their combined wisdom reveals healing techniques and approaches to health that can benefit everyone, whether the problem is weight control, anxiety, or physical illness. *Your Body, Your Diet* contains a powerful amount of knowledge culled from both Chinese and Western philosophies that will allow you for the first time to devise a *customized* weight-loss program—designed for you and you alone.

Uncontrollable weight gain—and loss—are symptoms of a deeper and more profound physical, emotional, and even spiritual change, but they are the symptoms that cause people to sit up and take notice that something is amiss. This means that by the time they become *visually* aware that they're putting on pounds, they're already in trouble. It is only then that they realize they haven't been feeling so well for the past few months; they've been catching a lot of colds; and they've been agitated or in the dumps. Women most likely have had uncomfortable periods and men may have lost their sex drive. Both men and women probably feel sluggish, may have lost their zest for life, or conversely have become so driven in their work that they've neglected the rest of their lives as the pounds keep piling on.

Let me repeat, the weight disorder is only a symptom. The primary problem is *metabolic imbalance*. In the following chapters of *Your Body, Your Diet*, you'll learn how this imbalance can be triggered by a variety of causes: physical or emotional stress; the power of the stress response; improper eating, especially of junk and processed foods; a burned-out modus operandi, in which rest becomes a luxury; dependence on alcohol, nicotine, sugar, or drugs (over-the-counter or prescribed); not enough or too much exercise; an overly sedentary or an excessively hyperactive lifestyle, which in turn can produce lethargy, depression, and weight gain—or fatigue, anxiety, and an abrupt weight shift up or down.

It might also interest you to know that metabolic imbalance can cause premature aging—and that correcting the imbalance can help turn back the clock, giving you a more youthful appearance—and outlook—to stay forever young.

1 Becoming a Great New You

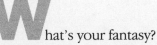hat's your fantasy?

Would you like to achieve your best weight and maintain it indefinitely with a diet and exercise regimen designed specifically for your body and your needs?

To do it all without horrible hunger pangs or killer cravings?

To protect yourself against the ravages of stress, aging, and disease—and learn exactly how not to get sick?

To maintain optimal energy and wellness for a lifetime—and never look your age?

To develop remarkable healing powers over your body, mind, emotions, and spirit (which is, of course, the key to it all)?

If you answer "yes" to even one of these questions, then my specialized weight-loss and regeneration program can help you turn your goals into reality. I'm Elizabeth Dane, O.M.D. and Ph.D. I'm a nutritionist and specialist in Eastern medicine who has learned, through years of experience solving my own health and weight problems and those of countless clients, that my unique plan can produce great results for anyone.

How can I be so sure? I'm not dealing in magic potions or secret elixirs. The Your Body, Your Diet system is based on a special recipe for success that I've developed. I've bridged two worlds, combining the concepts that have guided practitioners of Chinese medicine for thousands of years with the latest findings of Western medical science to create a weight-loss lifestyle strategy that is personalized for you. Just as we've learned that yoga and aerobics are both valuable, so is this East-West metabolic blend.

That's the key to it all—your metabolism. It's not just burning or storing fat. It's how you use it for quick bursts of energy and strength and how you calm, restore, and rejuvenate yourself to handle stress, avoid burnout or depression, and slow the aging process. Remember that playground seesaw? Balance is the name of the game here as well.

I'll show you how your cravings are the symptom, not the source, of your problem. How opposites really do attract. Why the very foods you've looked on as "comfort foods"—whether bread, cookies, or even lean steak or turkey—are likely to be most damaging to your body's unique metabolic needs. You'll see why, given your type, certain foods could even be causing unwanted facial hair or coarse skin. And you'll learn how your metabolic balance can affect your emotional health as well.

There are also some quick fixes. Find out how fresh juices, lemons, cranberries, and a blend of Eastern medicine's herbs and teas, along with a customized blend of vitamins and supplements, can jump-start your metabolic makeover. They will help you keep on track as you shed the sugar and caffeine and eat your way back to a balanced body. There are even "cheat" items for your special metabolism that can help you get through the tough times without tumbling off the wagon.

So forget calorie counting. It's not just your waistline or hips at stake here; it's the glow of your skin, the gleam in your eyes, the zest for living and loving. As you read this chapter, you will see that there's a great deal more to how and why your body holds on to those extra pounds than the fact that you can't keep your hands off your favorite snacks and desserts. But first, let me introduce you to one of my clients—Vicky. Her story will give you a firsthand look at why a tailor-made weight-loss plan, based on these ideas, can be so successful.

Vicky, forty-two, is a dynamic account executive at a major New York–based advertising agency, and she is great at her job. All her life she's had boundless energy and could eat practically anything she wanted without gaining a pound. She could also guzzle countless cups of coffee without getting wired and was also the only person in her office who never got the flu. Vicky came to me when her body began to change. She thought it might have been job pressure or the stress of juggling her career with being a wife and mom. Perhaps it was even her age.

Whatever the reasons, Vicky had begun catching bad colds all the time and feeling constantly exhausted and edgy. And even though she swore she was not necessarily eating more, she was putting on weight around her middle. With the specter of middle age looming, she decided to take action. She worked out five days a week at the gym with a personal trainer and religiously followed a popular low-carbohydrate, high-protein diet plan. But neither the exercise nor the weight-loss program made much of a difference. Then she really got frustrated because she and a coworker, Amanda, had embarked on the plan together, and Amanda was losing tons of weight.

Amanda, thirty-five, is a copywriter at the agency where Vicky works. The even bigger surprise is that Amanda was the type of person who constantly complained of being exhausted and depressed, and she was living with the fact that anything she ate (too often starches and sweets) landed directly on her hips and thighs. After trying an exercise regimen and the low-carbohydrate, high-protein plan (which cuts out virtually all starches and sweets), she's got more energy, she's in better spirits, and for six months she has kept off the twenty pounds she lost with minimal effort. For the first time she has no cause to complain about her ever-expanding hips and thighs.

Two women, one weight-loss plan. For one the low-carbohydrate, high-protein plan has been a major-league disappointment. For the other it's been virtually a miracle. How can we account for this mysterious disparity? It's no mystery—it's metabolism.

What works for Amanda doesn't work for Vicky because they are different metabolic types: Vicky has a classic fast metabolism. She's what I call an *accelerator*. Amanda, however, has a classic slow metabolism. She's a *synthesizer*.

Think about it. Two different metabolic types with one diet program just doesn't compute. The last thing accelerator Vicky's high-acid system needs is protein, whereas it's precisely what synthesizer Amanda's high-alkaline system must have to jump-start it back to balance.

Vicky's system requires a high-carbohydrate diet program to get her to where she wants to be. Amanda, on the other hand, could eat a high-carbohydrate diet forever and still not see results. In fact, it's a matter of apples (the basic shape of the overweight accelerator's body) and avocados (the basic shape of the overweight synthesizer's body).

The idea behind my Your Body, Your Diet system is to help you determine whether you're basically an accelerator or a synthesizer—or one of the variations of these two basic types—and provide you with a weight-loss program designed specifically for your metabolism. The key to the plan is that it has a special place for every metabolic type.

Overweight: Problem or Symptom?

How important is metabolism when it comes to weight and health? It's critical—which is why being overweight is just one symptom that tells you that your metabolic system is out of balance. Understanding your personal metabolic equation and working to balance it is what makes the Your Body, Your Diet plan so effective and unique.

Simply put, the low-carbohydrate, high-protein diet approach to weight loss is based solely on Western medical philosophy and limits its weight-loss regimen to the body. The entire concept is: if you're overweight, you're eating too many carbohydrates—period. If, however, you take a broader view of how the body works and include the principles of Eastern medicine—as I do in my work—you will discover that maintaining your optimum weight and achieving general well-being mean focusing on emotional and psychological concerns as well. Your body, mind, feelings, and belief systems all work together.

To Eastern-oriented physicians, overweight is not merely a hormonal or physical matter, since emotions and thought patterns are involved. It's not just psychological either. Our genetic predisposition is too strong to make it only an addiction. Finally, overweight can't be looked at as simply a situational problem (the "underloved, overfed" theory). It is a strong brew of physical (genetic), emotional, and spiritual elements.

So forget about your guilt and remorse. Controlling your weight is not just a matter of lack of self-control; it's a complex problem, which can be solved with surprising ease if you just learn to work with your mind and body. Weight problems reflect mental, emotional, spiritual, and physical imbalance and are magnified by stress.

All four of these aspects must be addressed, balanced, and nurtured for you to shed pounds while dealing with the additional pressures that customarily accompany dieting. That's why my unique plan is not only a chance to lose weight; it's an opportunity to achieve a happier and healthier body, mind, and spirit. Best of all, your body will work *with* you, not against you. That's because the body's most powerful drive is for regeneration—and this cell renewal, undoing the damage, is one of the important benefits you get from my Your Body, Your Diet approach.

Now even if you ate perfectly—all fresh foods, balanced for your metabolic requirements—you would still need help, especially when getting started on your new lifestyle and coping with new stresses. That's where vitamins and supplements come in. They provide a way to ensure that you have all the essentials for your body's chemistry as it boosts the fat-burning, cell-renewing campaign. Once you're in balance, you may not need that help on a daily basis. It's all designed to keep you in harmony as you re-build a happier, thinner, more energetic self.

Your Body, Your Diet is the result of my experiences working with clients as diverse as Broadway stars Bebe Neuwirth and Stockard Channing, actress Anjelica Huston, and singers James Taylor and Carly Simon—as well as dancers, carpenters, and others from all walks of life who balance the energy demands of hectic lives.

Metabolism and Weight Loss

Jennifer, a.k.a. "String Bean" to her friends, has always been in top physical shape and never had to worry about how much she ate. Now suddenly she can't keep her hands off the cookies and candy, and her new jeans are getting tight in the waist.

Melanie eats like a bird and puts in half an hour on the treadmill every day, yet she still finds keeping weight off her hips and thighs a terrible struggle.

Kevin follows a healthy diet augmented with vitamin and mineral supplements, but his allergies keep getting worse and worse, and at only twenty-five he's beginning to develop his father's spare tire around his middle.

Like Vicky and Amanda, Jennifer, Melanie, and Kevin are having trouble with their weight. But keep in mind that uncontrollable weight gain is only the symptom. The real problem behind their extra pounds is metabolic imbalance.

What Makes Your Metabolism Tick

The metabolic process is one of the ways, along with breathing, that our bodies produce all the types of energy we need to get through life.

This process is the sum of all the physical and chemical changes that take place in our bodies and all the transformations that occur within our cells. (*Metabolism,* in fact, comes from a Greek word meaning "state of change.") These transformations include the changes we naturally undergo during all our life stages (growth, maturity, and old age) that allow rest, repair, and regeneration. And on a more basic level, they control processes like the way we access energy from our food, how efficiently we burn calories, and how much get-up-and-go we have to work with when we start the day.

Your *personal* metabolic profile explains the unique ways in which *your* body breaks down food (and other ingested substances) into micronutrients—to be utilized for either tissue repair, cell regeneration, or energy.

Now those of you who've taken even the most elementary biology classes in school will probably say, "Come on now, it's common knowledge that everybody needs the same nutrients and breaks down and utilizes food in the same way. Did you forget we're all supposed to eat our way through the good old five food groups?"

Not true. Even though Western medicine employs some of the most advanced diagnostic techniques in the world, the body's abilities and processes, to a great extent, still remain a mystery. Yes, we do know a lot—but not enough to master easy, effective, long-lasting weight loss without paying attention to metabolism.

Achieving Balance

To understand how my Your Body, Your Diet plan teaches your metabolism to run like a well-honed machine, look at the forces that drive that metabolism. We'll begin in the East. Eastern philosophy teaches that the universe and the human body are composed of both male and female energy united as one. Male energy, as you may know, is referred to as *yang* and female energy as *yin*. Yin and yang are opposing forces, but they cannot exist without each other. Both forms of energy coexist in each of us.

According to this principle, Eastern philosophy regards every individual as operating according to his or her unique yin/yang balance—and that balance controls a large part of the workings of each person's metabolism. We each have our own specific nutritional requirements that guide the ways we break down our food—for tissue repair, cell regeneration, and energy.

Some people have stronger *yin-based energy*, and their metabolism is dominated by the need to rejuvenate or facilitate cell regeneration. These are people like Amanda, and I refer to them as synthesizers. The synthesizer represents one end of this spectrum of metabolic types.

Others carry primarily *yang-based energy*, with a metabolism dominated by the need to produce and utilize energy very quickly. These are people like Vicky, whom I call accelerators. They are the complete opposite of synthesizers.

This is why synthesizer vegetarians can seem sickly and weak, while accelerators on the same diet are robust and healthy—and why synthesizers who consume a steak a day remain in excellent physical shape, while accelerators on such a diet would suffer a cholesterol "blowout." It's also why fad diets work for a select group of people but definitely not for everyone.

Even if you are not a typical accelerator or synthesizer, your metabolism still carries many of the characteristics of the two types, and I promise that you will find yourself in the pages that follow.

Yin and yang affect your metabolism in two ways. The first type of action is the yin, or female, aspect. This is the process of synthesizing, assimilating, and building up your powers to regenerate. This phase sets the stage for the periods of rest that the body uses to repair itself. The other type of action represents the yang, or masculine, aspect. This includes all the processes that produce and expend energy and break down substances such as food, air, or water into the simplest components of pure energy.

Now let's see what we can learn from the West. Western medical science long ago revealed that our metabolisms were also driven by the nervous system. And much like the forces of yin and yang, it is divided into two parts—the central nervous system and the autonomic nervous system. The autonomic nervous system controls our metabolic processes and is divided into two parts—the parasympathetic and sympathetic.

The parasympathetic nervous system is responsible for keeping our bodies running smoothly. It's the source of the rhythm behind our breathing, the regularity of our heartbeat, the efficiency of our digestion, and many other everyday miracles. This part provides balance and stability. It helps us slow down, chill out, rest, and rejuvenate.

The sympathetic nervous system keeps us poised for action; it prepares the body for the activities of life. It gives us the ability to expend energy in situations that call for engaging in strenuous physical activity or enduring emotional stress and in emergencies that call for the body's "fight-or-flight" response. It speeds us up, moves us forward, and makes sure we get things done.

Much like the forces of yin and yang, these two interdependent parts of the autonomic nervous system are synchronized to work together. Impulses from one set of nerve fibers activate, while impulses from the other set inhibit. Again, the idea here is to create and maintain balance—the key to a slim, trim physique and good health.

As we bring together the philosophies of the Eastern and Western worlds about the way the body works, you can see how everyone is, to some degree, dominated by either parasympathetic/yin activity or sympathetic/yang activity.

The parasympathetic/yin metabolic profile is known as the synthesizer and is driven by the body's need to rest and regenerate.

The sympathetic/yang metabolic profile is known as the accelerator and is driven by the body's need to energize.

All of the metabolic types (or meta-types, as I call them) are based in these two master meta-types—the accelerator and the synthesizer.

This book addresses the six most common meta-types: the accelerator, the balanced accelerator, and the mixed accelerator; the synthesizer, the balanced synthesizer, and the mixed synthesizer.

Can you pinpoint your type? To help you along, let's return to the three examples I cited earlier:

Jennifer—the former "string bean" who is suddenly gaining weight from foods that aren't doing her body, mind, or emotions any good at all—used to be a well-balanced accelerator. However, extra stress from a high-pressure job, the breakup of a serious long-term romantic relationship, and an overly taxing social life designed to compensate for the loss of a steady love interest are forcing her metabolism way out of harmony. Fortunately the right diet for her meta-type can get her back on track.

Melanie—the perpetual dieter and exerciser who still can't keep the weight off her hips and thighs—is a synthesizer. What Melanie has yet to learn is that she may be eating too little of the food combinations she needs (since undernourishment also can be a cause of weight gain). She isn't availing herself of the vitamins, minerals, and herbs that can help speed up her metabolism healthily, and she might not even be doing the kinds of exercise that could benefit her the most. She'll be happy to learn that my Your Body, Your Diet plan can fix it so that she will never have to say "diet" again.

Kevin—who does everything right but is still developing his father's spare tire—is a more complex case. Whether he's really eating the right foods and taking the right vitamins and minerals depends on whether he's basically an accelerator or a synthesizer. Once he uses this book to find out just what his metabolic profile is, there'll be no guesswork. He'll know for sure what combinations of foods, minerals, vitamins, and herbs, along with exercise and stress-relaxing techniques such as massage and shiatsu, to use to stay trim and healthy. The Your Body, Your Diet plan will deflate his midriff bulge once and for all.

If you still cannot find yourself on the spectrum, don't worry. In the following pages, I'll show you exactly how to determine which forces are the most dominant in your system and how to work with those forces to achieve your best weight.

Now you understand some of the basics of how metabolism works, and you are well on your way to becoming an expert on your *own* metabolism. Once you comprehend that, you will discover how you can shed pounds through a customized, healthy, long-lasting method. Next, you'll learn all you need to know about what stress has to do with weight gain and how you can keep it under control—for good. Then you can identify your meta-type and select your personal diet, nutrition, and exercise program.

With my diet plan, your weight-loss program will be designed just for you and your best friend's just for her—and both of you will succeed. *You will get your metabolism back in balance and stay slim, fit, and great-looking—indefinitely.*

In only one short month, you'll feel like a million dollars, look like a million dollars, and have a million times more energy than you did before. You'll find yourself coping with stress in a healthy and productive way—and realizing that your secret dreams and goals really are within your reach. You'll begin weaning yourself off toxic substances such as alcohol and nicotine—without climbing the walls or screaming at your family and colleagues. And maybe best of all, you won't even have to *think* about your weight. Your program will put you on autopilot in days.

So here we go. This book gives you not only the benefit of my years of experience in clinical practice but also the actual knowledge you'll need to get—and keep—yourself whole.

2 How Energy Flows Run the Show

Now that you understand the unique characteristics of your metabolism, you are probably asking yourself a simple question: Once I know my metabolic type (meta-type), all I have to do is eat the right foods and my extra weight will magically disappear, right? Well, almost. That's one part of the weight-loss equation. Remember, Eastern medicine teaches us that managing your mental, emotional, and psychological states and getting the right amount of exercise is the other important part of the deal.

The key to taking weight off and *keeping* it off (while maintaining your health) is keeping your two types of energy—yin and yang—in balance, and it takes more than just eating the proper foods. Establishing and maintaining harmony between these two essential life forces in your body is the basic principle behind Eastern medicine and the Your Body, Your Diet plan.

Understanding Our Dual Nature

Energy is the movement of all life, but remember, it is divided into two basic types—that which is activated by very fast action (yang) and that which pulls that action back into a balanced rhythm (yin), that which throws out (yang) and that which regenerates (yin). Each depends on the other for existence.

Balancing these powerful, interdependent internal forces is critical to your health, well-being, and weight maintenance because whether you are a yin/synthesizer or a yang/accelerator, both types of energy are equally important to your body.

And by the way, this is not about the strengths or weaknesses of males and females. While the ancient terms that explain each type refer to yin as female and yang as male, the concepts have nothing to do with gender as we define it. Not all men are yang/accelerators, and not all women are yin/synthesizers (think of Vicky, the accelerator, in chapter 1). Every human body, male or female, is a system driven by these two forms of energy, which, under ideal circumstances, complement each other as they work together to give us strength to get through the day—or the serenity to calm down, rest, and rejuvenate when that day comes to an end.

What happens when energy balance becomes imbalance? Your body begins to overwork your nervous and endocrine systems in a fierce battle to set things right again. A moderate imbalance shows up as the beginning of weight gain and nagging, but not serious, health problems. A severe imbalance will produce significant weight gain, a loss of energy, and possibly a health crisis. That's when your system has slipped into a danger zone that I call the *stress response*—a hyperactive state that knocks your metabolism off track and guarantees you will put on weight no matter what you eat.

So if you thought the only problem in your struggle to slim your hips and trim your tummy was a simple lack of willpower when faced with a juicy burger or slab of chocolate cake—give yourself a break. Those cravings are the symptom, not the source, of your problem.

Your troubles do not begin when your girlfriend—who can eat just about anything and still fit into a size six—says, "Oh, have a little dessert. I'm going to have some." Your lack of resolve in the face of fatty or sugary foods is the natural response of a body lurching to regain its balance.

What triggers the loss of balance in the first place is a familiar culprit—everyday life. The alarm goes off, and your feet hit the floor at 7:00 A.M. Since you went to bed two hours late because you brought work home from the office, you still need at least two more hours of sleep. But there's no time for that—you've got a job to do. You may even have a toddler or a teenager to rouse and get ready, too. So you clear your house in record time, chugging coffee with milk and sugar, and make it to the office with barely a few minutes to choke down a bagel before the morning meeting. You're just in time to catch a sour look from your boss—and then the stress *really* begins.

Sound familiar? Your answer is probably "yes," since this is the way millions of men and women start the day, week after week, year after year. There is little time to manage emotions, catch up on rest, or give our bodies a moment to recover. We are creatures of the new millennium. No matter what the crisis, we flip open the cell phone, boot the computer, pour another cup of coffee, and rise to the occasion. It may *feel* as if we've got things under control, but racing through life as if it were a high-speed car chase is the quickest way to crash, to lapse into the stress response.

Obviously the solution is not to quit your job—or ditch your kids. The premise behind the Your Body, Your Diet plan is to learn to work *with* your body, not against it, and to give yourself the nutritional support you need to better manage stress and eliminate the crazy food cravings and up-and-down weight patterns that go along with it. Wouldn't you just love to stop losing those same ten pounds over and over again? It *is* possible. Read on.

All aspects of my program—food plans, nutritional supplements, exercise programs, and healing natural tonics—are designed to help you avoid the stress response. Or if you are like so many of my clients who arrive at my door overwhelmed by this metabolic state but unaware that it even exists, this program will help you *recover* from the stress response and return your system to its own healthy metabolic rhythm.

Why Stress Equals Distress

Anyone who has ever experienced the pressure of a bad day knows that stress can be felt deep in the pit of your stomach. It can leave you clammy, overwhelmed, and in need of a rest. But many of us become so accustomed to feeling bad that we begin to see it as normal—when our bodies are actually crying out for relief. Here's how it works:

Phase 1: Pick a scenario. You have a huge fight with your significant other that ends with slammed doors, crushed feelings, and worst of all, no resolution. Or your boss, an insensitive twit, has passed you over for a much-deserved promotion.

Since you're human, your response is distress and anger. As the rage builds, your pituitary gland snaps to attention and sends a massive dose of hormones to your adrenal glands. Your bloodstream floods with adrenaline, your heart rate increases, blood vessels dilate, and your blood pressure soars. This is why feeling bad emotionally leaves you feeling worn down physically.

When you absorb an emotional blow, your body goes into action—the fight-or-flight response. You're in pain, and your body is ready to do battle. As adrenaline and other hormones go to work, your pancreas (the organ that regulates your blood sugar) signals the liver to release its stored blood sugar to be used for the fight-or-flight energy. Your blood sugar rises. As the stress response continues, the adrenal hormones, especially *cortisol*, drive your hunger and food cravings, and you begin reaching for those starches and sugars. Your pancreas works harder as it releases insulin to offset your climbing blood sugar in a desperate attempt to stabilize your system. If phase 1 of your stress continues for a prolonged time, your pancreas can begin overproducing insulin, removing *too much* blood sugar and immediately converting this excess into your nemesis—fat—*not* back into stored energy. Then your blood sugar will plummet *below* normal levels, and you'll feel low on energy and desperate to stuff sugar, alcohol, other carbohydrates, and caffeine into your mouth to try to recapture balance.

Phase 2: All of this activity brews silently, below the surface, while you pace the floor or sit at your desk, wondering why you just can't calm down. Then the next stage of the cycle kicks in. You begin to emotionally and intellectually process what's just happened. In addition to blaming yourself for failing to win out over your boss or get the best of your spouse, you start feeding your body's need for energy and balance.

The problem is, your ricocheting metabolism takes over now, not your common sense. So rather than calming yourself with healing words and sitting down to a sensible salad, you let loose. You give in to the cravings that began in phase 1. You may soothe your soul with a box of Oreo cookies before moving on to potato chips with creamy dip and too much wine. These food choices may feel good at first, but in addition to being filled with empty calories, they send a message to your pancreas to keep working in overdrive. You end up stuffed, with your digestion stalled and your metabolism all but shut down.

You want to reach the healthy phase 3—rest and regeneration. But you have chosen the wrong route to success. If you're like most of us, the rage and recrimination keep coming, the adrenaline keeps pumping, and you keep feeding your emotions until your cravings become a matter of habit and your natural energy balance is so far off track that you can no longer recover on your own.

This process may set in over a matter of days, but it can quickly become a way of life. If the stress response ceases, your body should return to normal in about three days. What generally happens, however, is that you hold on to unresolved emotional issues (the key to illness and imbalance in the world of Eastern medicine), which are eventually exacerbated by other stressful events. Soon your body starts to *overreact* on a regular basis. The stress response becomes your typical response. In a word, your condition becomes chronic. Remember Jennifer, from chapter 1? Her attempts to heal her heart by tearing around town, until she was exhausted and her metabolism was off track, are a prime example. Whether you're a yin/

synthesizer or yang/accelerator, in this state, you stop eating the proper foods for your meta-type and create a vicious cycle of low energy, metabolic imbalance, and unwanted weight gain.

The Ideal Scenario

Phase 3: Stress—whether it's set off by an obnoxious boss, a fickle mate, or other bearers of bad news—is an unavoidable part of human life. So to keep your body in balance and your weight in check, you must become a master of the art of regeneration (cultivating the yin forces in your body). Relax. It's not as hard as it seems, and I'm here to help.

Remember what we learned in chapter 1 about the natural functions of the two types of energy—yin and yang? Yang is the force that heats, puts out, and pumps you up. Yin is the force that calms, heals, and evens things out. As long as they work in harmony, the needs of your meta-type will be met and your weight will stay within your healthiest and most attractive range. The minute one force or the other swings out of balance and begins to overtake your system (what the yang force is doing when your body starts to pump adrenaline and insulin), you slip out of metabolic balance. You gain weight and age faster.

Recovering means giving your body an opportunity to repair itself. In order to break the stress response cycle of adrenaline rush, insulin spike, fat storage, and metabolism shutdown, you need to let go of the painful emotions that set the whole process in motion in the first place. That is the only way to heal and reclaim your natural balance.

Even the world's best psychologist or psychotherapist cannot "talk" your metabolism back into line; you need a diet with the proper protein-carbohydrate-nutrient balance for your meta-type as well as emotional release.

Eating Your Way Back to a Healthy Weight

Understanding ways to create equilibrium between the yin (synthesizer) and yang (accelerator) energy forces in your body will put you on the road to your optimum weight. The Your Body, Your Diet plan helps you enjoy the best possible relationship between these two extremely powerful forces by managing your emotions and eating in accordance with your meta-type—stabilizing your metabolism in the bargain.

In the pages that follow, yang/accelerators will learn to calm and balance their need for carbohydrates and their tendency to go overboard on proteins while following a diet based primarily in fresh vegetables, fruits, and grains. Yin/synthesizers will figure out how to pump up their protein intake while reducing the carbohydrates they eat, as part of a diet based on meat, fresh fish, chicken, and vegetables. In addition, those elsewhere on the spectrum—the balanced and mixed accelerators and the balanced and mixed synthesizers—will learn to meet their metabolic needs so that they, too, can shed pounds in record time.

Along with your own personal meta-type diet, you'll have a carefully tailored selection of vitamins, minerals, and amino acid supplements that will help get your body in balance quickly—and keep it there—as you trim down. I promise you, after a few short weeks on my Your Body, Your Diet plan, you will discover a stronger, thinner you and will never again have to worry about giving in to the stress response or lugging around extra pounds. Your body will reestablish itself in the weight range Mother Nature intended just for you. Remember how great you looked in your twenties? Well, get ready to look that way again—and have energy to spare. Another important benefit is also guaranteed: you will develop a more resilient and responsive immune system.

After only one month you will be amazed at the change in your stamina and your body shape as well as the improvements in your skin and hair. You will definitely look and feel like a million dollars. So let's get started.

3 Cornerstones
of the Program

Before you take the test that will change your life and pinpoint your diet strategy, let's look at five cornerstones that make my program work. They'll spell success even if you've tried and failed repeatedly to control your weight.

Determining the Appropriate Diet for Your Meta-Type

The first cornerstone is to determine who can be a healthy vegetarian, who can be a healthy omnivore, and who can be a healthy protein-eating carnivore. This is how it works.

The accelerator categories incline toward a semivegetarian to vegetarian approach to eating, while the synthesizer categories lean toward semiomnivorous to carnivorous menus. Did you know that carbohydrates are the fastest-burning foods, animal proteins burn off very slowly, and fats are the slowest? This will help you understand why the metabolic types require different foods.

The accelerators tend to be *fast metabolizers*. They're driven by their strong energy-producing endocrine glands—the adrenals, thymus, and thyroid glands—which speed up the way their bodies break down, convert, and utilize energy. Since their food breaks down quickly, it mixes with less oxygen in the stomach. Consequently when the oxygen-free nutrients reach the cells to be transformed into *energy* (adenosine triphosphate, or ATP), they'll burn off at a slower pace, providing long-term energy (oxygen incites energy to burn at a rapid rate).

The accelerators also have less nerve stimulation to those organs of digestion and regeneration, so they'll tend to produce less stomach acid (hydrochloric acid, or HCl). Therefore, with their ability to burn off energy at a smoother pace and with a lower production of stomach acid, the accelerator categories can tolerate the lighter, faster-burning, and easier-to-digest carbohydrates. If the accelerators eat heavier proteins, they'll feel sluggish and lethargic. The leisurely digested proteins require ample stomach acid for digestion and burn off slowly as energy.

On the opposite side, the synthesizers tend to be *slow metabolizers*. The organs and endocrine glands of repair and regeneration motivate them: the pituitary, pancreas, and sex glands. They have little nerve stimulation to the powerful energy-producing glands that stimulate the fast breakdown of food and its transformation into energy. So their foods tend to digest at a slow pace and mix with ample oxygen in the stomach. By the time the oxygen-rich nutrients reach the cells to be converted into energy, they burn off at a rapid rate ("oxygen fans fire").

Unlike the accelerators, with abundant nerve stimulation to the digestive and regenerative organs, the synthesizers produce ample stomach acid. Therefore, the synthesizers need and require the slower-burning heavier proteins. If they gorge themselves on the lighter, fast-burning carbohydrates, the resultant energy burns too rapidly, triggering a swift energy spike followed by a rapid slump. They'll end up lethargic and fatigued, and cravings will begin in an effort to recapture that energy high.

The result: the pancreas overproduces *insulin*, which is the body's way of trying to maintain a steady flow of blood sugar. Instead of turning that blood sugar into stored energy in the liver or muscles, insulin's action turns it immediately into *fat*. You become an instant fat factory.

Here's an easy way to remember it: fast metabolizers break down their food quickly but use it slowly (slow oxidizers); slow metabolizers digest their food slowly but burn it off rapidly (fast oxidizers). Slow in, fast out; fast in, slow out. The accompanying table summarizes this process.

Meta-Type Food Breakdown and Utilization

TYPE	BREAKS DOWN FOOD	BURNS OFF ENERGY	FOOD NEEDED
Accelerators	**Quickly**	**Slowly**	**Carbohydrates**
Sympathetic nervous system dominant	Known as fast metabolizers. • They have medium amounts of stomach acid (HCl). • Food mixes with little oxygen in the stomach. • Food goes through the digestive process; nutrients enter the cells to be burned off as energy.	Known as slow oxidizers. • Nutrients reach the cells and are converted to energy by the cells' enzymes. • Since the nutrients have absorbed little oxygen from the digestive process, the energy burns off at a slower pace.	Can be semi- and full vegetarians. • Since carbohydrates are the fastest-burning foods, accelerators can tolerate them and will burn them at a slower pace. • The slower-burning proteins will make them feel sluggish.
Synthesizers	**Slowly**	**Quickly**	**Proteins**
Parasympathetic nervous system dominant	Known as slow metabolizers. • They have ample amounts of stomach acid (HCl). • Food mixes with a lot of oxygen during the slower breakdown of foods in the stomach. • Food goes through the digestive process, and nutrients enter the cells to be burned off as energy.	Known as fast oxidizers. • Nutrients reach the cells and are converted to energy by the cells' enzymes. • Nutrients are filled with ample amounts of oxygen from the digestive process and, when converted to energy, will burn off at a rapid pace. (Oxygen fans fire.)	Can be semi- and full carnivores. • Since carbohydrates are the fastest-burning foods, when mixed with a lot of oxygen they'll burn off immediately, causing a drop in blood sugar. This type of metabolism requires the slower-burning proteins.

When we look at the three accelerator meta-types and the three synthesizer meta-types, the percentage of animal proteins to carbohydrates for each would look something like the breakdown shown in the accompanying table.

Recommended Breakdown of Nutrients

META-TYPE	PROTEIN (%)	CARBOHYDRATES (%)	FAT (%)
Synthesizer: Carnivorous	55	30	15
Balanced synthesizer: ¾ Carnivorous ¼ Vegetarian	50	30	20
Mixed synthesizer: ½ Carnivorous ½ Vegetarian	45	40	15
Mixed accelerator: ½ Vegetarian ½ Carnivorous	40	45	15
Balanced accelerator: ¾ Vegetarian ¼ Carnivorous	30	50	20
Accelerator: Vegetarian	20	60	20

Establishing the Proper Acid-to-Alkaline Balance for Your Meta-Type

The second cornerstone is to establish the accurate acid-to-alkaline balance for your meta-type. As you've learned, each meta-type is controlled by a particular endocrine gland, which in turn controls certain organs of the body. For instance, the *regenerative* yin parasympathetic system stimulates the pituitary gland, which controls the whole repair and regeneration of the body. The pancreas gland rules digestion and blood sugar stability, and the sex glands are responsible for reproduction and sexuality.

The *powerful* yang sympathetic energy stimulates the adrenal glands, which are responsible for producing energy for the fight-or-flight stress response and our daily activity and for supporting the metabolism of our bodies. The thymus gland governs the immune system, while the thyroid gland is responsible for our basic metabolism (the way our bodies utilize energy) and energy production.

Together these functions control and are responsible for the different metabolic profiles.

Based on his or her genetic predisposition, each individual usually falls into one of these categories, exhibiting a dominant endocrine gland and an opposing weaker one. This helps to govern what people's preferences are with respect to certain interests, emotions, intellect, metabolism, and lifestyle—why some dance and others study math, why some are outgoing and others shy, why some eat for consolation and others forget food when they're upset.

According to Chinese medicine, the high-energy yang metabolism is *acid* by nature. People ruled by this energy can usually break down and utilize their foods quickly. The slower yin metabolism is *alkaline* by nature. People in this category usually break down and utilize their foods gradually. An individual's acid or alkaline nature indicates the acid or alkaline pH value of his or her blood, lymph, and tissue.

The pH values for the alkaline and acid natures run from approximately the 8–7.5 range to the 4.5–4 range. The alkaline nature has three divisions:

1. *Strong alkaline,* with a pH of 8–7.5
2. *Alkaline forming,* with a pH of 7.4 (the same as our blood)
3. *Weak alkaline,* with a pH of 6.8

The acid nature also has three divisions:

1. *Strong acid,* with a pH of 4.5–4
2. *Acid forming,* with a pH of 5
3. *Weak acid,* with a pH of 6.2

The table summarizes the metabolic profiles for the six meta-types.

Profiles of the Six Main Meta-Types

META-TYPE	DOMINANT NERVOUS SYSTEM	STRONG ENDOCRINE GLANDS	WEAK ENDOCRINE GLANDS	ACID/ ALKALINE NATURE	PH VALUE	BREAKS DOWN FOODS
Accelerator	Sympathetic	Adrenals	Sex glands	Strong acid	4.5–4	Very rapidly
Balanced accelerator	Sympathetic	Thymus	Pancreas	Acid forming	5	Rapidly; tends to burn off sugars more quickly
Mixed accelerator	Sympathetic	Thyroid	Pituitary	Weak acid	6.2	Less rapidly; burns sugars a bit faster
Mixed synthesizer	Parasympathetic	Sex glands	Adrenals	Weak alkaline	6.8	Slower; burns sugars more slowly
Balanced synthesizer	Parasympathetic	Pancreas	Thymus	Alkaline forming	7.4 (same as blood)	Slow; burns sugars fast
Synthesizer	Parasympathetic	Pituitary	Thyroid	Strong alkaline	8–7.5	Very slow; burns sugars very fast

Now *food* is also categorized as acid or alkaline, but when we speak of the acid or alkaline pH of foods, we're referring to the *nature of the end products* that foods leave in your body after they've been digested, *not* to foods in their uncooked or cooked state. For instance, lemons are more acid in their raw state, but their end product, or residue, is more alkaline. The residue refers to the "ash," or the end product of a food after it's been broken down in the body and stored in the cells. This, in turn, will create more acid or alkaline blood and body conditions, which can lead to either a healthy, slim, toned, and vibrant body or a body subject to disease.

One of the key secrets to losing weight and keeping it off permanently is to supply the right acid or alkaline foods to stabilize your meta-type's acid or alkaline balance. Accelerators tend to be acidic in varying degrees and require the more alkaline balancing foods found in green leafy vegetables and fruits, while the alkaline-producing synthesizers benefit from the more acid-forming foods found in proteins.

For instance, pure accelerators (very fast metabolism) are the most acid of all the meta-types and require the opposite foods of the pH spectrum—strong alkaline—to stabilize their metabolisms. As you'll see in the coming chapters, the accelerators' diet should mostly contain foods that are strong alkaline, alkaline, weak alkaline, and weak acid. Foods that are acid forming should be eaten seldom (once a week), and foods that are the same as their own pH values—strong acid—should be avoided.

The higher the calcium content, the more alkaline the food residue will be; and the higher the phosphorus content, the more acid the residue. Meat is high in acidic residue and is a perfect energetic food for the synthesizers, while leafy green vegetables are a great source of calcium—very alkaline in nature—and a perfect calming food for accelerators.

Knowing the Best Times to Eat

The third cornerstone establishes the best times to eat for each metabolic profile. The *time of day* as well as the *amount of food* are significant to losing those excess pounds quickly—and maintaining that desired new look for life. People of each meta-type have ample natural energy during the hours when their dominant endocrine gland is active (remember the larks and the night owls). During that time they don't need the additional energy liberated from food. But they will need to *eat for energy* when their strongest gland is at its weakest point, as well as for the body's regeneration. The accompanying table summarizes when and how much people of each meta-type should eat.

Appropriate Mealtimes and Amounts for Each Meta-Type

META-TYPE	STRONG GLAND	ACTIVE TIME	BREAKFAST	LUNCH	DINNER
Accelerator	Adrenals	Early morning to early afternoon	None or very light	Light to medium	Ample
Balanced accelerator	Thymus	Early morning to late afternoon	Very light	Medium	Ample
Mixed accelerator	Thyroid	Early morning to early afternoon to early evening	Light	Medium	Medium
Mixed synthesizer	Sex glands	Some mornings, early afternoon to late evening	Light	Ample	Medium
Balanced synthesizer	Pancreas	Midmorning, then evening	Moderate	Moderate	Moderate
Synthesizer	Pituitary	Early evening to night	Ample	Substantial	Very light

Learning How to Combine Foods Properly

The fourth cornerstone teaches people of each meta-type how to combine foods properly in order to facilitate rapid weight loss, avoid overburdening their digestion, and help them feel light and energetic.

Briefly, proteins don't combine well with grains or starchy vegetables; slightly starchy or nonstarchy vegetables can be eaten with grains or proteins; fruits should be eaten alone or at least half an hour before or after a meal. On some breakfasts I do include certain fruits that are rich in enzymes that help to break down foods. The principles of food combining are all explained in chapter 11, "Guidelines for Healthy Living."

Identifying the Appropriate Supplement and Lifestyle Regimens for Your Meta-Type

The fifth cornerstone is the vitamins, minerals, herbs, aromatherapy, and Bach flower remedies for each individual metabolic type. These balance, harmonize, and stabilize each type's dominant endocrine gland, keeping it from over- or underacting while stimulating and supporting the corresponding weaker gland. In turn, this helps to eliminate food cravings while normalizing and stimulating the body's regeneration and weight loss.

You'll also discover how to use simple, ancient arts, such as acupressure, to lose weight and keep it off, and you'll discover what exercises are best not only for your meta-type but for your personality.

Part two

Identifying
Your Meta-Type

The next step is to determine your meta-type so that you can select the proper diet plan. Read the personality sketches in chapters 4–9, then take the Meta-Type Profile Questionnaire in chapter 10. If you are still a little unsure of your meta-type after reading the profiles, you can double-check your personality attributes against the checklist of ten basic meta-type characteristics that follows each personality sketch. Keep in mind that no one fits every aspect of every meta-type. Look for the profile that seems the *most familiar* and then compare that with your highest questionnaire score to make the right decision. The science of metabolic types is accurate, but, of course, there are always some crossover characteristics.

Most diet plans are one-size-fits-all. They assume we all have the same metabolism, calorie-burning rate, and ability to manage stress. Obviously nothing could be further from the truth. Within your own family, you can probably see dramatic differences in the way you, your parents, your siblings, or your children gain and lose weight, maintain health, and handle stress. That's because you all have your own unique ways of using energy.

My plan works because it recognizes that when it comes to weight maintenance, we all have distinct needs. *Your Body, Your Diet* is the result of my years of experience applying the principles of Eastern medicine to the health and weight problems so often created by our traditional Western diet. So you are sure to discover your type—and maybe even a few pleasant surprises about your personality—in this plan.

4 The Classic Yang/Accelerator

My client Ellen is exactly what people think of when they hear the phrase "type A personality." She works twelve-hour days, races to meet the needs of a five-ton client load, and takes great pride in her skills at litigation. And that's just her day job. The rest of her time is spent keeping up with her two daughters (Kathy, age six, and Joanna, eleven) and building a life with her husband, Jack. Ellen lives her life full speed ahead, seven days a week. She is a classic example of the accelerator meta-type—a person driven by the body's yang forces. Eastern medical practitioners learned thousands of years ago that accelerators, like Ellen, draw their tremendous drive and energy from a metabolism dominated by the sympathetic nervous system and activated by the adrenal glands.

The gland that dominates the accelerators' high-energy system is the adrenals—their master gland—the source of adrenaline. The accelerators' weaker glands are the sex organs, the origin of the body's sex hormone (estrogen and testosterone) supply. As with all the meta-types, keeping these two glandular systems in balance and working in harmony is the key to keeping accelerators at their healthiest weight.

If you are an accelerator, your motto is "I think first, then act." You love to get things done, whether it's building a business, climbing a mountain, or renovating your home. If you're not careful, you tend to be a workaholic, and the words you hear most often from concerned pals and family members are "Slow down. Take it easy." But of course, *easy* is not in your vocabulary.

You stay on the go, but you're not reed-thin. Your natural body type tends to be strong, sometimes squareish, and perhaps a bit stocky, yet on the slender side when your system is in balance. But no matter how fast you move, if you slip into the stress response, or ignore your body's natural eating cues, you start to pile on the pounds. Ellen's inability to avoid the stress response and keep her weight under control after having two children is what made her decide to come to me.

Accelerators—male or female—love to achieve. At work they are savvy enough to employ the skills of outlaw entrepreneurs or corporate team players. It just depends on the scenario. They seldom back away from tough problems. And they are generally great at making difficult decisions. The left side of the accelerators' brains dominates the thought processes, so the search for logic and reason often rules their lives.

At play accelerators are usually the competitors on the field. Whether cheering a son's peewee-league game from the sidelines or taking on the opposing team in their own game of basketball, accelerators take challenge *very* seriously. When an accelerator does slow down, "relaxing" is likely to include rearranging the furniture or landscaping the yard.

This meta-type loves the limelight. For some examples, just pick up the newspaper or turn on the TV: Hillary Rodham Clinton, Madonna, Madeleine Albright, Donald Trump, and Danny DeVito—all are classic accelerators.

If this is your meta-type, you are most likely to be a powerhouse in the morning. You wake up early, raring to go, and tend to wind down early, running out of steam about 10:00 P.M. From 6:00 to 8:00 A.M., you're roaring ahead with plans for the day, while your neighbors have just begun to stir.

Your natural habitat is warm weather. Sunshine stimulates your energy-producing adrenals. Life in a sunny climate, preferably near the ocean, is ideal for you. So even if your career keeps you city-centered, you'll crave those wide-open, sunny spaces.

If you are saying, "This is my life" (except for the movie star part, perhaps), you are an accelerator—the living embodiment of yang energy. When your brain desires action, your body is quick to release the adrenaline you need to get going. Your metabolism burns calories fast and—if your system *stays* in balance—you seldom have to worry about your weight. But if stress gets the best of you, you will find yourself battling weight gain and eventually health problems.

Spinning Out of Control

Accelerators are driven by the intellect—a tremendous gift. They are determined to get the job done—at almost any cost—and they rarely let anything get in their way. The stress response surfaces when the accelerators' efforts to maintain that urgent pace are blocked.

Faced with adverse or illogical circumstances, accelerators tend not to adjust well. They push, channeling all their energy into controlling and reshaping what may be an uncontrollable situation. When that happens, an already sensitive sympathetic nervous system clicks into overdrive, sending the message to the adrenal glands to pump out more adrenaline to fuel the fight. As you're now learning, this is the beginning of the stress response. But for accelerators, who naturally live at high speeds, these early stages of trouble feel like business as usual. So they just push harder.

The pancreas gets further into the act. As larger and larger doses of insulin are pushed into the bloodstream, the accelerators' high-speed metabolism starts to flip out of balance. You begin storing fat to compensate for the extra blood sugar. Once your metabolism enters this stage, weight gain is just the first sign that you are out of balance. Within weeks your cholesterol levels begin to climb, it's increasingly difficult for your blood pressure to stabilize, and your body starts to crave the high-sugar, high-fat foods that are guaranteed to make things even worse.

People with this meta-type often end up completely mystified by the fact that even as they continue to move fast, they put on weight. They are unaware that they are caught in an almost constant stress response state while eating all the wrong foods for their system. This chain of events is easily explained by one of the most basic theories of Eastern medicine. Simply put: poorly managed emotions lead to chemical reactions that lead to imbalances in the body. Imbalances equal weight gain, out-of-control eating habits, and eventually poor health. That's why eating right for your meta-type is crucial.

Basics of the Accelerator Food Plan

The Your Body, Your Diet plan is based on the simplest principles of yin and yang, hot and cold, acid and alkaline. It works to create and maintain the balance between these opposing yet interdependent forces in your body. That is why learning to eat the proper amount—and combination—of natural foods at each meal gives you the power to control your weight and your health. To make things as easy as possible, I've done the work for you. No calorie counting. The meals, recipes, suggested herbal and nutritional supplements—and even the cheat sheet (a list of snacks for days when you want a little something extra) in the accelerator diet section—have all been prepared to fit the needs of your meta-type.

If you are an accelerator, your focus is speed and energy, made possible by your extremely active adrenal glands. You have a fast metabolism. You're able to break down your foods quickly into the energy that you need to fuel your high-powered lifestyle. This, however, tends to give you more of an acid body chemistry, which means that in order to stay in balance so that you can control your weight, you need to keep the acid foods in your diet to a minimum and concentrate on more alkalinizing foods. Whole grains, fresh vegetables and fruits, and moderate amounts of unsaturated fats are the foundation of your diet plan. High-acid foods—such as the proteins found in meats and refined carbohydrates like sugars, starches, and alcohol—should be consumed in *very* limited amounts.

Your accelerator food formula should look something like this:

- Carbohydrates: 60 percent
- Fats: 20 percent (unsaturated fat only)
- Proteins: 20 percent

One more thing. If you think that you fit this profile, take a few minutes to work through the questionnaire in chapter 10 and look at the checklist at the end of this chapter to be sure. The questions are designed to confirm your meta-type selection. Think of the questionnaire as just one small step toward a great dieting and lifestyle success story.

Accelerator Body Basics

- Dominant glands: adrenals
- Weakest glands: sex organs
- Most likely to gain weight in: upper body (tends to be apple-shaped)
- Physical type: stocky, but slender when in type

The Gender Difference

Since our model accelerator is a woman, male readers may need a little assistance recognizing themselves. Men and women who share the same meta-type also share the same basic metabolic body chemistry. Since each sex possesses a different mixture of hormones, however, men and women may gain weight in similar patterns but express other aspects of their meta-type *very* differently.

If you are a male accelerator, people probably notice you immediately, because you won't have it any other way. The male accelerator tends to be an empire builder—a self-starter who fights and works hard to achieve positions of great power and prominence. Two examples that come to mind easily are Bill Clinton and his inspiration, John F. Kennedy. The male accelerator is the classic patriarchal father, provider, and protector. He is:

- *Ambitious*. His tremendous need to succeed may lead to fame and power from even the most humble beginnings.
- *Confident*. He believes in himself and his dreams.
- *Domineering*. When out of metabolic balance, he has to be careful to know when to take control and when to respect others.
- *Energetic*. When in meta-balance, this is the one with nearly boundless energy—the worker at his desk at 8:00 A.M., ready to go after only four hours of sleep.
- *Fearless*. He knows when to take on risks and simply sees them as an entertaining challenge.
- *Insensitive*. Again, out of balance, he can become hyperfocused on work or his own needs to the detriment of his relationships with family and friends.
- *Intellectual*. Like the female accelerator, he is dominated by his intellect, with little input from his emotional side.
- *Realistic*. The male accelerator is not usually an idealist. He accepts the world more or less as it is and wants to find his own fast-moving path through the system.
- *Strong*. Men of this meta-type tend to be stocky and muscular rather than lean. When they are out of balance, excess pounds generally settle on the upper torso and around the face, or in the worst cases, they tend toward potbellies.

Checklist: Ten Basic Characteristics of Accelerators

❑ Psychological inclination	More intellectual than emotional. May "live in the head" and be emotionally closed.
❑ Motto	"I think, then act decisively."
❑ Life's direction	Competitive and workaholic. Ambitious in life and driven to accomplish and acquire.
❑ Energy	Extremely active. Usually has a whole day's work done before most people get up. Doesn't require food for energy, especially in the mornings.

❑ **Reaction to stress**   Anxiety. Likes to work under pressure and usually lives on the stress response.

❑ **Best energy time**   Early morning to late afternoon. Begins to fade when the sun goes down.

❑ **Puts weight on**   Stomach and upper body—the "apple."

❑ **Sleep pattern**   Usually has a hard time falling asleep; may have a tendency toward insomnia.

❑ **Exercise**   Loves exercise, especially sports.

❑ **Food cravings**   Sugar, salt, starches, and sometimes meat.

5 The Yang/Balanced Accelerator

No one can keep an office moving at a smooth pace like my client Julie. Her sharp intellect and decisive way of handling the million and one problems that come her way daily, as the office manager at a fairly large Long Island–based insurance company, are critical to her company's success—and she knows it.

Julie's meta-type—the balanced accelerator—is exactly what the name implies, the center of the accelerator metabolic scale. As with all accelerators, her incredibly abundant energy comes from the yang forces in her body, which work with the sympathetic nervous system and the thymus gland to keep Julie centered and healthy.

The gland that works the hardest to keep the balanced accelerators' health and weight under control is the thymus, their master gland. The thymus's most important function in the body, however, is guiding the activities of the immune system. The weaker gland in the balanced accelerators' bodies is the pancreas, which controls—among other things—the ebb and flow of blood sugar. As you read more about this type, you'll come to understand how supporting and balancing these two glands is critical to the balanced accelerators' good health and ability to maintain a proper weight.

If you share Julie's balanced accelerator meta-type, then your motto is most likely to be "I think, I intuit, then I take decisive action." You just might be famous among your coworkers and family members for your ability to focus on a problem and stick with it until the best possible solution is found. Your considerable powers of concentration and insistence on meeting your goals are most likely your greatest gifts.

Like most balanced accelerators, Julie has a pale to rosy complexion and bright, clear eyes, and she's medium to tall in height. She had been somewhat slender but not particularly lean-muscled. She came to me because she had begun to gain weight in her stomach, hips, and upper body, where balanced accelerators are most likely to put on the pounds.

Julie has an engaging personality. But as we talked, I became aware that she was genuinely frustrated about her inability to keep her weight down. She had applied her considerable balanced accelerator intellect to the project and tried several popular diets, only to find that when she dropped a few pounds, they seemed to creep back on within weeks.

True to her meta-type, Julie began doing meticulous research to find a more effective program. Eventually a friend recommended her to me. She was more than happy to make the long drive from her Long Island home to see if we could discover the root of her problem and help her regain her great figure. After all, she was only thirty-six. There was no reason for her to suddenly get fat—or was there?

Balanced accelerators, when in type, tend to be exactly that—balanced, happy, type A personalities. It was clear, however, from looking at Julie's expanding figure and listening to her talk about her newly out-of-control eating habits that something had flipped her out of balance. So we began examining her life, not her appetite, for clues.

Julie's career choice—office manager, responsible for the total reorganization of her enormous department—was a good fit for someone with her meta-type. Balanced accelerators are most often masters of organization and detail and gifted with an ability to truly understand other people's problems. She was well suited to the task of handling her coworkers and the ups and downs of the office.

She also possessed other common balanced accelerator traits. She was in good spirits on most days, and her favorite time to accomplish her goals was early morning to early afternoon, when her energy was at its peak. Her powerful personality—an almost perfect mixture of beauty, brains, and heart—is also something commonly found among people of her meta-type. They often come across as in charge and on top of things, but also warm and sincere. Goldie Hawn, Cameron Diaz, and Cindy Crawford are great examples of balanced accelerators.

Pushing the Envelope

After we chatted for a while, it became clear that although Julie was blessed with superior problem-solving skills, she was also burdened with another trait—the inability to relax or let go. Like the accelerators, balanced accelerators tend to grab on to an issue or a problem and push with all their might until it's resolved. Balanced accelerators can have an even tougher time because they usually find it difficult to take a breather until everything on their list is completed. Sound stressful? Well, it is, and that's exactly what had hold of Julie—a self-imposed version of the stress response.

Her company was in the midst of a yearlong reorganization. She was swamped with more work than even the most competent person could handle but would not ask for help. She pressed on, and the pounds piled on, as her system flipped further and further out of type. To aggravate the situation even more, she was incredibly cranky at work and home (something most balanced accelerators struggle with when out of type). So the people who would normally support her were keeping a safe distance, lest they get their heads snapped off when Julie was in one of her moods.

Her office was the perfect place for binges, too. Many coworkers were skilled in the kitchen and thought that the way to ease the pain of the long work hours was to bake cookies, brownies, and even cream puffs for their office mates. Nice sentiment, but the sugar and fat were absolutely the last things Julie's balanced accelerator metabolism needed. The calories were a problem, of course. But more important, for Julie's particular system, the sugar and dairy products helped exacerbate her body's natural imbalances. Her pancreas (the weakest link in the chain for most balanced accelerators) and related organs were overwhelmed by all the extra fat and sugar she was pouring into her system. That meant they were doing a poor job of managing her blood sugar and breaking down the fat.

And one more problem surfaced. Balanced accelerators love the light and always feel best in southern latitudes. Sunlight stimulates their adrenals and thymus glands. So the dreary Long Island winter was draining Julie's energy and initiative as well.

She saw only a slow but steady weight gain that seemed focused on her stomach and hips, but there was a lot more going on there.

To help Julie get her situation under control and rescue her health, despite what was happening at work, I suggested some important adjustments in her eating and exercise habits. But a little sugar detox was in order first.

Basics of the Balanced Accelerator Food Plan

For Julie, and other folks with her meta-type, the Your Body, Your Diet solution is based on this principle: the balanced accelerator is an acid meta-type and requires alkaline foods to stay in balance and deal with stress. Sugar was the worst thing for Julie to eat, and fat a close second. As with all meta-types, calorie counting was not the most important element of her healthy eating plan; proper nutritional balance was the key.

A semivegetarian diet, with a smaller amount of fish and chicken, was the most likely solution for Julie and others with this meta-type. A good complement of vegetables and fruits would also help.

Your balanced accelerator food formula should look something like this:

- Carbohydrates: 50 percent
- Proteins: 30 percent
- Fat: 20 percent

It's that simple. Julie found the answer to her weight problem with my Your Body, Your Diet plan, and so can you. If Julie seems familiar to you and you suspect that balanced accelerator is your meta-type, turn to the questionnaire in chapter 10 and the checklist at the end of this chapter to be sure. Remember, each diet plan is carefully calibrated to suit the needs of each meta-type, so you want to be certain to select the right one. It's the best way to ensure your success on the Your Body, Your Diet plan.

Balanced Accelerator Body Basics

- Dominant gland: thymus
- Weakest gland: pancreas
- Most likely to gain weight in: stomach first, then hips
- Physical characteristics: medium to tall height and medium build

The Gender Difference

Male readers may need a little help recognizing their meta-type, since our balanced accelerator profile features a woman. The news is the same for every type: except for the ways that certain hormones behave in our bodies, the men and women of each type share the same fundamental characteristics.

The personalities, however, may be a little bit different. While for most of the six meta-types there are significant differences between the behavioral characteristics of the men and women, those who fall under the balanced accelerator heading actually have a great deal in common. The men of this meta-type also tend to be deeply intellectual, intuitive, and excellent problem solvers. And they tend to be truly nice guys: think of Mel Gibson and Tom Hanks, two classic balanced accelerators, and you'll have the right idea. The balanced accelerator male may also be:

• *Bold.* Many in this meta-type have the ability to make grand gestures or take dramatic public stands with ease.

• *Creative.* They are often known for their agile minds. Many gifted musicians fit this type.

• *Clever.* Native Americans would call this type of man a "shapeshifter." He would make a superb diplomat or actor.

• *Cunning.* You might think of this as the flip side of clever. When out of type, Mr. Balanced Accelerator can focus his considerable intellectual energy on the darker side of life.

• *Decisive.* Like their female counterparts, men of this meta-type are great at making tough decisions.

• *Energetic.* He can be like spring, full of energy, activity, and ideas. When he is balanced, he can really brighten your day.

• *Insensitive.* At their worst (but only on truly bad days), men of this meta-type have a difficult time respecting the property and rights of other people.

• *Romantic.* This is the one who can, without a doubt, steal your heart. But keep an eye on him: he just might stray.

• *Shrewd.* Nice guy or not, he's not to be taken lightly.

• *Spiritual.* Men of this meta-type are often drawn to the larger questions in life and driven to understand mysticism and religion.

Checklist: Ten Basic Characteristics of Balanced Accelerators

❏ Psychological inclination	Intellectually dominant, strong intuition, access to emotions, but "rules" from the mind.
❏ Motto	"I think, I intuit, then act decisively."
❏ Life's direction	Focus, concentration, clarity, and intense commitment to goals.
❏ Energy	Very active, with abundant energy, especially in the morning. Needs little food for energy production. Has abundant stored energy.

❑ **Reaction to stress**   Anxiety. Doesn't like pressure but lives on intensity. Usually is very happy.

❑ **Best energy time**   Early morning, morning to late afternoon. Feels the effect of the midafternoon "adrenal crash."

❑ **Puts weight on**   Stomach first, then hips.

❑ **Sleep pattern**   If anxious, wakes during the night or has insomnia. Falls asleep easily and sleeps well when not under stress.

❑ **Exercise**   Loves Dancercise; hates repetitious exercise. Needs to keep the mind active and entertained.

❑ **Food cravings**   Starches (breads, crackers), sugar, and fats.

6 The Yang/Mixed Accelerator

The differences among meta-types can be surprisingly subtle. Yet recognizing the small variations that make your metabolism different from mine or from your older sister's is an important part of managing your weight.

In a world that moves as quickly as ours, it may seem as if everyone were an accelerator. But the fact is, you may live a life as fast-paced as that of Ellen (the accelerator we met in chapter 4) without realizing that the pace may be all wrong for you. You may be even more likely to make this mistake if you have some of the basic characteristics of an accelerator mixed with aspects of another metabolic type. If that's the case, you're a yang/mixed accelerator.

If you're a mixed accelerator, your system is primarily driven by yang energy and the sympathetic nervous system. The key difference between you and an accelerator is the fact that yin energy plays a larger role in how your metabolism functions. This slight shift in emphasis—from a system completely dominated by yang influences to a system moderately dominated by yang and a healthy dose of yin—means that mixed accelerators experience short, unstable bursts of energy and have moderately slower metabolisms than balanced accelerators or accelerators.

The other significant force in a mixed accelerator's body is the thyroid gland—the master gland for people of this meta-type. The thyroid produces thyroxine, the hormone that speeds the body's metabolism. When things are working smoothly, this system keeps weight in balance. If the thyroid is out of balance, however, it can be hyperactive (overactive) or hypoactive (underactive). The weakest gland in the mixed accelerator's body is the pituitary, which is responsible for producing and regulating the flow of *all* the body's hormones.

Your mixed accelerator path through life is guided by the rational influence of the left brain, but the right brain plays just enough of a role to ensure that you are deeply emotional as well. The result is your motto: "I think, then I act—but only if I'm sure and I know what to feel."

An old friend of mine, who eventually became a client, is a quintessential mixed accelerator. Jeff is a popular, Chicago-based pediatrician who passionately enjoys his work. He is blessed with one of the mixed accelerator's greatest gifts—a warm, winning personality. For all the years I've known him, Jeff has always been the guy whom everyone loved to be around—the consummate golden boy, without the cocky edge. Jeff, like most mixed accelerators, is deeply compassionate *and* competent. He has a knack for getting right to the heart of his young patients' concerns at times when even the most astute parents cannot figure out the source of their child's sniffles or tears.

Under normal circumstances, Jeff is also an expert at making the best use of his unpredictable but nonetheless formidable mixed accelerator energy stores. He seems to instinctively understand that he needs to slow down occasionally and take a breather. So he divides his long hours spent at work with time spent feeding the yin side of his nature with more creative pursuits.

Mixed accelerators often take great pleasure in the arts—whether it's ballet, opera, rock music, or viewing abstract paintings. Even better, Jeff often travels from his Chicago home for a little R and R in a warm, sunny, and dry locale like Arizona. It's the perfect mixed accelerator vacation spot because of the arid climate.

Like most happy people, Jeff took his slim physique and good spirits for granted. He had no idea that he owed this pleasant state to a metabolism that was getting exactly what it needed most of the time. You see, the mixed accelerator's dominant gland—the thyroid—is on call all day and all night, but it does most of its work in short intervals. It delivers brief, unstable spurts of energy that don't have much staying power. That means that if you're a mixed accelerator, your energy is high in the early morning, early afternoon, and early evening. Late afternoon is when you are most likely to run out of fuel.

By eating right for his meta-type, balancing his stressful and nonstressful activities, and getting regular exercise, Jeff easily maintained his natural mixed accelerator body shape—slim, not quite lanky, and muscular in the chest and arms. When in balance, this meta-type has the kind of build that makes women stare and men sneak a second glance. Mixed accelerators are long and lean in the torso and legs but have just enough curve where it counts. For an almost perfect picture, think of these four very hot mixed accelerator hunks: actors Clint Eastwood, Pierce Brosnan, Brad Pitt, and Tom Cruise.

Jeff found he could almost effortlessly maintain his weight by occasionally playing a long, hard game of tennis or sweating out eighteen holes of golf (he walked—no cart), the type of skill-focused sports that mixed accelerators most often find challenging. He was also naturally drawn to a diet with a heavy emphasis on grains and vegetables, with small amounts of fish, poultry, and at times meat. The small, healthy meals and snacks that he munched during the day were perfect for his meta-type.

From early adulthood well into his thirties—as he married, developed his professional life, and became a father—Jeff kept his emotions, his unpredictable energy levels, and his weight in balance. His close friends and family were so accustomed to his amiable, steady presence that I think, at least at first, we failed to even notice when things began to change.

Dealing with the Hidden Side

Even with all his years of medical experience, Jeff made the mistake that most of us make when our waistlines begin to thicken. He saw his increasing weight as the source of his problem rather than a symptom. It never dawned on him that all these changes might have a deeper cause.

He was slipping into the most common mixed accelerator response to stress—the dark side. When exposed to long periods of aggravation or disappointment, mixed accelerators do not usually become crazed, type A personalities, like accelerators. Rather, they are likely to repress their emotions and live in a state of nervous tension, obsessive worry, and anger. In Jeff's case this meant that he was irritable and surly a good deal of the time. And he confessed during our first consultation that he was finding it tough to connect with his young patients for the first time in his career. He and his wife, Jody, had even begun to argue and snap at each other over minor things. She said Jeff always seemed to be on edge and had no interest in sex.

Jeff also recognized one other, very significant change: he was craving and eating all the wrong foods. As a physician, he certainly knew that it was inappropriate to trade in his morning bowl of granola and fruit for a big, gooey cinnamon bun. But once he gave in, he just couldn't help himself. "It's only an extra two hundred calories or so, and I easily work that off in a day," he rationalized. He was right about the calorie load, but what he *didn't* know was that for his meta-type one of his greatest enemies was the incredible amount of sugar packed into those buns. In addition, he had replaced his afternoon apple or banana with a bag of potato chips or a candy bar and started eating heavier midday and evening meals. The more he gave in to his desires and ignored his healthy eating habits, the more he contributed to his sugar cravings, knocking his system off balance and piling on the excess pounds.

By eating all the wrong foods while enduring a period of prolonged stress, he was slowing his thyroid gland activity far below normal levels and slowing his metabolism. He was caught in a vicious cycle—gaining weight, upsetting his family and coworkers, becoming increasingly grouchy and unhappy. And he was completely confused about how he got into this shape or how to get out.

Like Ellen, Jeff was experiencing his own version of the stress response. By the time he came to me, he had put on fifteen pounds—mostly around his middle and hips—the typical mixed accelerator pattern. Jody was about to pack up and leave him, and he was doing far less than his best work with his patients.

When I asked what was wrong, he immediately replied from his intellectual side (the forces of yang), neatly listing all of his symptoms—weight gain, irritability, food cravings. "Gaining the weight," he said, "was the source" of his problems. I explained that he was only skimming the surface of the issue. He had to dig deeper. "What," I asked, "is really going on in your life? What has changed besides your body? Was there trouble at home, work, or both? Was something else at risk?"

It took him a moment, and then he just dropped his head and said, "We're headed in the wrong direction. It's just a huge mistake." What, I asked, was going in the wrong direction? Our discussion? "No," he replied. "It's what's happening at the hospital and in my practice."

Like millions of physicians nationwide, Jeff was dealing with HMOs for the first time. As a result, he had lost something tremendously important to him—control over the quantity and quality of care he offered his patients.

He was also experiencing one of the mixed accelerator's worst nightmares: a loss of control over his life and one of the very things that helped him keep the yin and yang parts of his nature in balance—his career. Things were truly spiraling out of control, precisely because he was giving in to his out-of-whack system. The frustrations at work fed the sugar cravings, which wreaked havoc with his nervous and endocrine systems and produced more irritability and sugar cravings. All of that sapped his energy for exercise (further contributing to his weight gain).

My challenge was to use my Your Body, Your Diet plan to help Jeff get his weight, and his life, under control.

Basics of the Mixed Accelerator Food Plan

The essential truth for every meta-type is that healing (and successful weight loss) begins in the mind, not in the body. With Jeff my first task was to get him to address all that pent-up emotion. He had to acknowledge that he could not change the medical world by himself and resolve to work with his new boss on some level.

The next step was to drop those cinnamon buns and resist those afternoon candy bar attacks. As a mixed accelerator, you "burn off" food fairly quickly but digest food more slowly than accelerators do, because the more prominent yin influence speeds up the way you burn off energy. Metabolically speaking, then, that means you need adequate amounts of alkaline foods, such as vegetables, fruits, and grains, well balanced by semi-acid foods, such as fish, chicken, and small amounts of red meat.

Your mixed accelerator food formula looks something like this:

- Carbohydrates: 45 percent
- Protein: 40 percent
- Fat: 15 percent

If reading Jeff's story has convinced you that the mixed accelerator is definitely your meta-type, double-check your conclusion by taking the questionnaire in chapter 10 and reviewing the checklist at the end of this chapter. If you're still not sure where you fit on the metabolic spectrum, read on.

Mixed Accelerator Body Basics

- Dominant gland: thyroid
- Weakest gland: pituitary
- Most likely to gain weight in: stomach first, then hips and thighs
- Physical characteristics: long, lean body; broad or full chest

The Gender Difference

Since our mixed accelerator profile features a man, the following list of characteristics should help female mixed accelerators better recognize their unique qualities. As with all meta-types, mixed accelerator men and women are basically the same when it comes to metabolism, but there are a few other important differences that need to be noted.

If you are a female mixed accelerator, you are probably extremely smart and accomplished. Women of this meta-type are likely to achieve great things while maintaining their independence and femininity. Jane Fonda, Michelle Pfeiffer, Heather Locklear, and Anjelica Huston are prime examples of this meta-type. The female mixed accelerator tends to be:

• *Ageless.* The kind of woman who seldom seems to add a year to her face or body.

• *Compassionate.* No matter what type of work she does, she usually takes time out to do something to make the world a better place.

• *Driven.* If she wants something, she seldom stops until she has it all under control.

• *Energetic.* She has lots of energy, but even when she feels invincible, her energy levels are unpredictable. She is a type A personality with strong type B influences.

• *Insensitive.* No, this is not a contradiction. It's characteristic of a female mixed accelerator who has flipped out of type. When she turns to her dark side, she can be contemptuous of people who are vulnerable and become emotionally remote.

• *Intuitive.* Like the mixed accelerator male, she has an almost uncanny ability to guide herself through hunches or dreams.

• *Maternal.* She can be a protective mom, skilled at teaching independence, but not an intense earth mother.

• *Strong-willed.* "My Way" could easily be her theme song.

• *Slender.* When in balance, firmly living within the guidelines for her meta-type, she tends to have a leggy, lithe figure.

Checklist: Ten Basic Characteristics of Mixed Accelerators

❏ Psychological inclination — Intellectually dominant, with a strong emotional tendency. When torn between emotion and intellect, rationalization wins.

❏ Motto — "I think, I feel, then act when I'm sure."

❑ **Life's direction**   Professionally, family, and socially oriented. Her life's work is exceptionally important to her and must be fulfilling.

❑ **Energy**   Active energy, usually in short bursts and with little endurance. Tires easily. Needs three meals to help stabilize energy.

❑ **Reaction to stress**   Anxiety first, then depression if in a prolonged stress response.

❑ **Best energy time**   Early morning to early afternoon, then again in the early evening.

❑ **Puts weight on**   Stomach, hips, then thighs.

❑ **Sleep pattern**   Falls asleep very easily and requires considerable sleep. If hyperactive, may tend toward restlessness or insomnia.

❑ **Exercise**   Needs exercise to keep the thyroid stimulated—although she doesn't necessarily *like* to do it.

❑ **Food cravings**   Starches (breads, pastry, pasta) and sugar.

7 The Classic Yin/Synthesizer

The synthesizer is the accelerator's polar opposite—the anchor at the other end of the metabolic spectrum. If you found it impossible to relate to the accelerator's high-speed, no-time-to-stop-and-smell-the-roses approach to life, it may be because you are a classic synthesizer—a smooth-moving, magically creative, earthbound type B personality who relishes passion, beauty, and family. The synthesizer is the earth mother (or earth father) of the metabolic spectrum.

Sophia, a young woman who arrived in my office complaining about weight gain and suffering from deep depression a few months ago, is a true synthesizer. The forces of yin/female energy drive her system, with intense stimulation from the parasympathetic nervous system.

The gland that works the hardest (is the most dominant) at helping the synthesizer maintain a healthy weight is the pituitary—the tiny but extremely powerful regulator of all the body's hormones, especially the growth and sex hormones. It also stimulates the adrenal glands and has a lot to do with how your body distributes fat. The weakest gland in the synthesizer's system is the thyroid—which holds the key to metabolism. Some synthesizers also experience weakness in the sex glands (which may cause an irregular or low sex drive) and the thymus (which stimulates the immune system), since these glands are related to the thyroid's activity.

If you are a true synthesizer, you probably already know that your meta-type's battle cry is "I feel." Synthesizers are the world's great creators, builders, and romantics. While you may fail to notice your special gifts, the people who share your life have undoubtedly noted your talents as a great and generous lover, parent, friend, or even philanthropist.

Medium tall, with a full, curvaceous figure and thick, healthy auburn hair, Sophia was beautiful even with the extra forty pounds she was lugging around. And as is so often the case, she thought her depression had been brought on by her inability to lose weight. But before I even attempted to design a weight-loss program for her, I asked her to tell me about her life.

Not surprisingly, Sophia was a musician—a great career choice for a synthesizer. At the age of twenty-eight, she had already established a solid reputation not only as a pianist but as a music therapist—someone who helps people overcome psychological or physical problems through artistic expression. Like most true synthesizers, she described her creativity, as well as her desire to nurture and support others, as the driving force in her life. But her work was not the source of her problem.

About a year before her visit to my office, she had suffered a tremendous loss—the breakup with her boyfriend, Cliff, after four years together and a yearlong engagement. After I listened to her for a few moments, it was clear that she had lost not only a relationship but many of her hopes for the future as well. The wedding had been planned, the invitations were out, and Sophia was thrilled about the prospect of starting a family (synthesizers tend to be very maternal). Suddenly her groom-to-be admitted to a continuing relationship with another woman and called the whole thing off.

Sophia was devastated, as most would be, but she also failed to realize that people with her meta-type have a particularly difficult time healing and moving on after romantic or emotional crises. To make things worse, she was blaming herself, mourning the loss slowly, *and* gaining weight. Here was a lovely young woman with *great* insight—like most synthesizers—into the mysteries of life, music, and her many clients but no clue to her own basic metabolic rhythm.

Synthesizers can become engulfed in emotional intensity and lapse into depression, becoming "emotional eaters," especially when faced with betrayals from the people they love and depend on. This triggered Sophia's depression and inability to move forward after her split with Cliff as well as her rapid weight gain. She had unwittingly run headlong down her own road to the stress response and flipped her metabolism out of type—without ever knowing what hit her.

Stuck in Second Gear

When Sophia discovered that she had given years of her life to a guy who was hardly worth sixty seconds, she went through the typical stages—shock, hurt, and anger. Then she got stuck in that anger mode and could not move on to healing. Feeding an almost endless effort to feel needed—the mechanism synthesizers often use to feel secure when things are out of sync—Sophia stepped up her schedule by adding volunteer activities. Her motive was to take her mind off Cliff, but she was pushing toward extremes—rapidly flipping out of type.

Rather than sticking to her normal diet of protein (fish, chicken, or meat) with vegetables and very little grain or fruit, she began to indulge in buttery casseroles laden with cheese, cream-sauce-covered pasta dishes, and gooey desserts. She worked herself into near exhaustion with charity work. And she spun so out of control, she no longer had time for even moderate exercise. Naturally the weight piled on, but by that time, she was too deep into the synthesizer stress response cycle to get out by herself.

Sophia's blood sugar was low, her thyroid had slowed to a standstill in response to her frenetic behavior, and her diet was no longer fulfilling her nutritional needs.

This last point is particularly important for this meta-type, because the synthesizers' somewhat slow metabolism is focused on growth and regeneration. They have small natural energy stores and need to draw all their energy from each day's food intake. If a diet is inadequate and filled with sugar and fat, the body lacks the proper fuel to go forward. Rather than revving up all systems, the synthesizers' metabolism slows to a crawl, and a natural tendency to gain weight kicks in.

Givers Who Go the Distance

Don't waste a minute mistaking the synthesizer for a flaky, creative type. Despite profoundly artistic natures, people with this meta-type are also blessed with exceptionally sharp minds and an ability to achieve. If they are not in the arts, they are often in the healing professions, and not in a passive role. Male or female, the synthesizer is the friend who will listen to your sad story until even you are sick of hearing yourself talk, the nurse who will watch over the patient long after her shift is over to quell a family's fears. Singer Dolly Parton, talk show hostess Rosie O'Donnell, and actress Roseanne fit this profile well.

The force behind this extraordinary group of people is, as I said earlier, yin/female energy, dominated by the parasympathetic nervous system.

They tend to have slower metabolisms and digest and break down foods at a relatively slow pace. And as Sophia discovered when she increased the fat and sugar content of her diet, synthesizers have a strong tendency to be overweight. Once they slip out of type, their thyroid glands simply cease to function efficiently. With this meta-type the body is constantly striving to synthesize, assimilate, and build—taking food and almost immediately converting it into flesh, not energy.

These basically gifted, calm, right brain–dominant folks tend to love cool weather, and they don't really mind a gray day or two. With little prompting a synthesizer can happily blow a whole weekend watching videos or old movies or buried in a good book, while munching on any-thing from gourmet food to corn chips (synthesizers just love to eat). The desire for R and R is not complete laziness; synthesizers are naturally given to periods of tiredness and fatigue. And even though they need exercise to stay in balance more than any other meta-types, synthesizers are not keen about a physically active lifestyle.

These charming conversationalists are seldom angry, except when out of type, and tend to be slow and cautious about making important deci-sions. If overextended, they'll become weak, quickly overwhelmed by stress and prone to quickly burn out. They have to watch out for low blood sugar (which can lead to hypoglycemia) and be vigilant about keeping their strong appetites under control.

Basics of the Synthesizer Food Plan

The synthesizers' recommended diet is based on the principle that people of this meta-type are extremely alkaline. They need more acid and slow-burning foods, such as meat and fish (low-fat dishes, of course), to keep their bodies in balance. And like most meta-types, the less refined sugar they eat, the better. The synthesizers' natural intolerance for carbo-hydrates leads to severe fatigue and weight gain when they fill up on these foods.

Your synthesizer food formula should look something like this:

- Protein: 55 percent
- Carbohydrates: 30 percent
- Fat: 15 percent

If you think you see yourself in the description of Sophia or these basic characteristics of the synthesizer, then congratulations, you may have found your meta-type. To be absolutely sure, however, check your choice by taking the questionnaire in chapter 10 and reviewing the checklist at the end of this chapter.

> ## Synthesizer Body Basics
>
> * Dominant gland: pituitary
> * Weakest gland: thyroid
> * Most likely to gain weight: evenly, all over the body
> * Physical characteristics: medium to tall, often voluptuous

The Gender Difference

Here is some information to help male synthesizers recognize themselves. As with all meta-types, men and women who share the same type have the same basic metabolic chemistry, but there are differences in how each gender expresses feelings and handles emotional situations.

The ebbs and flows of the male synthesizer's emotional and physical states are also controlled by yin/female energy, with the primary support of the parasympathetic nervous system. While most in this meta-type tend to be amazingly creative, men of this meta-type need to guard against the potentially volatile male synthesizer nature. If you are a male synthesizer, you can probably be nightmarishly temperamental when you flip out of type, even if you are very caring when in metabolic balance. For almost perfect male synthesizers, think of singers Elton John and Luciano Pavarotti, the late comedian Jackie Gleason, or actor Paul Sorvino.

The male synthesizer tends to be:

* *Compassionate.* He's most often a bighearted guy.
* *Creative.* Like his female counterpart, this is a man who wants to make his living in some creative or artistic fashion.
* *Disorganized.* When overly focused on his emotions, he may have a tendency to forget about time and organization as he concentrates intently on creative projects.
* *Difficult.* Heaven help the person who must tell Mr. Male Synthesizer what to do when he is having a bad day. Taking direction is not his thing.
* *Intuitive.* His quick insight into almost any situation often enhances his creativity.

• *Moody.* When out of type, he is prone to dark, angry fits of temper, which can cost him important relationships.

• *Nurturing.* Even though he can be a little tough to get along with, he is also quick to make chicken soup for a sick friend or be there when a friend or loved one is down.

• *Sexy.* He is probably the most passionate male in the metabolic spectrum.

• *Spiritual.* Whether in or out of type, this man is always willing to look for the greater and finer meaning in life.

Checklist: Ten Basic Characteristics of Synthesizers

❑ Psychological inclination	Emotionally dominant, highly creative. Warm and generous; emotions win over intellect.
❑ Motto	"I feel"; may turn inward rather than acting.
❑ Life's direction	Empathetic and loving, driven to feel and create with a deep spiritual bent. Loves family, children, friends, animals, the arts, cooking, and crafts.
❑ Energy	Slower and more passive but may display endurance. Slow to get started. Requires food for daily energy production.
❑ Reaction to stress	Depression—usually causing an emotional implosion or repression.
❑ Best energy time	Early evening to late night.
❑ Puts weight on	All over the body.
❑ Sleep pattern	Falls asleep very easlly and can sleep for long periods. If depressed or under stress, may wake during the night.
❑ Exercise	Doesn't like exercise, and may even hate it, but really needs it.
❑ Food cravings	Dairy, creams, ice cream, and sugar.

8 The Yin/Balanced Synthesizer

Emily is the old-fashioned type. In an era when most women are fighting to cram careers, kids, and happy relationships into their lives and still have time to make it to the gym, Emily has decided to make her family—especially her marriage—the center of her world. Her choice may seem surprising to lots of today's women, but it's not unusual for a female balanced synthesizer.

As with each meta-type in the synthesizer spectrum, Emily's system is dominated by the forces of yin/female energy, with a great deal of support from the parasympathetic nervous system to keep her in balance and at an optimum weight.

The dominant gland for balanced synthesizers is the pancreas, which is responsible for the enzyme production that helps the body use proteins, fats, and carbohydrates. It also produces insulin, which helps keep blood sugar under control.

The balanced synthesizers' weakest gland is the thymus, the gland that guides the body's immune system and keeps it strong. Protecting both of these glandular systems from stress and the wrong foods (especially sugar) is the key to keeping this meta-type slender and in good health.

If you are a true balanced synthesizer like Emily, then the words "I feel, I intuit, then I'll act if I'm sure—emotionally" ring true. Emotions are most often the driving force behind your actions, even though you have considerable intellectual gifts and amazing creative abilities.

While she had put on weight (the reason she was in my office), Emily was still attractive. She had long hair, a medium build, and an hourglass figure. Like most balanced synthesizers, she had to work hard to maintain that shape, so her recent loss of interest in fitness and many other important things only made the battle of the bulge tougher to win. With just a little nudge from pasta, a few cakes, pies, or pastries, balanced synthesizers are likely to develop a pear shape—gaining weight first in their hips and especially their thighs, which can be tough to reverse. That was exactly what was going on with Emily.

Emily expressed herself with enormous power and was naturally dramatic. She was fascinating to watch as she explained her feelings and frustrations. Her femininity and appearance were extremely important to her, so she was furious at herself for letting go of her once-careful eating regimen. I reminded her that getting heavy was not a sign of some fatal flaw in her personality but more likely an indication that something had thrown her system off balance, increasing her appetite and cravings for foods that were wrong for her system, especially sugar and starches. Since she was depressed and uninterested in exercise, it was natural to see a weight change.

The source of that depression was also a very important part of Emily's story. She had always worked hard to keep her weight down. After each of her three pregnancies, Emily adhered to exercise and diet routines that would have given a supermodel pause, but now even those methods seemed to fail her. She confessed to a weakness for breads, pasta, and pastries, but even when she ate little else and did her best to keep her calorie intake under control, the pounds stayed glued to her body.

Drowning in a Tide of Emotion

As always, the answer was not in Emily's kitchen. Food and "the art of eating" were a ritual to her psyche and healing. This time the answer was in her heart and her head. This gracious, engaging woman had spent more than a decade and the lion's share of her incredible creativity building a wonderful life for her husband and children. Their Manhattan apartment—while decorated on a reasonable budget—was worthy of a magazine spread. Her children had never known what it was like to come home to an empty house, because she was always available to hear the latest tales about school, add her unique touch to their homework, and prepare for bake sales, parents' night, and other activities. And most important, she was *always* there for Greg, her husband.

Emily had been a successful florist early in their marriage, using her flair for color and texture to create popular arrangements. But she felt that family should come first, so she closed up shop as soon as Greg began to earn enough money to support the family.

Her trust was well placed in that regard. Greg was successful in the corporate world, even though the endless traveling, long hours, and almost constant stress sapped most of his energy. Emily felt she understood his sacrifices, so she worked overtime to lighten his burden. She was the superwife, supermom—dedicated to her husband's career, her children's success and happiness, and the serenity of her home.

So what threw her world out of whack? The answers were common: her husband's infidelity and her daughter's adolescence. Her eldest girl, formerly a sweet-natured, cooperative child, hit puberty and became a rebel.

Her "little" girl (no matter how tall she got) was cutting classes, showing up at odd hours with alcohol on her breath, and hanging out with kids Emily found absolutely frightening. Emily felt guilty because she regarded her daughter's problems as having been caused at least partly by the tension at home. Emily had discovered that Greg had had several affairs. He called them "business-trip flings." Greg and Emily were in counseling, but Emily was almost beside herself with rage and shock. They fought constantly.

Emily suddenly found that the people to whom she had dedicated her life were not behaving in ways she expected. She was devastated, and for balanced synthesizers that meant her emotions were running hot, raw, and out of control a good deal of the time.

A Body Out of Balance

Emily understood that there was a connection between her weight gain and her family problems, but she could not understand why the weight stayed on and on—even after she tried her old diet methods.

The answer was simple. Emily's metabolism had been slowed because her hormones and blood sugar were spiking and dipping well beyond normal levels with each of those emotional outbursts and rages. The pastries just exacerbated the crisis. She was dealing with her own version of the stress response.

Balanced synthesizers are generally peaceful, calm, type B personalities. But when faced with betrayals, they flip into extremely volatile bouts of anger followed by depression. That was Emily's way of getting back at Greg. But she was actually causing her digestive system to shut down and slack off on its insulin-regulating responsibilities. It also meant that her already weak thymus gland was working at about half strength, weakening her immune system and draining her energy.

Emily was almost overcome by frustration and heartache but unable to move beyond her anger. She needed to forgive herself for the things that had happened in her family (none of which were actually her fault)—and she needed to undo the damage done to her system.

Basics of the Balanced Synthesizer Food Plan

For Emily and other balanced synthesizers, the diet formula that works best is primarily composed of the slower-burning acidic foods that work to neutralize the balanced synthesizers' alkaline system. She also needed to avoid excess sugar and follow a diet focused on protein, vegetables, some fruit, and small amounts of grains to get her body's insulin levels back in balance, her sugar cravings under control, and her metabolism up and running properly again.

If you are a balanced synthesizer, your food formula looks something like this:

- Carbohydrates: 30 percent
- Protein: 50 percent
- Fat: 20 percent

Now if you think the characteristics of the balanced synthesizer sound like a page out of your life story, then you've probably found your meta-type. But just to be sure, take the questionnaire in chapter 10 and consult the checklist at the end of this chapter.

Balanced Synthesizer Body Basics

- Dominant gland: pancreas
- Weakest gland: thymus
- Most likely to gain weight in: hips and thighs
- Physical characteristics: lovely skin, curvaceous figure

The Gender Difference

Since our balanced synthesizer profile features a woman, male readers who fit this meta-type may need a little assistance recognizing their own unique balanced synthesizer characteristics. As with all meta-types, the basic metabolic functions are the same for men and women, but the personalities might be a bit different.

The men of this meta-type, much like the women, are very passionate, dramatic, and creative. They, too, are driven by their emotions, but not nearly as focused on family and relationships. They can view the corporate world as their "family." Their eyes are on work—which they tend to regard as a calling. Almost all their energy is channeled into pursuing their goals and achieving their dreams. Great artists such as Vincent van Gogh and compelling actors like Laurence Fishburne, the late Richard Burton, Jerry Orbach, and Robert De Niro are excellent examples. A man who is a balanced synthesizer may also be:

* *Earthy.* These men tend to like real people and things of substance. They have little interest in appearances.
* *Humane.* These are men with big hearts (even though they may try to hide it) who will go the distance for others.
* *Intense.* Balanced synthesizer men are often very focused and serious about all aspects of life.
* *Introverted.* Though many great actors fit this meta-type, balanced synthesizer men are often quite shy at heart. They really like to keep some part of themselves hidden and maintain privacy.
* *Nonconformist.* Balanced synthesizer men most often march to their own beat—do things their own way.
* *Physical.* Men of this meta-type tend to like to get their hands dirty—to really become physically involved in their work or other activities.
* *Productive.* Balanced synthesizer men are hard workers who can accomplish a great deal in a short amount of time.
* *Sad.* They are prone to depression, especially if they fail to find satisfying work or are subjected to a continual stress response.
* *Sensitive.* Guys who fall under this meta-type are often very sensitive. They do not take criticism well.
* *Stubborn.* Heaven help those who have to tell this fellow what to do. He does not take orders easily, especially if he has flipped out of metabolic type.

Checklist: Ten Basic Characteristics of Balanced Synthesizers

❑ Psychological inclination	Emotionally dominant, strong intuition, capable of powerful intellect. Emotional needs win over the mind.
❑ Motto	"I feel, I intuit, then I'll act—with emotional forcefulness—when I'm sure."
❑ Life's direction	Usually needs a partner, resides in feelings, needs to create, has a dramatic flair.

❑ **Energy** Tends to be a bit slow in the morning, gaining momentum as the day progresses. Needs to eat regularly to have energy.

❑ **Reaction to stress** Depression to anxiety to depression. Usually internalizes anxieties.

❑ **Best energy time** Mid- to late morning, then early to late evening.

❑ **Puts weight on** Hips and thighs—the "avocado."

❑ **Sleep pattern** Falls asleep easily and needs sleep. Unlike the accelerator, the balanced synthesizer needs sleep to regenerate and function in the daily world.

❑ **Exercise** Requires robust exercise and feels better, but doesn't like it.

❑ **Food cravings** Sugar and starches.

9 The Yin/Mixed Synthesizer

f you've read this far and become convinced that I've forgotten all about your meta-type, have patience. The mixed synthesizer is the last of the six meta-types, but it's just as important as all the types you've read about earlier. Although you may think you have already discovered your meta-type, the mixed synthesizer profile might be a better fit, so please read on.

A few years ago I met an artist and craftsman named Alec who is a perfect mixed synthesizer. He made intriguing things from wood and stone, in addition to being a fairly successful painter. I discovered him after admiring his work in a gallery show. We became friends, and he eventually became a client.

There is no doubt that mixed synthesizers, like Alec, share many of the basic characteristics of the synthesizer. As with the synthesizer, this meta-type is dominated by the forces of yin/female energy, with powerful support from the parasympathetic nervous system as well as strong stimulation from the sympathetic nervous system.

The dominant glands for people of this meta-type, however, are the sex glands, the master glands of creativity and, of course, the glands that control the body's flow of testosterone, estrogen, and progesterone. The mixed synthesizers' weakest glands are the adrenals, which control the activities of the sympathetic nervous system and the body's energy flows.

If this is your meta-type, then you share Alec's motto: "I feel, I think, then I'll act." Sensuous and stunningly creative, mixed synthesizers are also likely to be known for intense sexuality, impassioned support of important issues or causes, and their flair for the dramatic. In Alec's case drama was his calling card—especially under stress.

Alec became a client because he wanted to lose weight. But typical of a mixed synthesizer, he was not suffering from the fallout of any special life crisis. He had so many emotional ups and downs—accompanied by bingeing on food and drink, of course—that he came to see if I could help him achieve some lasting balance. He had put on quite a few pounds because he was out of balance so much of the time. He was concerned about his appearance, since he wanted to remain attractive for his wife, Sandy, and he recognized that his moods were becoming a problem for many people he dealt with each day.

Alec has the classic mixed synthesizer body type—just enough over six feet that you would think of him as tall, with a muscular build. His deep-set eyes and thick hair are among his best features, but when he was out of type, his hips would spread.

Getting Off the Roller Coaster

Alec's problems were really common for a mixed synthesizer: whenever he was feeling insecure or slighted ("feeling like a loser," as he put it), he would become angry, depressed, and extremely argumentative. His problems had become chronic, since in the art world he always faced some form of criticism (of his work or his behavior) and regular rejection. For every fifty people who loved a painting, there was routinely at least one snide critic.

This situation might have been easier on a hardier soul. But since he was a supersensitive mixed synthesizer who was out of type about 90 percent of the time, Alec did not toughen up as he became more successful; he developed an even *thinner* skin. Like the synthesizer, he kept his true emotions bottled up—at first. People with this meta-type often find it painful to talk about their feelings. Alec would spend days stomping around with boiling rage and resentment locked inside. Then, since he was always afraid of letting the anger surface and seriously damaging a work relationship or his marriage, he would start to drink and eat carbohydrates—especially refined sugar and alcohol—in an attempt to keep his emotions under control. Of course, those two things are guaranteed to dump a massive amount of sugar into your bloodstream.

His other tactic: he'd decide that sex was the solution. Not a great idea, since Sandy was often on the receiving end of his hostilities and therefore seldom in the "mood"—in which case he would find "satisfaction" in the "outside world."

As you can imagine, after Alec had a few drinks, his feelings would swing from one extreme to the other, and he would tumble into a deep, brooding depression or lose his temper at some innocent bystander. Alec was giving in to the very behavior he was originally trying to avoid by drinking or binge-eating. He hated this cycle but had no idea where it came from or how to stop it. Helping him find those answers was my job.

First, he had to understand the mixed synthesizer's unique body chemistry. People who share this meta-type lapse into the stress response faster than any other meta-type in the group. Their relatively weak adrenal glands fail them when they're needed most—to combat stress—leaving them open to a roller coaster of emotions. When a mixed synthesizer experiences stress, the breathing and heart rate shoot up almost immediately. This is followed by the release of blood sugar by the liver. Simultaneously digestion starts to shut down. The blood sugar then spikes and begins to drop. A mixed synthesizer will respond by frantically gobbling sugar products. Now, obviously, if this happens once or twice, it's no big deal. But for the average mixed synthesizer living with the stress response, it becomes a way of life. It certainly did for poor Alec.

After a while a mixed synthesizer's metabolism develops a hypersensitivity to carbohydrates: everything—wine, scotch, doughnuts, or candy—slows the system down. Next, the weight balloons at an amazing rate.

Balancing the blood sugar—and the emotions—is the key. The metabolism simply can't work smoothly unless both are in sync. I'll tell you a little more about the dietary balance that now keeps Alec on an even keel shortly, but first look at some of the other aspects of this meta-type.

Powered by Passion

Both Sandy and Alec were fortunate that he recognized that his life was out of control. Mixed synthesizers—especially men—are pleasure seekers who can be extremely physical. In type they can be great lovers and extremely empathetic friends. But when they start down the road that Alec was on, there's trouble.

Their tendency to find solutions in erotic relationships frequently leads to extramarital affairs. Their desire for intensity and excitement can lead to substance abuse and temper tantrums. To get an idea of the perfect male mixed synthesizer, think of Sylvester Stallone, Bruce Willis, Jack Nicholson, Don Johnson, or Darryl Strawberry.

Alec, however, was a man who knew himself well enough to realize that he needed a change. So I introduced him to my Your Body, Your Diet plan.

Basics of the Mixed Synthesizer Food Plan

Like most truly sensual people, mixed synthesizers love to eat. Food to them is like love. But that's fine, because the Your Body, Your Diet plan turns this into an advantage. The mixed synthesizers' system tends to be semialkaline, but it can become extremely acid when out of type. For that reason this meta-type's diet must strike a careful balance of vegetables, fruits, and proteins (but not red meat, fats, or sugar). The idea is to get the weight and the mood swings under control.

Your mixed synthesizer formula should look something like this:

- Protein: 45 percent
- Carbohydrates: 40 percent
- Fat: 15 percent

That's it. This is the final meta-type. Again, even if you are certain that this is where you fit on the metabolic spectrum, take the questionnaire in the next chapter and review the checklist at the end of this chapter to be sure that you've made the right decision.

Now you're ready for the details of your personal Your Body, Your Diet plan.

Mixed Synthesizer Body Basics

- Dominant glands: sex glands
- Weakest gland: adrenals
- Most likely to gain weight in: hips, especially the buttocks
- Physical characteristics: medium to tall in height; slender when in type

The Gender Difference

Since our classic mixed synthesizer profile focuses on a man, this section will help female mixed synthesizers recognize their meta-type, if this is the chapter for them. As I mentioned in previous chapters, the basic metabolic chemistry of each meta-type is the same—whether you are male or female. But when it comes to personality characteristics and other small details to help determine your meta-type, there are several differences that you need to take into consideration.

If you are a female mixed synthesizer, you also want love to be the center of your life, and sexuality is just a piece of the puzzle—not the main event. You probably prefer relationships in which there is romance and lots of give-and-take. Four classic mixed synthesizer females are Elizabeth Taylor, Melanie Griffith, Marilyn Monroe, and Oprah Winfrey. Women with this meta-type may tend to be:

• *Angry.* Much like their male counterparts, when women of this meta-type are out of balance, their considerable passion may turn to anger.
• *Bright.* The mixed synthesizer female most often has a lively, active mind.
• *Beautiful.* Keeping herself looking great for the special person in her life is a natural activity for women of this meta-type.
• *Creative.* This woman's wonderful mix of intellect and emotional passion is often expressed in artistic pursuits.
• *Extroverted.* Mixed synthesizer females are not shrinking violets, although they may have a shy side to their personality. They usually love relationships, people, and contact.
• *Heartbreaking.* This lady tends to expect a lot from her men—like perfection. She can love them and leave them fast when things are not as she wants.
• *Independent.* As much as mixed synthesizer women love relationships, they are also quite independent. They can take care of themselves.
• *Receptive.* Women of this meta-type tend to be very open-minded.
• *Sensuous.* Men can barely keep their minds off women of this meta-type.
• *Strong.* These women are usually in control of themselves and handle difficult situations well.
• *Warm.* Some female mixed synthesizers almost have a glow. They may also have a gift for making people feel comfortable.

Checklist: Ten Basic Characteristics of Mixed Synthesizers

❑ Psychological inclination   Emotionally dominant, with a strong intellect. May get pulled between the mind and emotions but usually follows the heart.

❑ Motto   "I feel, I think, then I'll act."

❑ **Life's direction**   Warm and sensuous nature, feels and expresses emotional and creative intensity. Highly creative, with a strong dramatic flair.

❑ **Energy**   Slow to get started but once in gear goes all the way until the project is done. Requires regular food for energy production.

❑ **Reaction to stress**   Anxiety to depression. Responds to stress with anxiety but can easily fall into depression if emotional needs aren't expressed or heard.

❑ **Best energy time**   Sometimes late morning, early to late evening.

❑ **Puts weight on**   Hips and especially the buttocks; sometimes the thighs.

❑ **Sleep pattern**   Falls asleep easily, loves to sleep, and sleeps through the night, but wakeful if under stress.

❑ **Exercise**   Definitely needs exercise but dislikes it or finds it a chore.

❑ **Food cravings**   Spicy foods, cream, fats, oils; sometimes sugar.

10 Meta-Type Profile Questionnaire

The questionnaire in this chapter is designed to help you determine your specific metabolic type. It is followed by a table that summarizes the characteristics of each meta-type.

The questions evaluate the most basic aspects of your metabolism and in turn indicate your ability to produce energy. The essential difference between the *slow* and *fast* meta-types is in their *energy levels*. Therefore, the questions are primarily energy-related.

The questionnaire is divided into five sections dealing with you and your life. The topics covered in each section are *energetically* influenced by your dominant endocrine gland. Follow the instructions at the start of each section. When you've finished answering the questions in each section, add up your score at the end of the section. Then tally up the scores for all the sections at the end of the questionnaire to discover your meta-type.

Once you've determined which metabolic category you fit into, you'll quickly be able to find which diet, nutritional supplements, and herbs are appropriate for you.

A history of eating the wrong foods for your type, eating processed and chemically preserved foods, suffering from illness, aging prematurely, or being overshadowed by a continued stress response can easily cause you to flip out of your own basic metabolism and into one of the other categories. For instance, a person with chronic low blood pressure may suddenly develop high blood pressure. Therefore, answer the questions based on your conditions *today*.

Your body has a remarkable ability to regenerate itself, and given the right foods, your metabolism will begin to move back into its natural category.

Meta-Type Profile Questionnaire

1. Energy Patterns

Pick out the response in each group that you relate to most strongly and put the number 2 in the blank to the right of that response.

Energy level:

I'm exceptionally active; I don't stop.	A. _____
I have great energy.	B. _____
I'm fairly active.	C. _____
I have good energy.	D. _____
I can be lethargic.	E. _____
I'm very lethargic.	F. _____

Best energy time:

I'm up early and do half my work before others are out of bed.	A. _____
I always rise early.	B. _____
Morning is my best energy time.	C. _____
I don't operate well until midmorning or noon.	D. _____
I'm most active in the late afternoon and evening.	E. _____
Nighttime is my best energy time.	F. _____

Amount of sleep needed:

I can thrive on very little sleep.	A. _____
I need five to six hours' sleep.	B. _____
I need a normal amount of sleep (seven to eight hours).	C. _____
I sometimes need extra sleep.	D. _____
I repeatedly need extra sleep.	E. _____
I need a lot of extra sleep.	F. _____

Falling asleep:

I fall asleep with difficulty—may have insomnia.	A. _____
I can have a hard time falling asleep.	B. _____
I fall asleep with difficulty sometimes.	C. _____
I normally fall asleep easily.	D. _____
I fall asleep effortlessly at bedtime.	E. _____
I fall asleep extremely easily and at any time.	F. _____

Dreaming:

I don't dream.	A. _____
I dream rarely and can't remember much.	B. _____
I dream sporadically but don't recall my dreams well.	C. _____
I sometimes dream.	D. _____
I dream on a recurrent basis and remember my dreams well.	E. _____
I dream often and remember my dreams vividly.	F. _____

Exercise:

I love to exercise all the time.	A. _____
I enjoy exercise and do it as often as I can.	B. _____
I feel better when I exercise.	C. _____
I don't have time for exercise but *try* to enjoy it.	D. _____
I enjoy exercise on an occasional basis.	E. _____
I hate exercising and avoid it at all costs.	F. _____

TOTALS A: ____ B: ____ C: ____ D: ____ E: ____ F: ____

2. Personality

Pick out the response in each group that you relate to most strongly and put the number 2 in the blank to the right of that response.

Handling stress:

I always handle stress excellently.	A. _____
I have a great ability to handle stress.	B. _____
I handle stress well most of the time.	C. _____
I normally handle stress pretty well.	D. _____
I have a hard time with stress.	E. _____
I don't handle stress well at all.	F. _____

Dealing with anxiety:

I can become anxious easily.	A. _____
I often have anxiety reactions to stress.	B. _____
I become anxious rather than depressed.	C. _____
I'll have intermittent periods of fatigue if I'm anxious.	D. _____
I get tired if I'm under stress.	E. _____
I'll become lethargic if I'm anxious.	F. _____

Dealing with depression:

I'm ordinarily happy and don't get depressed.　　A. _____

I hardly ever get depressed.　　B. _____

Sometimes I'll be depressed.　　C. _____

I have ups and downs.　　D. _____

I get depressed easily.　　E. _____

I'm frequently depressed.　　F. _____

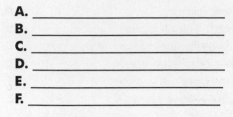

Handling emotional energy:

I get upset very easily if things don't go my way.　　A. _____

I can regularly get upset if things don't go right.　　B. _____

I'm predisposed to be upset easily.　　C. _____

Once in a while I get upset.　　D. _____

I'm usually emotionally stable.　　E. _____

I hardly ever get upset.　　F. _____

My moods can fluctuate between highs and lows:

Regularly.　　A. _____

Easily.　　B. _____

Repeatedly.　　C. _____

Fairly often.　　D. _____

Once in a while.　　E. _____

Rarely.　　F. _____

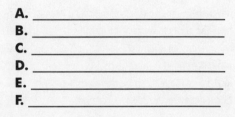

Dealing with anger:

I have a temper and can get extremely angry.　　A. _____

I can easily get angry, and I express it.　　B. _____

I get upset inside but usually don't show my anger.　　C. _____

At times I get angry.　　D. _____

It takes a lot to get me angry.　　E. _____

I never get angry.　　F. _____

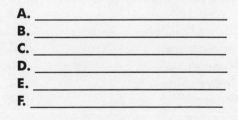

Dealing with fears:

I hardly fear anything.　　A. _____

I'm seldom fearful.　　B. _____

I'm sometimes fearful.　　C. _____

I have a predisposition to fearfulness.　　D. _____

I'm often fearful.　　E. _____

I'm fearful most of the time.　　F. _____

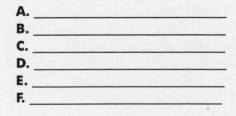

Patience:

I'm extremely impatient.   **A.** _____

I regularly become impatient.   **B.** _____

I can get impatient easily.   **C.** _____

I'm usually a patient person.   **D.** _____

I have a great deal of patience.   **E.** _____

I never become impatient.   **F.** _____

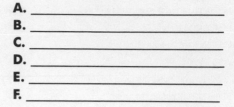

Handling intellectual energy and making decisions:

I make instantaneous decisions.   **A.** _____

I'm decisive and can make quick decisions.   **B.** _____

I have no problems making decisions.   **C.** _____

I'll have backup plans if I make a decision.   **D.** _____

I think very carefully before making any decisions.   **E.** _____

I have a difficult time making decisions.   **F.** _____

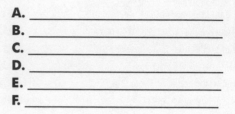

Ability to concentrate:

I have a heightened gift for concentrating intently.   **A.** _____

I have the ability to concentrate intently.   **B.** _____

My concentration is normal.   **C.** _____

I can concentrate for short spurts.   **D.** _____

I lack the skill to concentrate intently.   **E.** _____

I find it almost impossible to concentrate.   **F.** _____

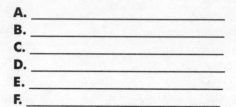

Dealing with concerns and worries:

I worry most of the time.   **A.** _____

I worry regularly if things don't go right.   **B.** _____

I can be a worrywart.   **C.** _____

I'll worry occasionally.   **D.** _____

I hardly ever worry.   **E.** _____

Why worry?   **F.** _____

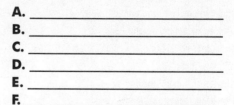

"Drive" in life:

I'm determined and intense.   **A.** _____

I'm focused and goal-oriented.   **B.** _____

I have a heightened sense of drive toward goals.   **C.** _____

My drive is average.   **D.** _____

I have a predisposition toward indifference.   **E.** _____

My drive is weak.   **F.** _____

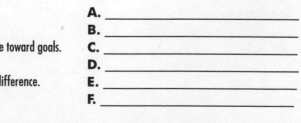

TOTALS A: _____ **B:** _____ **C:** _____ **D:** _____ **E:** _____ **F:** _____

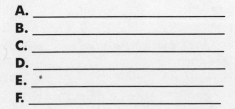

3. Appearance

Pick out the response in each group that you relate to most strongly and put the number 1 in the blank to the right of that response.

Skin tone:

My skin is usually on the paler
   side but could become ruddy.   **A.** _____

I have a pale complexion.   **B.** _____

I can become pale easily.   **C.** _____

I look fairly normal.   **D.** _____

I can get somewhat red.   **E.** _____

I'm usually red.   **F.** _____

My eyes:

Are bright and active.   **A.** _____

Are large and open.   **B.** _____

Are large.   **C.** _____

Are normal.   **D.** _____

Are set back in my head.   **E.** _____

Look sunken in my face.   **F.** _____

Hair:

My hair is dry and breaks easily.   **A.** _____

My hair is thin and often dry.   **B.** _____

My hair tends to be dry.   **C.** _____

My hair is normal.   **D.** _____

My hair tends to be oily.   **E.** _____

My hair is oily.   **F.** _____

Skin:

My skin is remarkably dry.   **A.** _____

My skin is quite dry.   **B.** _____

My skin is on the dry side.   **C.** _____

My skin is healthy and moist.   **D.** _____

My skin is moist but has a predisposition to be oily.   **E.** _____

My skin is oily.   **F.** _____

Nails:

My nails are split and thin all the time.   **A.** _____

My nails will often be thin and break easily.   **B.** _____

I'm predisposed to breaking nails.   **C.** _____

My nails will sometimes become thin.   **D.** _____
I have strong nails, which break infrequently.   **E.** _____
I have very strong nails.   **F.** _____

Distribution of fat on my body:
I hold the fat on my stomach and upper torso.   **A.** _____
I usually hold the fat on my stomach first.   **B.** _____
I hold the fat on my waist, and hips.   **C.** _____
I hold the fat on my derriere.   **D.** _____
I hold the fat on "saddlebags" on my thighs.   **E.** _____
I hold the fat all over.   **F.** _____

TOTALS A: _____ **B:** _____ **C:** _____ **D:** _____ **E:** _____ **F:** _____

4. Functioning in Life

Pick out the response in each group that you relate to most strongly and put the number 1 in the blank to the right of that response.

My blood pressure:
Is generally low but can rise if I'm upset.   **A.** _____
Is usually low.   **B.** _____
Is constantly low.   **C.** _____
Is fairly normal.   **D.** _____
Can periodically be high.   **E.** _____
Can easily go high.   **F.** _____

Body temperature:
I like sun.   **A.** _____
I need the sun.   **B.** _____
I like summer.   **C.** _____
I can take either winter or summer.   **D.** _____
I like the cold.   **E.** _____
I love winter.   **F.** _____

Immunity to colds and flu:
I never get the flu or colds.   **A.** _____
I seldom get sick.   **B.** _____
My resistance is above average.   **C.** _____
My resistance is normal.   **D.** _____

I usually get a cold or the flu in the winter.　　　　E. _____

I catch colds or have the flu a lot.　　　　F. _____

Reaction to allergens:

I never have allergic reactions.　　　　A. _____

I can sometimes have allergic reactions.　　　　B. _____

If under stress, I can have allergic reactions.　　　　C. _____

I'm predisposed to allergies.　　　　D. _____

I have recurring reactions.　　　　E. _____

I have extreme reactions.　　　　F. _____

Weight fluctuations:

I can keep my weight stable unless I'm under stress.　　A. _____

If I gain weight, I can lose it easily.　　　　B. _____

It's easy for me to gain weight if I'm under stress.　　C. _____

I gain weight extremely easily.　　　　D. _____

I'm always a bit overweight; I love food.　　　　E. _____

I'm always overweight.　　　　F. _____

In the morning:

I don't want to eat.　　　　A. _____

I want nothing or may have a roll or coffee.　　　　B. _____

Sometimes I want a very small breakfast.　　　　C. _____

I love a breakfast of French toast.　　　　D. _____

I love juice, coffee, cereal, and bread.　　　　E. _____

I like breakfast.　　　　F. _____

I prefer my biggest meal to be:

Definitely dinner　　　　A. _____

Dinner　　　　B. _____

Lunch or dinner　　　　C. _____

Definitely lunch or breakfast　　　　D. _____

Breakfast　　　　E. _____

Snacks　　　　F. _____

If I eat late or just before I go to bed, I'll:

Toss, turn, and either sleep restlessly or
　　get no sleep.　　　　A. _____

Feel extremely uncomfortable and wake.　　　　B. _____

Feel uneasy.　　　　C. _____

Often feel better.　　　　D. _____

Usually feel better.   **E.** _____

Always feel better.   **F.** _____

I have gas two to three hours after I eat:

All the time.   **A.** _____

Regularly.   **B.** _____

Fairly often.   **C.** _____

From time to time.   **D.** _____

Hardly ever.   **E.** _____

Never.   **F.** _____

I move my bowels:

Maybe every one to three days.   **A.** _____

Usually every other day.   **B.** _____

Infrequently; I usually tend toward constipation.   **C.** _____

Normally once a day.   **D.** _____

Once or twice a day.   **E.** _____

Often during the day.   **F.** _____

Tendency to energy drops or low blood sugar:

I have energy all day long and get tired only at night. **A.** _____

I usually have stable energy until about 4:00 P.M.   **B.** _____

I definitely "crash" in the afternoon.   **C.** _____

I must be careful to eat or I have energy drops.   **D.** _____

I have regular blood sugar drops,
   especially if I've eaten "carbs."   **E.** _____

I have serious blood sugar and energy drops.   **F.** _____

Foods I love or crave:

Red meat and salt   **A.** _____

Sugar and desserts   **B.** _____

Breads and sweets   **C.** _____

Rich and spicy dishes   **D.** _____

Bread   **E.** _____

Dairy products and chocolate   **F.** _____

TOTALS A: _____ **B:** _____ **C:** _____ **D:** _____ **E:** _____ **F:** _____

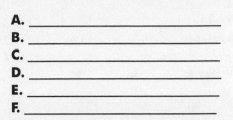

5. Dealing with Sexuality

Pick out the response in each group that you relate to most strongly and put the number 1 in the blank to the right of that response.

Subject matter I really love to talk about:

Business, organization, and how to make money. **A.** _____

Achieving goals and having monetary success. **B.** _____

Current news, entertainment, or my own projects. **C.** _____

My family, sexuality, food. **D.** _____

Politics, organization, food. **E.** _____

Philosophical ideals, the occult and mystical. **F.** _____

How I relate intimately with another person:

I'm a great friend, very open but practical. **A.** _____

I'm careful and open; being a friend is important. **B.** _____

I'm changeable; I like action and get bored easily. **C.** _____

I'm extremely sensuous, inviting, and warm. **D.** _____

I'm warm, caring, and have great empathy. **E.** _____

I'm cool, detached but really "earthy." **F.** _____

How often I would like to have sex:

At least two or three times per week. **A.** _____

Once or twice a week is fine for me. **B.** _____

It's erratic: maybe a lot, then nothing for a while. **C.** _____

As often as I can—daily. **D.** _____

When I'm not tired, very often. **E.** _____

Two or three times a month is fine with me. **F.** _____

Passions:

I don't think I have emotional passions. **A.** _____

I easily suppress my passions. **B.** _____

I can take or leave emotional passion. **C.** _____

I thrive on emotional and sexual passion. **D.** _____

I love passion and sex. **E.** _____

I'm extremely passionate about what I believe in. **F.** _____

TOTALS A: _____ **B:** _____ **C:** _____ **D:** _____ **E:** _____ **F:** _____

Now add up all your scores:

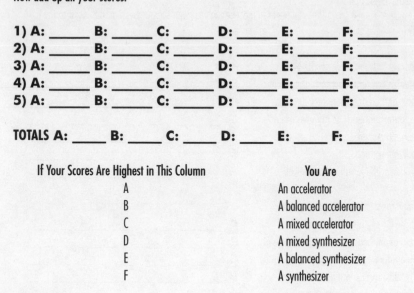

1) **A:** _____ **B:** _____ **C:** _____ **D:** _____ **E:** _____ **F:** _____
2) **A:** _____ **B:** _____ **C:** _____ **D:** _____ **E:** _____ **F:** _____
3) **A:** _____ **B:** _____ **C:** _____ **D:** _____ **E:** _____ **F:** _____
4) **A:** _____ **B:** _____ **C:** _____ **D:** _____ **E:** _____ **F:** _____
5) **A:** _____ **B:** _____ **C:** _____ **D:** _____ **E:** _____ **F:** _____

TOTALS A: _____ **B:** _____ **C:** _____ **D:** _____ **E:** _____ **F:** _____

If Your Scores Are Highest in This Column	You Are
A	An accelerator
B	A balanced accelerator
C	A mixed accelerator
D	A mixed synthesizer
E	A balanced synthesizer
F	A synthesizer

Meta-Type Characteristic Checklist

TENDENCIES	ACCELERATOR	BALANCED ACCELERATOR	MIXED ACCELERATOR	SYNTHESIZER	BALANCED SYNTHESIZER	MIXED SYNTHESIZER
Psychological inclination	Intellectually dominant; rational and linear thinking; hard time getting to their emotions	Intellectually dominant; strong intuition; deep emotions; rules from their head	Intellectually dominant; strong emotions; may "stuff" down feelings	Emotionally dominant; lives in their feelings; highly creative	Emotionally dominant; strong intuition; can have strong intellect	Emotionally dominant; strong intellect; gets pulled between both
Motto	"I think—then act decisively."	"I think, I intuit—then act decisively."	"I think—feel then act only when I'm sure."	"I feel—and I may not even act!"	"I feel, I intuit—then act—only when I'm sure."	"I feel, I think through things, then I'll act."
Life's direction	Ambitious, competitive, and workaholic	Focus, concentration, clarity, intensity, driven	Professionally, family, and socially oriented	Empathic; needs to create and feel	Lives in their feelings; needs to partner	Warm and sensuous nature; must create
Energy	Extremely active and doesn't stop	Very active; abundant stored energy	Active energy in short spurts; little endurance	Slow and passive	Slow morning; builds throughout the day	Slow to get started, then goes until done
Reaction to stress	Anxiety; uses it to fuel their energy	Anxiety; lives on intensity	Anxiety; depression if under prolonged stress	Depression	Depression to anxiety to depression	Anxiety to depression
Best energy time	Early morning to late afternoon	Morning to late afternoon	Morning to early afternoon; early evening	Evening to night	Midmorning, then early to late evening	Sometimes mornings; early to late evenings
Weather preference	Loves the sun; warm, warm, warm	Hot and tropical	Warm	Gray, cloudy, cool	Cool	Mild; not too cold, not too hot
Strong endocrine gland	Adrenals	Thymus	Thyroid	Pituitary	Pancreas	Sex glands
Weak endocrine gland	Sex glands	Pancreas	Pituitary	Thyroid	Thymus	Adrenals
Gains weight	Slowly unless under stress	Slowly, loses easily unless eating fats	Easily if under stress or their thyroid is low	Extremely easily	Very easily	Easily

TENDENCIES	ACCELERATOR	BALANCED ACCELERATOR	MIXED ACCELERATOR	SYNTHESIZER	BALANCED SYNTHESIZER	MIXED SYNTHESIZER
Puts weight on:	Upper torso	Stomach, upper torso, then hips	Stomach first, then hips and thighs	All over the body	Thighs and hips	Buttocks and hips
Thinks of food as:	Functional	Functional; may use as a reward factor	Enjoys; may eat to repress their emotions	A ritual	Pleasure; loves their three meals a day	Is a sensuous eater; loves to eat
Food Cravings:	Sugar, salt, starches, and sometimes meat	Sugar and fats	Breads, pasta, sugar	Creams, dairy, sugar	Sugar, starches	Spices, oils, fats, sugar
Metabolism type: (Oxidize = burns off energy)	Fast metabolizer; fairly slow oxidizer	Fairly fast metabolizer; slow oxidizer	Semifast metabolizer; semifast oxidizer	Very slow metabolizer; speedy oxidizer	Slow metabolizer; rapid oxidizer	Fairly slow metabolizer; quick oxidizer
Cellular pH range:	Strong acid, 4.5–4	Acid forming, 5	Weak acid, 6.2	Strong alkaline, 8–7.5	Alkaline forming, 7.4	Weak alkaline, 6.8
Needs type of foods:	Vegetarian	Semivegetarian	Omnivore	Carnivore	Semicarnivore	Omnivore; no red meat
Exercise:	Loves their exercise; an exercise "fiend"	Hates repetitive exercise; bores easily; loves Dancercize	Needs exercise; likes it most of the time	Dislikes it but really needs it	Needs "robust" exercise	May dislike; definitely needs it
Sleep pattern	Has a hard time falling asleep; often insomnia	Can fall asleep easily; has insomnia or wakes if stressed	Falls asleep easily, sleeps through the night	"Out like a light"; needs a lot of sleep	Falls asleep quickly; needs over eight hours rest	Effortlessly falls asleep; may wake with anxiety

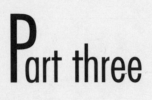

Part three

Making the Plan Work for You

Now before you skip ahead to part four and jump right into your metabolic diet and food plans to create that fantastic new you, read chapters 11 through 13. Chapter 11 contains absolutely *essential* guidelines for using this program, chapter 12 introduces you to some beverages that can make the difference when it comes to quick weight loss and high energy, and chapter 13 shows you how to jump-start your nutrition plan by balancing your foods with the correct vitamins and supplements. These chapters will give you the controls, impetus, and information you need in order to make this program stick everlastingly as a new, lifelong way of existing—and feel exhilarated, full of energy, and sublimely thin and fit for a powerful life.

11 Guidelines for Healthy Living

As you have probably discovered by now, the Your Body, Your Diet plan is far more than just a weight-loss program; it's your road map to a healthier, more vibrant, more energetic life. Imagine the power of not only controlling your weight but also finding effective new ways to manage stress, banish depression, and feel absolutely wonderful, day after day. With *Your Body, Your Diet* all of this is easily within your reach. To be sure that you get the most out of the plan, however, I've filled this chapter with important advice—little markers to help you find your way as you embark on your journey.

No matter what meta-type you are, your body repairs, regenerates, transforms, or destroys itself as a result of what you eat, drink, think, and feel each day. Now this may sound oversimplified, but it's true. If you eat dead foods, your body and mind will die in many small ways, far before your time. You will actually speed up the aging process.

Living foods, alive with their own natural enzymes, are the fuel on which your body depends for the powerful amino acids, vitamins, and minerals needed to repair itself and keep you strong. These wonderful foods encourage and nurture the natural rhythms and flow of life, and that's why they are the basis of the plan. And I'll show you a formula for combining foods that will put a stop to bloating, gas, and other dietary discomforts.

What you eat and how you eat it will determine whether your body ages quickly or barely ages at all. Remember, beauty really does begin deep within. I know you're eager to turn to your actual diet plan, but take a few more moments to look over these plan basics.

Understanding the Basics

Relax

Taking it easy before you eat helps all the organs of your digestion—the stomach, small intestines, pancreas, liver, and gallbladder—release their precious enzymes and juices. This in turn enables you to break down, absorb, and assimilate your foods *completely*, which eliminates gases produced by incompletely digested or undigested foods.

Dine Stress-Free

Never eat in a stressful or tense environment. The stress response causes your parasympathetic nervous system's vagus nerve—in the middle of your solar plexus—to literally shut down, stopping you from digesting anything. Its closed-down circuitry inhibits the release of essential pancreatic enzymes (as well as other digestive juices) and puts a halt to your digestive and regenerative abilities. Food ends up feeling like a rock in your stomach. It won't be digested or eliminated quickly and turns to fat more easily.

Be Patient

Don't gulp your meals. Chew your food slowly. Digestion begins inside the mouth as the enzyme *ptyalin* in the saliva starts the digestive process. So take your time; chew and mix well.

Don't Stuff Yourself

Eat no more than what you need at each meal. Your body can produce only a certain amount of enzymes and digestive juices at a time, so your system can handle a limited amount of food at a time. When you feel pleasantly full—stop. Don't continue eating out of emotional need.

Be Conscious of What You'll Need

Make your week's food plan ahead of time and shop in advance. If you stock your kitchen with the items you'll be needing, you'll eliminate that temptation to "grab anything." Then when you've just gotten home, tired from a day's work, and have only a short time to prepare your meal, you'll have all the essential ingredients.

Stay on Track

Eat regular meals and don't eat late at night (unless the information in your meta-type meal plan says this is okay). Eating late keeps the body busy digesting that food rather than cleaning out the day's toxic residue and waste, repairing your cells, and redistributing existing fat. Unfortunately the food you've just eaten will only turn to new fat.

Late meals also regularly cause you to have a restless night's sleep or to wake three to four hours into your sleep cycle. Food takes time to digest, so shortly after you fall asleep, the energy released from those late foods will flood your bloodstream, raising your blood sugar level sky-high and waking you.

Outsmart Food Cravings

Each meta-type is dominated by a specific endocrine gland, which governs that meta-type's metabolism and provides most of its energy. Whatever your meta-type, you'll find that you've had a natural affinity for the food groups that stimulate your strongest gland. The trouble starts when you develop the habit of overindulging in foods from that particular group when you are tired, sick, or under stress. Then these specific foods become your comfort foods, the ones you just can't turn down even when you really want to drop a few pounds. In addition to thickening your waistline, overeating those foods that stimulate your dominant gland is like getting the gas pedal stuck. It floods your engine, overstimulating the gland and often causing allergic reactions. To banish these cravings, you must eliminate the foods that needlessly stimulate your dominant endocrine gland. That gives your key gland a chance to rest and repair.

Work with Your Body Clock

When it comes to getting rid of fat, your metabolism has its own way of ensuring that it does not have to work overtime. The two most dominant alkaline times for the body to regenerate and burn fat are:

1. 3:30 A.M., lasting about two to three hours
2. 2:30 P.M., lasting for about two hours

If you take just a few minutes to relax during these periods, your body's mechanisms can take over and quickly stimulate a rapid turnover of your fat molecules to energy molecules to be burned up, especially in the late afternoon. Then you can *see* your fat melt away.

Understand Your Body's Balance

Each layer of the body has a different acid-alkaline makeup, known as the pH value. The skin and saliva are slightly acid; the stomach is more acid; the small intestine is slightly acid; urine is acid. Your blood, cells, and large intestine are slightly more alkaline, and your body regenerates and transforms cellular tissue in those two more alkaline time phases mentioned in the preceding subsection. So an extremely acid state interferes with the healing and repair of the body.

Excess sugar (glucose) creates a very acid environment, as do caffeine, alcohol, refined carbohydrates, and nicotine. That means that along with eliminating those toxifying acid producers, it's also necessary to eat foods that have a low sugar content or low glycemic index and are absorbed more slowly. That maintains the harmonious balance of your alkaline and acid environments, allowing your body to regenerate.

Now each metabolic profile tends to be more acid or alkaline based on how the autonomic nervous system functions, as explained in chapter 3. So by choosing foods from the opposite end of the spectrum, you can achieve that perfect balance of yin and yang.

Appendix 5 lists the full spectrum of foods and their pH values.

Know Your Nutrients

Remember, proteins are utilized for cell repair, carbohydrates are used for energy, and fats are employed for energy, padding, and insulation around your body, as well as for hormones.

How and when food can *energize* or *regenerate* your body depends on how long it takes for each category of food to be digested—broken down, absorbed, then utilized by the body. Knowing these times (which are shown in the accompanying table) gives you a better understanding of when to eat to get a boost of energy or to repair your cells.

Fruits are the body's scrubbers and cleansers; proteins are the building blocks of your cellular structure; carbohydrates energize and provide the vitamins and minerals that hold the building blocks together; fats lubricate and insulate.

Digestion Times for the Principal Categories of Foods

TYPE OF FOOD	TIME (HOURS)
Protein	
Meat, fish, fowl, seeds, nuts, dairy	12
Protein starch: some legumes	12
Fats	
Oils, creams	12
Carbohydrates	
Legumes	6
Grains	5
Starchy vegetables (such as potatoes)	5
Nonstarchy vegetables (such as leafy greens)	5
Fruits: Sweet—fresh or dried	3
Acid or subacid	2
Melons	2
Refined sugar and starches	2

Remember, eat just what you need to be comfortable; any food—protein, carbohydrates, or fat—will turn into fat if it's not utilized properly.

Shop for the Best

Your foods should be fresh and as close to their natural state as possible. Never use canned foods. They will be contaminated from the can itself. Then you will be eating food that is not only dead but also laced with an enormous amount of aluminum, which is not conducive to regeneration. Frozen foods also lose nutrients, so whenever possible, opt for the fresh version.

Eat for Variety

Make wide selections from the foods listed for your meta-type. The more color, the better. It's simple to remember: the greater the color variety of your foods, the more abundant the mineral content you take into your body. If it's on your specific health plan, use one to two root vegetables (such as carrots, beets, and parsnips) to two to three above-ground vegetables (spinach, broccoli, escarole, squash, and the like) and follow the food-combining instructions discussed later in this chapter.

Cook with Care

Cooking methods play an important role in protecting the enzyme, vitamin, mineral, or fatty acid content of the foods you eat. Boiling for any length of time destroys all active enzymes. Frying transforms valuable unsaturated fatty acids into destructive saturated fat. So preparing your food the right way is essential. Here are some tips for how to prepare foods properly:

- *Proteins* should be baked, broiled, or steamed—*never* fried.
- *Vegetables* should be barely steamed or baked to ensure their enzyme life.
- *Fruits* should be eaten in their natural, raw state if possible.
- *Fats* should be taken as oils. The way fats are at room temperature is the way they will reside in your body. Oils (unsaturated fats) are liquid and shift easily inside the body, whereas saturated fats (such as butter) remain solid and can easily clog your arteries. Try *never* to fry with oils. The heat turns the chemical components of unsaturated fats *into* the harmful saturated fats.
- *Honey* should be used only in small amounts.

Balance Your Supplements

One day per week eliminate the supplements from your program. They strongly stimulate your body to regenerate and repair itself. Skipping your amino acids, vitamins, or minerals for this one day will give your body a day in which it can just relax and not worry about having to work at regeneration. Sunday is always a good day for rest and recreation.

Understand Food Combining

Food combining is an essential and indispensable part of your program. It's one of the keys to staying young. Why? Because it's based on the digestive requirements of each food group. You've seen how long it takes each food group to be digested. If you use this knowledge to combine your foods properly, you will ensure that every bit of food you take in will be absorbed and utilized properly. This will liberate your food's vast storehouse of precious vitamins, minerals, and amino acids. And on a more "social" comfort level, it can reduce gas and bloating.

If your program consists of a more vegetarian eating plan, on certain days or throughout, be sure to *mix 60 percent grains to 40 percent legumes or tofu* (steamed) for a complete protein balance. Animal protein is the only protein that contains all the essential amino acids we need to get from outside sources. Our bodies manufacture the rest. Grains are deficient in lysine, one of the most essential of the amino acid building blocks, but high in methionine, a key amino acid for energizing the body as well as making the essential neurotransmitter of the parasympathetic nervous system—acetylcholine. Conversely, the starchy vegetable proteins—such as soybeans, dried beans, and peas—are rich in lysine but much lower in methionine. Combining these two food groups of carbohydrates provides the total complement of proteins we need from outside food sources.

Principles like these, along with the timing of food digestion, are the fundamentals of food combining. Just follow these guidelines and you'll get the idea:

• *Only one type of protein should be eaten at a time.* This allows the single protein to have ample amounts of hydrochloric acid so it can be completely digested. Otherwise, two or more proteins would "compete" for the stomach acids, and there would always be a "loser," creating bloating, abdominal distension, and gas.

• *Proteins and fats shouldn't be eaten together.* Proteins and fats break down and oxidize, or "burn," slowly and require the same amount of digestive time. Therefore, if they are eaten together, one will "compete" with the other for the digestive enzymes, which leaves the "loser"—the one with less enzymes—improperly broken down. A domino effect starts, creating a myriad of problems, and you begin building fat.

• *Proteins and grains shouldn't be eaten together.* As you've seen, protein requires the acid medium of the stomach (aerobic environment—with air) to break down slowly, while grains break down rapidly and go right through the stomach acid directly to the small intestines (anaerobic environment—without air), where they require the more alkaline medium to be absorbed into the body. If they are eaten together, either the grains will get caught with the proteins in the stomach and not digest, causing gas and bloating, or the grains will rob the proteins of their hydrochloric acid. In turn, the proteins will break down incompletely, resulting in heartburn, bloating, gas, and a buildup of toxins.

• *Fruits and simple sugars should be eaten by themselves.* Because their digestive time is so rapid, fruits and simple sugars should be eaten independently of any other foods. Acid and subacid fruits can be eaten together, while sweet fruits and melons should be eaten by themselves—all based on the digestive timing of the different food categories.

Combining foods isn't as hard as it sounds. Actually it's pretty simple. Keep the accompanying food-combining chart on hand for use as an easy reference.

Dane's Simple-to-Use Food-Combining Chart

EAT GRAINS (RICE, WHEAT, COUSCOUS, ETC.) WITH	EAT ANIMAL PROTEINS (MEAT, CHICKEN, FOWL, FISH) WITH	EAT FRUITS BY THEMSELVES
Nonanimal proteins (dairy, seeds, nuts, etc.) Vegetable-starch proteins (dry beans, peas, etc.) Leafy green above-ground vegetables (spinach, broccoli, kale, etc.) Starchy vegetables (potatoes, corn, squash, etc.) Mildly starchy vegetables (carrots, beets, turnips, etc.) Fats (oils)	Leafy green above-ground vegetables (spinach, broccoli, kale, etc.) Starchy vegetables (potatoes, corn, squash, etc.) Mildly starchy vegetables (carrots, beets, turnips, etc.)	Acid and sub-acid fruits can be eaten together Sweet and dried fruits can be eaten together Melons should be eaten by themselves Leave *simple sugars* alone

Note: Do not combine grains and fats with animal proteins.

Clean House

Now, as you suspected, there are certain foods in your diet that just have to go. If you're really *serious* about looking and feeling your best, then foods that are denatured and/or filled with additives and chemicals are out. They fill your body with toxic substances and make you old far before your time. So here goes:

GIVE IT UP
- Foods sprayed with pesticides
- Foods filled with additives
- All canned and packaged foods
- All foods made from refined white flour—cakes, cookies, white-flour pasta, and so forth
- All foods made from refined white sugar—breads, pastries, and so on
- Refined sugar and artificial sweeteners—especially candy
- All artificially processed foods
- Salt and foods with salt added
- All fried foods
- Soft drinks, canned drinks, and pasteurized juices
- Commercial cereals

- High-fat dairy products
- Hydrogenated fats and oils
- Excess chocolate
- Caffeine
- Smoked meat and fish
- Pork and fatty beef
- Excess alcohol
- Fluoridated water

Now for the good news. Along with the foods selected for your individual diet program, you can:

FEEL FREE TO
- Spice things up with a variety of fresh and dried herbs.
- Enjoy delicious herbal teas and fresh juices.
- Indulge in an abundance of fresh vegetables and legumes, grains, fresh fruits, and proteins (vegetable proteins mixed with grains, nuts, and seeds; low-fat dairy; fish; poultry; and lean beef or lamb).

Facing Down Food Allergies

Now we come to the issue of allergies. Once you're well on the road to your new way of eating, most of your symptoms should disappear, as long as you haven't succumbed to a continuous or prolonged stress response. But even then your allergies can be licked.

The tables in this section will help you avoid trigger foods and those awful attacks. Food allergies can be of varying degrees of severity. Symptoms may not arise if only one food is eaten. If a number of trigger foods are eaten at one time or in large quantities, however, an allergic reaction can develop in minutes.

The speed and severity of the reaction also depend on how rapidly your food is absorbed into your bloodstream from your digestive tract. *The faster the absorption rate, the faster the allergic reaction.* For instance, a carbohydrate with a high glycemic index (sugar content) will be absorbed almost immediately and can cause an allergic reaction in a flash.

In addition to the foods themselves, some food additives may also cause allergic reactions. The accompanying table lists foods that commonly cause problems. Shellfish, for example, is a prime culprit. If you think you are having a reaction to a food or group of foods, test yourself by eating that food alone and monitoring your body's response.

Foods That Can Cause Allergic Reactions

DAIRY PRODUCTS	PROTEINS		GRAINS (CONTAINING GLUTEN)
	Fowl	Fish	

Milk
Butter
Cream
Yogurt
Cheese
Ice cream
Milk additives:
   calcium caseinate,
   casein, caseinate,
   casein hydrolysate,
   dried milk solids (DMS),
   lactalbumin, lactate
   solids, milk solid
   pastes, sweetened
   condensed milk,
   whey solids
	Eggs
	Egg derivatives:
	   albumin, dried egg
	   solids, egg solids,
	   globulin, ovomucin,
	   and vitellin
		Shellfish, especially:
		• Fresh, canned,
		  smoked, or pickled
		  fish
		• Fish-liver oils and
		  concentrates
		• Stews, broth,
		  chowders, soups,
		  salads with shellfish
			Wheat—the biggest
			  offender
			Corn
			Oats
			Rye
			Barley
			Grain derivatives:
			  enriched flour, flour,
			  hydrolyzed flour,
			  modified food
			  starch, MSG
			  (monosodium
			  glutamate), self-
			  rising flour, sodium
			  glutamate

NUTS AND SOME SEEDS	LEGUMES (BEANS)	HIGH-STARCH VEGETABLES	FOODS CONTAINING THE *POISONOUS* SOLANINE ALKALOID

Peanuts—most
  common (really a
  legume)
Peanut oil
Walnuts
Pecans
Brazil nuts
Filberts (hazelnuts)
Coconut
	Alfalfa
	Beans: green, kidney,
	  lima, mung, navy, wax
	Soybeans: soya flour,
	  oil, tofu (bean curd)
	Carob
	Lentils
	Licorice
	Peas: black-eyed, chick,
	  green, split
	Peanuts (see "Nuts")
	Legume derivatives:
	  hydrolyzed
	  vegetable protein,
	  soy flour and
	  concentrate,
	  textured vegetable
	  protein, concentrated
	  "vege" protein
		Corn
		Corn derivatives: corn
		  solids, corn starch,
		  corn syrup,
		  vegetable starch
			Nightshade plants:
			• Tomatoes
			• Red peppers
			• Eggplants
			• Potatoes
			• Tobacco plant
			
			Small amount in:
			• Apples
			• Sugar beets

Medical research has also shown that if you are allergic to one food, you may be allergic to all foods in that particular family of foods. The connections may seem obvious, like shrimp and scallops, but they aren't always that simple. Onion and asparagus, for example, are in the same family. The most common trigger foods, and their relatives, are listed in the accompanying table.

Families of Foods That Can Trigger an Allergic Reaction

NIGHTSHADE FAMILY	CEREAL FAMILY	PEA FAMILY	PALM FAMILY	LILY FAMILY
Bell peppers	Barley	Black-eyed	Coconut	Asparagus
Cayenne peppers	Cane sugar	Chick	Dates	Chives
Eggplants	Corn	Navy	Olive palm	Garlic
Potatoes	Malt	Kidney		Leeks
Tomatoes	Millet	Pinto		Onions
	Oats	Lentils		Shallots
	Popcorn	Licorice		
	Rice	Peas		
	Rye	Peanuts		
	Sorghum	Soybeans		
	Wheat			
	Wild rice			

GOURD FAMILY	PARSLEY FAMILY	PLUM FAMILY	SUNFLOWER FAMILY	CABBAGE AND MUSTARD FAMILY
Cantaloupes	Anise	Almonds	Artichokes	Broccoli
Cucumbers	Caraway seeds	Apricots	Dandelions	Brussels sprouts
Pumpkin	Carrots	Cherries	Endives	Cabbage
Squash	Celery	Nectarines	Jerusalem	Chinese cabbage
Watermelon	Parsley	Peaches	artichokes	Cauliflower
	Parsnips	Plums	Lettuce	Collards
			Safflower	Horseradish
			Sunflower seeds	Kale
				Mustard greens
				Radishes
				Turnips
				Watercress

As I mentioned earlier, foods with a high glycemic index—those that have a high concentration of sugar or glucose—are absorbed into your bloodstream almost immediately and can cause an instant allergic reaction as well as an immediate increase in insulin. Therefore, the following foods should be scrupulously avoided if you are suffering from any degree of allergies, low blood sugar, or weight problems:

- Alcohol of any kind
- Artificial sweeteners
- Caffeinated coffee or even tea
- Some fruits: bananas, raisins, and mangoes
- Dry breakfast cereals of any kind, even granola
- Dried fruit and fruit juices
- Ice cream
- Jams and jellies, even fruit-sweetened
- Pastry: cake, cookies, pie, and the like
- Sodas, even diet soda
- Sugars of any kind: honey, syrup, molasses, brown sugar, and the like
- White-flour products: rolls, bread, flour, bagels, muffins, pasta, chips, pretzels
- White rice and white potatoes
- Yogurt, flavored or frozen

Chemical processing as well as the fiber content in each food alters the food's glycemic index. Increased fiber lowers the glycemic index, while chemical processing increases it. So white rice has a glycemic index of 70, while brown rice has a glycemic index of 50. Guess which one is better for you? The accompanying table will help you choose the appropriate foods, based on their glucose content.

Foods Ranked by Their Glycemic Index

FOOD	GLYCEMIC INDEX
High Glycemic Index (110–51)	
Alcohol	110
Glucose	110
White bread	95
Honey, jam	90
Packaged cereals and popcorn	85
Carrots	85
Refined sugar	75
Corn	70
Beets	70

FOOD	GLYCEMIC INDEX
White rice	70
Cookies	70
Boiled potatoes	70
White-flour pasta	65
Bananas, raisins	60
Mangoes	60
Low Glycemic Index (50–10)	
Whole or brown rice	50
Whole wheat bread/pasta	50
White beans, fresh	40
Oatmeal	40
Rye bread	40
Green peas, fresh	40
Whole cereals—not wheat or oats	35
Dairy products	35
Wild rice	35
Fruits, fresh	35
Lentils	30
Chickpeas	30
Beans, dried	30
Peas, dried	30
Fructose	20
Soya	15
Green vegetables	<15

To simplify matters, the accompanying table gives a quick summary of the "good guys" and the "bad guys." It will help jog your memory when you're out and about.

What to Avoid and What to Enjoy

BAD GUYS	GOOD GUYS
All sugar: cane, beet, brown, maple syrup, molasses	Whole cereals: oats, barley, millet, wheat
Honey	Whole-grain products: flour, bread, pasta, bran
Jams, jellies	Rice: brown and wild
Soft drinks	Beans
White-flour products—any and all: bread, pasta, cakes, cookies, rolls, muffins, bagels, pretzels, chips, pizza, croissants, quiche	Legumes
	Most fruits

BAD GUYS	GOOD GUYS
White rice Potatoes, even sweet potatoes (Darn!) Corn Carrots Beets Bananas Raisins Mangoes Semolina, even couscous Packaged cereals Alcohol	And the really good guys Mom demanded you eat: all vegetables—especially the green leafy ones—except the starchy vegetables listed in the "bad guys" column

Kicking Caffeine

Last but certainly not least on the list of things that can throw your body out of balance is caffeine, whether we're talking coffee or those often misleading "diet" colas.

I had a client who said in despair that she just *hated* to give up her beloved morning espresso because of "the awful headaches, nausea, and queasiness I experience every time I stop drinking coffee." No wonder she had headaches—with a *daily* morning ritual of *three cups of espresso*.

"Suffer not," I told her. "I have the perfect plan to rid your body of that noxious caffeine without the 'headache special.' It's called the 'James Taylor remedy.'"

Years ago, when James first came to me, we devised a plan to *wean* him off caffeine, so he wouldn't fall prey to those awful withdrawal headaches, which terribly inhibited his creativity and performances.

Now you can have the benefit of his experience and save yourself all the wear and tear of caffeine withdrawal. You might be surprised to learn that the coffee bean is an herb and can be used the way we use herbs—a little at a time or on the special occasions when it's required for certain types of healing. But taken on a continual basis, it creates a terrible addiction, in which the body begins to rely on false stimulation to get itself going.

Diet colas can be a real stumbling block. They're packed with even more chemicals and sodium than those espressos and may actually trigger a sweet tooth.

Once you're into caffeine addiction, it begins to mask the serious deficiencies in the body while stimulating and pumping your glands even further to produce those hormones from an already exhausted endocrine system. So it's best to give up caffeine altogether, and the accompanying chart shows you how to do it. You can take one to three weeks—but *no longer* than three weeks.

Kicking Caffeine: The Three-Week Plan

WEEK	CAFFEINE INTAKE
1	Give up all caffeine-laced foods except coffee (but including chocolate and diet colas) and drink *plenty* of water.
2	Limit your caffeine intake to only one cup of coffee per day.
3	Days 1–3: Drink ¾ cup of coffee diluted with ¼ water.
	Days 4–5: Drink ½ cup coffee diluted with ½ cup water.
	Days 6–7: Drink ¼ cup coffee diluted with ¾ cup water.
	Day 8: Give it up.

Whenever you have questions about keeping your diet on track, just turn back to this chapter for a refresher on those tips that will help you move toward safe weight loss and a stronger, healthier you.

12 Elegant Elixirs: Drinking Your Way to Energetic Health

Water is the best tonic for health, no secret there. Drinking six to eight glasses a day will put you on the road to real success. But depending on your meta-type, fresh juices, cranberry juice (the concentrated kind, with no added sugars), and herbal teas can give you such a high-energy, low-fat boost, you'll really be drinking to your health.

Melting Weight Away with Herbs

Eastern medicine's famous herbal remedies work to maintain the body's energy balance—the forces of yin and yang. I've created a mixture of some of the most powerful and effective herbs to help you achieve this balance while on the Your Body, Your Diet plan. For centuries healers have dispensed flowers, seeds, stems, bark, and roots of plants and trees. The first written herbal formula dates from 5000 B.C., and ancient Chinese doctors customarily paid their patients if any fell ill while under their care. From early Egypt and Greece to modern Europe, herbal remedies and homeopathic formulas have been widely accepted. And U.S. scientists today are turning to the South American rain forests to find therapies for cancer and other diseases.

My Master Weight-Loss Tea, chock-full of these healing herbs, can be used by every meta-type. There are small variations (explained in the diet chapters for each type), but the basic formula appears in the accompanying table.

Unless I'm making a decoction for medicine, I generally prepare my herbs the European way rather than the Eastern way (both methods are described later in this section). But many clients like to be able to choose which approach to use, so I always send their teas with the roots and seeds in one package and the flowers and leaves in a separate bag.

The great thing about these techniques is that you can make up extra tea in advance, keep it in the refrigerator, and use it as needed. For instance, prepare enough over the weekend to get you through your busy week.

It's best to drink one to three cupfuls per day—but *not* late in the evening.

Master Weight-Loss Tea Formula

NAME			FUNCTION
Common	Latin	Eastern	
Alisma: water-plantain tuber	*Alisma plantage aquatica*	Ze xie	Regulates water metabolism and reduces fat, especially in the liver.
Poria (mushrooms): Indian bread	*Poria cocus*	Fu ling	Regulates water metabolism; reduces abdominal distension.
Rhubarb root	*Rheum plamatum*	Da huang	Regulates the intestines; cleans the liver.
Red clover tops	*Trifolium pratense*	—	Powerful blood cleanser; also cleans out the lymphatic system.
Alfalfa leaf	*Medicago sativa*	—	The "great healer"— cleanses blood and reduces cholesterol and fatty plaque.
Hawthorn berry	*Crataegus pinnatifida oxycantha*	Shan za	Regulates digestion; reduces cholesterol, fatty tissue, and abdominal distension.
Radish seed	*Raphanus* seed: *Semen raphani*	Lai fu zi	Regulates digestion; reduces fat.
Sargassum: kelp, sea wrack	*Sargassum fusiforme*	Hai zao	Regulates the body's basal metabolic rate by balancing the thyroid gland.

NAME			FUNCTION
Common	Latin	Eastern	
Indian chickweed: starwort	*Stellaria media*	—	Dissolves fat; stops food cravings.
Evergreen artemesia	*Artemisia capillaris*	Yin chen hao	Dissolves fatty tissue.
Astragalus root	*Astragalus membranaceus*	Huang qi	Balances the yang energy; regenerates the endocrine system.
Fleeceflower root	*Radix polygoni multiflori, Polygonum multiflorum*	He shou wu, fo ti tieng	Balances the yin energy; reduces cholesterol; prevents aging.
Citrus peel	*Citrus reticulata*	Chen pi	Spreads the energy throughout the body; eliminates abdominal fullness.

Note: If you are pregnant, have high blood pressure, or are allergic to grasses or flowers, it's suggested that these teas not be used.

The required herbs can be found at your local health-food store or ordered from the places listed in appendix 2, "Shopping Guide."

Preparing the herbs is a simple matter. You can choose to use all of them or just the ones that seem to fit your individual needs. Mix *equal* parts of the roots, seeds, bark, and woody parts of the herbs together and store them in an airtight plastic container or bag. Do the same thing for the flowers or leaves of the herbs. The *European technique* is as follows:

1. Take ½ ounce of the combination of the roots, stems, and seeds for each glass of tea. Put it into a stainless steel pan and cover it with 10 to 12 ounces of water (a little more than a large glass). Cover the pan and let the mixture soak for about ten minutes. Then bring the mixture to a boil and simmer gently for about ten minutes.

2. Add the flowers or leaves of the herbs—½ ounce for each glass of tea—and let steep, with the lid on tightly, for another ten to fifteen minutes. Strain off the herbs, cool, and drink the tea warm or at room temperature.

The Eastern technique is a bit different. Although the roots aren't separated from the flowers, the cooking time tends to be a bit longer. When Eastern physicians prepare their herbs as medicine, they put them in a round ceramic pot, cover them with water (about 1 quart), and boil—fairly rapidly—until only one cup of the "brew" is left. That can be pretty intense, so that's *not* what we're doing here. This is going to be a pleasant experience. So to prepare your weight-loss tea my *modified Eastern way*, use the following techniques:

• *To make a light, refreshing herbal tea:* Mix equal parts of the herbs together. When ready to use, put one to two tablespoons of the mixed herbs into a stainless steel or ceramic pot—*not aluminum*—as you boil a separate pot of water. Pour the boiling water—about two to three cupfuls—over the herbs until they're completely covered. Cover the pot of herbs and let them steep seven to ten minutes. Strain out the herbs, then drink the tea warm. You can repeat this process a second time, although the herbs will be less strong. (With this preparation method, you won't get all the benefits from the roots.)

• *To make a stronger "herbal brew":* Mix equal parts of the herbs together. Put about ½ to 1 ounce of the mixed herbs into a stainless steel or ceramic pot—*never aluminum*. Cover them with twice as much water as you'll need. (If you want an 8-ounce cup of tea, use 16 ounces of water.) Bring the mixture to a boil, then cover and slowly simmer for about twenty-five minutes, depending on the strength you desire. (You can add more water if the mixture seems too strong for your taste.) Strain off the water and drink the tea warm or at room temperature. You can repeat this process a second time, although the tea will be less strong.

The Benefits of Green Tea

While the herbal teas are designed especially for your meta-type, the other types of tea are universal in their appeal and benefits. After centuries of use in Eastern lifestyles, green tea is getting applause from Western medicine these days.

Green tea is made by lightly steaming or gently heating newly picked tea leaves to stop the oxidizing process as the fresh leaves' enzymes are exposed to air. This gentle action retains the active *polyphenols*—the miracle ingredients—and the tea can be drunk the same day the leaves are picked. (Black tea goes through further processes in which the leaves are allowed to oxidize and even fermented. That destroys the polyphenols but provides the distinctive taste and blackened look.)

Polyphenols, known as *catechins*, are a group of powerful antioxidants—similar to, but stronger than, vitamins C and E—that are highly acclaimed for inhibiting the devastating impact of *free radicals* in the body. Those free radicals are highly reactive molecules or fragments of molecules that can latch on to and damage healthy cells and even damage the DNA structure. Then every time that once-healthy cell reproduces, it reproduces in a disfigured form, paving the way for many serious degenerative diseases, such as cancer and heart disease. (You can read more about the action of free radicals in chapter 15, "The Balanced Accelerator Diet.")

A quick way to spot free-radical damage in your body is to check your skin for those ugly brown spots, known as "old-age" or "liver" spots. Polyphenols have the amazing ability to deactivate those vicious free radicals, stopping them in their tracks and helping protect the body from disease and aging.

These polyphenols are in a large class of antioxidants and are also found in many other plants besides tea plants. Antioxidants as a whole are in vitamins, minerals, and enzymes.

But what about caffeine? Green tea does have some, but in very small amounts compared to coffee, colas, and chocolate. Here's how the caffeine content of green tea stacks up against that of other sources of caffeine:

- Green tea: 10 to 40 milligrams per cup
- Black tea: 20 to 90 milligrams per cup
- Cola: 50 milligrams per glass
- Instant or iced tea: 10 to 45 milligrams per cup
- Chocolate: 8 to 120 milligrams per 8-ounce bar
- Coffee: 76 to 155 milligrams per cup

As you might imagine, brewing tea for only a short time lessens the caffeine content. Steeping the tea for one minute, rather than the more common three minutes, lowers the amount of caffeine but keeps the antioxidants intact, and the benefits of those antioxidants outweigh the bit of caffeine.

Green tea has also been known to be effective in weight loss. It's believed to have the ability to slow down and regulate the fast carbohydrate burn-off in cells, which stops the high blood insulin spike that turns many meta-types into fat factories. And the small amount of caffeine can boost your body's metabolic rate, making it a good reward for the synthesizer categories.

Again, Western science is underscoring what practitioners of Chinese medicine have shown for centuries: green tea can tip the scales toward weight loss and good health.

Raw Vegetable Juices—Your Magic Mixes

Are you ready for that gorgeous body, that clear complexion, those toned and tight muscles? Great, because here's another easy secret to help you achieve your goal with guaranteed results—raw vegetable juices. They're powerhouses of precious vitamins and minerals, but most of all, they supply the missing enzymes that are crucial to weight loss and regeneration. Adding specific juice formulas for your own metabolic type can speed up your weight loss in a matter of days or weeks—not months.

You've seen or heard about Mr. Juiceman on television. He has such exuberance when he expounds on his theories about raw vegetable juices—and he's right. They fill your body with the natural form of the very enzymes needed for losing weight as well as repairing your body as you sleep. They're what helps tone that sagging skin and tighten those muscles while your fat is burning away. They fill in those gaunt facial lines as the bloat disappears. Raw vegetable juices, full of life-giving enzymes, are truly miracle workers. Think of them as a liquid face-lift, only for the whole body.

Raw vegetable juices go straight into your digestive system. They immediately begin repairing and rejuvenating your body, all the while burning away that excess fat. Extracting the juices from vegetables gives you just their precious nutrients, in full bloom, while saving your body the time-consuming job of having to digest and break down all that fibrous material. Vegetable fibers are extremely important, of course: they sweep through your intestinal tract. But you'll get enough of these fibers from the foods in your diet plan. These juices have great benefits. They enable you to absorb food enzymes in their natural form—alive. And those enzymes, which are precious fat burners, are killed by cooking.

The vegetables are easy to get at the supermarket, but be sure to scrub them well. You can easily find a vegetable juicer at your local health-food store or at most large department stores.

For each specific meta-type, I recommend certain juices and juice combinations—I call them *elixirs*—which you'll find in your individual food program. Take them one to three times per week, depending on your particular plan. They'll help stabilize and strengthen both your weaker and stronger endocrine glands while bringing balance and harmony to your body as you burn off those excess pounds.

It's best to alternate the juice combinations so that your body can absorb all the available nutrients. Here are some important hints regarding raw vegetable juices:

- Mix water with each juice to help it break down quickly and be absorbed almost immediately in the body.
- Drink juices as close to the time of their preparation as possible, while the enzymes are still active. (Enzymes last from about twenty minutes to one hour after a juice is prepared.)

• Remember, vegetable juices are food, and although they've shed their heavy fiber, they still need to be digested as food. Digestion starts in your mouth, activated by the enzyme *ptyalin*, which begins the food's initial breakdown in the body. Ptyalin is active in your saliva and is increased by your chewing process, so it's a smart idea to *chew your juices* before swallowing them. Don't gulp your juices but just swish them around in your mouth, mixing them gently with your saliva, and then swallow.

Concentrating on the "Berry" Best

Cranberry juice can be a great slimming aid for many meta-types, helping to flush out toxins and squeeze out excess water retention. But the particular cranberry juice I suggest is not the familiar prepackaged, bottled juice bought in your favorite supermarket. That's loaded with sugar or fructose. Do *not* use juices made with fructose, glucose, grape juice, or pear juice. I'm suggesting the pure concentrate cranberry juice found in health-food stores. The formula is usually one part cranberry juice to five to seven parts water—depending on how you like the taste.

You're about to turn back the clock and feel better than you ever imagined. Happy regeneration!

13 Helpers and Healers: Supplements

In our hectic lives of work, family, and fun, the chances of finding all the right foods, in the right combinations, on a daily basis are slim. So along with your meta-type's diet plan, you can get a jump start to a new life by balancing your foods with additional vitamins and food supplements. These will help you lose weight even faster, boost your brainpower, and improve your overall health and well-being.

Some are herbs that have proved themselves through centuries of use; some are new formulations that modern science uses to capture the essential healing ingredients. Today it's becoming easier to select the best of both the Eastern and Western worlds.

A person's *individual metabolism plays a primary role* in determining which nutrients he or she needs. But whatever your meta-type, you need two simple sets of amino acids, vitamins, and minerals—pure, concentrated, natural food supplements—to maintain balance. One set helps restore the balance of your master gland. Your controlling endocrine gland, governed by your dominant nervous system, can easily be overworked and get out of balance. It can become either too revved up or sluggish (hyperactive or hypoactive).

At the same time, the second set is for your opposite nervous system, which needs a full-spectrum formula of amino acids, vitamins, and minerals to support it.

The strategies: soothe and restore your dominant glands while bolstering the weaker alternative ones. It may sound complicated—and there may be a wide variety of pills for you to sort and swallow—but it's the way to guarantee your body's quick switchover to a happy, humming, well-balanced machine.

In the half century since the pioneering research on vitamins by Nobel Prize winner Dr. Linus Pauling, we've come a long way toward understanding how additional doses of vitamins and minerals can make our bodies resist illness and aging.

But extra amino acids, those proteins that are the body's cellular building blocks (like the Tinkertoys and LEGOs of childhood), have special talents—busting fat, toning muscles, and boosting both your memory and your power to think quickly, without that addictive caffeine jolt. The bottom line: you'll enjoy wonderful health while shedding those unwanted pounds.

As with the foods you eat and the times at which you eat them, these vitamins and supplements are all tailored to your own special meta-type. One size, again, just cannot fit all. When you turn to your meta-type's specially designed diet, you'll also find the recommended vitamins, minerals, amino acids, and fatty acids.

Appendixes 3 and 4 provide detailed information on the actions of key vitamins, minerals, and amino acids, and appendix 2 lists companies where you can purchase the ones that are right for you. If you prefer to get all your nutrients from foods, I've listed the foods highest in each of the vitamins, minerals, and amino acids in your diet chapter and have also included this information in appendixes 3 and 4.

Let's take a moment to look at these supplements. They enable you to give your body some pure food components—while you're learning to shed old habits and old pounds. Since it's difficult these days to find food that has not been exposed to pesticides, animal-growth hormones, or preservative chemicals, these supplements can help you fill in the nutrient gaps.

Those with fast metabolisms, the accelerators, are genetically geared to draw energy from their more active sympathetic nervous system, so they need the vitamins, minerals, and amino acids that enhance the calming, sedating, and regenerating role of their weaker parasympathetic nervous system. Otherwise, accelerators can be extremely vulnerable to stress and anxiety attacks.

The flip side of the coin is needed for the synthesizers, those powerhouses of regeneration. They most need those extra nutrients that can energize their sympathetic nervous system. Without the more energizing nutrients, these people can easily develop low blood pressure, lethargy, lack of ambition, and fatigue, and may even be quite susceptible to depression.

And your meta-type is important. Some supplements act as "fat burners," for example—but the supplements that perform this function are not the same for accelerators as for synthesizers. Even such familiar substances as calcium and the B vitamins play different roles for different meta-types.

A word more about those amino acids: there are around eighty, but only twenty of them regenerate or repair the body. Some, called essential amino acids, must come from outside food sources. Animal proteins—meat, fowl, dairy, and fish—contain the whole complement; soy does also, but in a much weaker balance; grains and legumes lack some. So a blend of supplements—which round out your food intake and counterbalance your body's natural tendencies—can help speed you toward a new body, brimming with good health and energy.

Another reason for turning to supplements is stress. This inescapable part of daily life not only gobbles up nutrients but also makes the body *retain* the minerals that stimulate or excite it while *inhibiting* the substances that calm and regenerate. If regeneration is impaired, the immune system loses its ability to defend the body, so it's essential to boost your nutrient levels to support the overnight repair process that can spell the difference when it comes to aging and good health.

In the *alarm stage* of stress, vitamins C, D, E, B_1, B_6, and B_{12} and the minerals calcium, copper, cobalt, and selenium are literally burned up in a flash. Unless they're replenished, you slide into nutritional trouble.

In the second stage of stress, the *resistance stage*, vitamins A, B_2, B_3 (niacin), and B_5 (pantothenic acid) and the minerals potassium, zinc, manganese, iron, and magnesium are abruptly liberated into the bloodstream and utilized quickly. Unless these nutrients are replenished regularly, your immune function becomes suppressed, you slip deeper into fatigue, and you're fair game for the next cold, virus, or serious illness lurking around.

If you make it to the third stage of stress, the *recovery stage*, your body now requires many more of those nutrients to heal, plus another more crucial one: folic acid.

This is when, for example, accelerators can quickly become addicted to those "easy-to-grab" substances that slow or calm the body—alcohol, cigarettes, or drugs—opening the way for destructive complications, such as heart attacks, ulcers, allergies, arthritis, and diabetes.

It's not just a scare story, however. The positive results are dramatic. In days you'll find that bolstering your metabolic thermostat will help burn excess pounds and intensify your body's rejuvenation—producing toned muscles and brighter, tighter skin. Irritability disappears, too.

I have designed two very specific formulas based on either the accelerator or the synthesizer metabolism. These are your basics. Other nutrients can be added for the metabolic subcategory, determined by the dominant or weak endocrine glands.

For instance, extra nutrients known as the fat burners can be added to the accelerator's program, such as the vitamins choline and inositol and the amino acid carnitine. The extra nutrient fat burners that energize the synthesizer's program include vitamins B_1 and B_2 and the amino acid methionine.

Remember, you'll want to get a complete amino acid, vitamin, and mineral multiple combination supplement, so try to find one that meets the requirements for your meta-type. Accelerators don't want to be gulping down lots of the energizing Bs when their real need is for the calming Bs.

Be sure to obtain the highest quality of amino acids, vitamins, and minerals from a top-name company. You can purchase them at your health-food store or vitamin shop or order them from the companies listed in appendix 2.

I've done long, hard research to find the best-quality ingredients for my formulas and know there's a significant difference between high-quality supplements and those weakened by inferior ingredients. It's like the difference between nutrient-rich whole-grain sprouted bread and super-refined white bread.

If you're taking the right nutrients, you'll feel the difference within the first week—none of this six to eight weeks to feel better as other programs claim.

Even the best of diets can be improved with the addition of the basic nutrients needed by your individual metabolic type, but in a weight-loss and regeneration program, those extra nutrients can spell real success.

There are a few easy things to remember about taking the supplements:

• Try to take amino acids on an empty stomach or by themselves (they need adequate amounts of stomach enzymes to be broken down properly).
• If possible, take enzymes with your meals to aid in your food digestion.
• Take vitamins and minerals after you've eaten, which helps their assimilation.
• The water-soluble vitamins—the B-complex vitamins and vitamins C and P (bioflavonoids)—can be taken at any time.
• Your body isn't used to concentrated food substances, so I recom-

mend that you introduce one type of amino acid, vitamin, or mineral into your regimen every few days. Gently and easily is the name of the game.

• And as I discussed in chapter 11 (see page 92), it's a good idea to eliminate the supplements from your program one day per week.

As the preceding tips suggest, certain food supplements shouldn't be taken on an empty stomach. If you're required to take some supplements before you eat, this means *no longer* than ten to fifteen minutes before your meal—not between meals. Some nutrients, like the amino acids, require much more stomach acid to break down, so they need an empty stomach environment filled with ample amounts of hydrochloric acid all to themselves. But in general, supplements should be taken just before, with, or just after eating your meal to help them assimilate more easily and be absorbed into the body more quickly. Remember, amino acids, fatty acids, vitamins, and minerals are food.

Part four

The Meta-Type Diets

Yes, I know you're anxious to get to your diet plan, but before you begin, there are just a few quick things I want to share. Whether you're an accelerator, a balanced accelerator, a mixed accelerator, a synthesizer, a balanced synthesizer, or a mixed synthesizer, one of the most important things you can do for yourself in the next four weeks is decide to be a little bit selfish. It's time to focus on your needs for a change and let some of your other obligations take care of themselves, as much as you possibly can. This is a time to put your energies into rejuvenating yourself. You'll love the results. Here are some specific tips:

- *Don't look back.* If you slip up and eat foods that aren't on your program—and you certainly will—*don't beat yourself up*. Get right back into the swing of things and begin again.
- *Make time to meet your needs.* Set aside time to shop for fresh fruits and veggies and to make your fresh juices. Don't forget to get regular exercise and the proper amount of rest as well.
- *Be kind to yourself.* Become your own best friend. Give yourself a pep talk each day. Remind yourself of all the good things in your life and don't waste time focusing on fat. Your special diet will take care of that.
- *Get happy.* At least once a week, do something that really brings you joy. Listen to music, take a bicycle ride in the country, go shopping (just not for junk food).
- *Hold a weekend revival.* When Sunday rolls around and you've completed another successful week on the program, reward yourself. Get a massage or facial or indulge in some other little luxury.

• *Don't worry if you hit the wall.* Old habits die hard. If friends get upset because you're not eating pizza or chugging beer with them, relax. You don't need to give in to that pressure. Take some quiet time and list your feelings about why friends or certain foods challenge you—and when. Look at your list again the next morning. You'll discover what pushes your buttons and what *triggers* may lead you to overeat or reach for foods that are wrong for your meta-type.

Try to create three guidelines you can follow comfortably, which will help keep your feelings of frustration from coming back. First, if everyone's drinking, don't sulk with an empty glass. Enjoy a fruit-juice spritzer or an iced herbal tea and still be part of the group's fun. Second, if you know that pizza is your weakness, ask your friends to have dinner at a restaurant with a more diverse menu. Odds are they'll be glad to go along with your request. Last, find new ways to eliminate food cravings. Look in the aromatherapy section of chapter 20 and find an exotic or calming scent, tailored to your meta-type, that will take your mind off food.

• *Take a night off.* When you've completed three weeks on the program, then celebrate with a night out (to dinner, that is). Have one meal of anything you want. It's a chance to relax the rules and see how much your tastes, and your body, have changed. You may find that your old fatty favorites are no longer favorites after all.

• *Expand your weekly diet to a 28-day plan.* I've designed a weekly menu plan for each meta-type from the individual food choices listed at the end of each menu plan. For your one-month program, you may repeat this same menu each week for four weeks. Alternatively, you may vary your menu plan by picking from the food choices listed for your meta-type and adhering to the food combination guidelines followed in your individual menu and described in detail in chapter 11, "Guidelines for Healthy Living."

Now you're well on the road to creating a fantastic new, slender, healthy you. And you're about to learn to turn back the clock on the aging process as well. Enjoy it—as so many of my clients have over the past twenty years.

Let's get started!

14 The Accelerator Diet

If your questionnaire results in chapter 10 revealed that you are an accelerator, this chapter is just for you. Weight is not always a problem for you, but it can certainly become an issue when you're operating out of your metabolic type. I am going introduce you to a whole new way of eating, living, and feeling great. Just a few quick words on how your personal accelerator diet works, then on to the menus.

As you read, remember:

- Your dominant glands are the adrenals.
- Your weakest glands are your sex organs.
- You are most likely to gain weight in the upper body.

The Science behind Your System

Although I explained a good deal about your unique body chemistry in chapter 4, I'm going to remind you of a few important facts so that you fully understand why your food plan features certain foods and excludes others.

Remember, since you are an accelerator, your system is dominated by the sympathetic nervous system, so you receive more nerve stimulation to those glands and organs responsible for energy production—primarily your adrenal glands, which perch atop your kidneys. You know them best for providing adrenaline, the jolt that ranges from your morning wake-up to skiing the slopes, racing for Olympic gold, or the superstrength of a mother lifting an automobile to free her trapped child. It's that famous "fight-or-flight" capacity. But they also produce hormones that trigger both your digestive system and your sex glands.

An accelerator's stimulus also goes readily to the thyroid gland, along with the thymus gland, spleen, lungs, and heart. With your meta-type, less nerve stimulation goes to the glands of digestion—the salivary glands, stomach, pancreas, small intestine, liver, large intestine, kidneys, and bladder. Your natural metabolic action is the breakdown and utilization of carbohydrates, fats, and proteins to be employed for your favorite thing—*energy*.

Since your focus is speed and energy, heightened by your extremely active adrenal and thyroid glands, you tend to be a *fast metabolizer*. This enables you to break down your foods quickly and turn them into energy in a flash.

In fact, you have the fastest metabolic rate of all of the six meta-types (except for the mixed accelerator if he or she has flipped into hyperactivity). So with more nerve stimulation to your energy-producing glands and less to your digestive organs, you will tend to have:

- Low production of stomach acid (HCl, or hydrochloric acid), which may be decreased further if the stress response suppresses it
- Tissue acidity
- Low production of pancreatic enzymes
- Probable high production of pancreatic insulin

Since your food breaks down quickly, the oxygen taken into your stomach as you eat is limited, creating an anaerobic environment that slows the way you burn off, or oxidize, your blood sugar energy. We talked about this in chapter 3.

This simply means that you need the faster-burning, more *alkalinizing* foods because you'll burn them off at a slower pace. These are the complex carbohydrates in grains, vegetables, and fruits. You'll also need a moderate amount of unsaturated oil—*not* saturated fats. You don't need the acid-forming foods that you're probably most attracted to—meats and especially refined carbohydrates, like sugars, starches, and alcohol. These just overload your already supercharged system. Slow-burning meats will make you sluggish.

Accelerators have a tendency toward high insulin levels, so this means that pounds can pile on when you eat the "cheap carbs," those refined ones. Another undesirable side effect is higher levels of toxic waste in your cells—the culprits behind illness and aging. It all conspires against your body's efforts to rejuvenate.

For your faster accelerator metabolism, you need to put more emphasis on a vegetarian approach to eating, so your accelerator food formula looks like this:

- Carbohydrates: 60 percent
- Protein: 20 percent
- Fat: 20 percent

Accelerator Food Choices

Complicated? Not at all. It's simply a matter of giving your body what it needs to function smoothly and efficiently. After twenty-eight days on the Your Body, Your Diet plan, you will drop excess fat and be introduced to a level of vitality and good health that you never dreamed possible. Once you have looked at the basic menus, you will find lists that will show you the wide variety of delicious foods that are best for you. Vitamins and supplements will help boost your fat burning and balance your system, especially as you reorganize your eating habits. I've included a suggested list of vitamins and supplements for your meta-type. The next three subsections give you an overview of the basic principles you'll be following.

What to Avoid

Steer clear of fatty foods, red meats, starches, salty foods, and sugars. These are the high-speed foods that will jolt your already accelerated metabolism—by as much as 30 to 60 percent. If you eat them, you may feel an initial surge of energy, but then you'll crash and find yourself sleepy and even lower on energy, keeping the adrenaline cycle spinning further out of control. The cholesterol in the meat stimulates the adrenal hormones, as does sodium, or salt.

Note some surprises here. Asparagus, salmon, shrimp, and mushrooms may sound like diet freebies. But they're not for your acid system. They're called purine foods and—like organ meats, shellfish, and others—produce large amounts of uric acid in your already high-acid system. They're a big reason why those "all-protein, all-the-time" diets do their damage.

Caffeine, that herbal stimulant beloved of coffee fanatics and diet-soda fans alike, pushes your already revved-up adrenal glands to produce even more hormones, adds acid, and can boost anxiety levels into "adrenal burnout." It also triggers the liver to release stored blood sugar. Then, when you grab those extra-refined carbohydrates—like candy, cakes, and even bread and pasta—your insulin level leaps, the blood sugar converts to fat, and you get that sudden energy crash. You wind up depleted or trapped in an ever-escalating cycle of dependency.

The accompanying table gives you an overview of the foods that do *not* suit your meta-type.

Your *Never* Foods

MEAT	PURINE FOODS	REFINED STARCH AND SUGAR	SALT
Beef	Organ meats	White sugar	MSG (monosodium
Lamb	Mincemeats	White flour	glutamate)
Venison	Sardines	Processed syrups	Salty foods
Veal	Herring	Refined foods	Olives
Fatty meats	Anchovies	Any refined products	Pretzels
Processed meats	Salmon	Synthetic additives or	Potato chips
Bacon	Shellfish (especially	sweeteners	Peanuts
Sausage	oysters)		Salted nuts
Pork	Asparagus	**FATS**	
	Mushrooms	Butter	
	Caffeine	Margarine	
		Mayonnaise	

What to Fill Up On

Think of yourself as a planet whirling in space. You need a balancing gravitational pull to keep you in orbit and avoid burnout. Therefore, foods that are more alkaline in nature (*light* proteins, vegetables, fruits, and grains) balance your naturally acid system. These are also complementary yin foods—the foods of the earth. Think grains—and greens to offset your high-acid system. These foods will help calm your adrenal glands and boost your already high metabolic rate by a mild 4 to 15 percent. You'll burn your food more efficiently, delivering it to your body for quick action and cell rejuvenation, without triggering the extra insulin that your body reads as a signal to store fat. Spicy foods stimulate estrogen and testosterone and dilate your blood vessels, letting more of your precious hormones race through your pelvic area.

The accompanying table lists the foods that best suit your meta-type.

Your *Always* Foods

PROTEINS		CARBOHYDRATES		FATS
Food	Times per Week	Food	Times per Week	
Fowl: eggs	1–2	Grains: variety	3	*Moderate* amount
Fish: small variety	2	Legumes: variety	3	of unsaturated fatty
Dairy: abundant low-fat		Starchy vegetables: variety	3	acids—cold-pressed
(if you have *no* allergies)	4–5	Slightly starchy vegetables:		vegetable or nut oils
Seeds/nuts: variety of nuts	2–3	variety	3–4	Choose from your
No seeds	—	Nonstarchy vegetables:		food plan
Legume protein: abundant		abundant	Daily	
tofu, variety of beans	2–3	Fruit: abundant	Daily	

The foods required by your specific metabolic type include unsaturated fatty acids and spices—exactly the ones that feed and support your weaker endocrine glands, primarily the sex glands (ovaries and testes).

How to Speed Up Weight Loss

Here are a few other tips to stimulate faster weight loss:

• When eating a vegetarian meal, mix 60 percent grains to 40 percent legumes (beans) or tofu (soybean curd) for a complete protein complement. Tofu is an excellent accompaniment to grains.
• Chew your food slowly and well.
• Try to avoid drinking more than one glass of water or liquid during your meals. Drinking large amounts of liquid during meals dilutes the precious enzymes needed for your digestion.
• Have at least six to eight glasses of water during the day, *not* at mealtimes.

Keeping Your Adrenals in Balance

As you've learned, the adrenals are your superchargers, triggering both your energy and your digestion. They're twin triangles, sitting on your kidneys. Your meta-type tends to have adrenal overdrive. It's easy to burn out under your constant mental and emotional stimulation—whether self-induced (that constant drive to succeed) or triggered by your boss, your bills, or your kids.

There's also the hormone crunch here. As you pack on the fat, your already supercharged adrenal glands can overproduce androgens (primarily male hormones), and since your sex glands are less active, this can cause women to be low on estrogen. It's a combination that can even cause you to sprout unwanted, excess facial hair and make your skin rougher.

That's why getting hooked on high-acid, adrenal-stimulating meats, excess fats, refined sugars, starch, and salt has been your downfall—and why skipping those gives an immediate beauty dividend while you shed those pounds. The adrenals' inner core has a reversed yang role, producing hormones from your daily wake-up to your stress response, dopamine, norepinephrine, and epinephrine (better known as adrenaline).

The outer core, the yin, produces three potent sets of hormones from cholesterol and steroid compounds. Cortisol stimulates the thyroid and liver to convert carbohydrates, fats, and protein to energy. It also metabolizes into cortisone. Aldosterone controls blood pressure and fluid retention by balancing your sodium and potassium levels. Finally, androgens convert into varying degrees of the sex hormones, testosterone and estrogen.

Acid-generating foods, the yang types you "crave" to continue revving your engine, will just guarantee burnout. These glands must get a chance to rest and regenerate with more calming alkaline foods. Remember, there is a direct relationship among foods, your mind, and your emotions. You know that "adrenaline high" can be addictive. That's why your meta-type tends to include plenty of workaholics.

You reach for the foods that keep you hyped, and under stress your digestive system shuts down, your pancreas goes into overdrive, producing excess insulin, and you become "carbohydrate-intolerant." The blood flow to your skin is cut back, and along with cold hands and feet, you develop broken blood vessels in your face and legs or varicose veins.

It's also the start of high blood pressure as you retain water, as well as the start of new allergies. As the pounds pack on, your cortisol levels put you on the road to obesity, and you start developing that "buffalo hump" on the back of your neck and shoulders.

Your out-of-control adrenals will pump out an excess of androgens— predominantly male hormones—which can also lead to angry outbursts.

Now extra male hormones might sound good, since your weakest glands tend to be the sex organs, but not so. You need to support your weaker glands (testes for men, ovaries for women) and not overload your once-strong ones.

A variety of medical problems can be linked to your sex-hormone functions.

For men an androgen overload might give a "King Kong" effect for a time as testosterone rises, but when the crash comes, impotence could follow. Baldness and acne are also on the list of side effects from adrenal burnout. Your weaker sex glands can also spell prostate problems.

For women the androgen overload eventually blocks your natural estrogen being produced from your weaker ovaries, making you infertile or causing you to develop more masculine traits, such as excess hair and lower voice. Your weaker sex-hormone output also affects menstrual cramps, menopausal hot flashes, and your sex drive.

But you can learn to calm the "speed demons," and boost your sex glands, to find a balance—not forfeiting your high energy but keeping calmer as you avoid those undesirable side effects and shed those unwanted pounds.

And as you've seen, spices—the flavorings and foods needed to stimulate the sex glands—can even spice up your sex life.

Later in this chapter you can find specific ways to support your adrenals—and your weaker sex glands.

Your Accelerator Secret Weapons

Now I know—from firsthand experience—just how tough it can be to switch to a whole new way of eating. In addition to having to apply a lot of willpower, you have to give your body time to adjust to your new lifestyle. But even if you find yourself feeling cranky or frustrated, relax; it's par for the course. It's just a sign that you're shedding those extra pounds and getting back into balance.

The teas, elixirs, and snacking suggestions in this chapter were created to help you sail through the transition phase of your meta-type diet while making the pounds melt away even faster.

Fantastic Fruits

For each meta-type, there is one food or group of foods that helps to speed the weight-loss process. For you those foods are *fruits*—especially *citrus fruits*. Not only will they help you squeeze out the excess toxins from the day before, but they'll also jump-start your weight-loss process by supplying you with valuable enzymes that break down excess flab. While citrus fruits sound like acid, the way your body breaks them down is not. These essential fruits provide your body with a more alkaline environment, help keep you calm, and rebalance your glands. In addition citrus fruits are loaded with valuable vitamin C, the nutrient that helps to feed, calm, and restore balance to your adrenal glands. So these enzymes will literally liquefy that excess fat. There's a bonus, too: they give you a radiant glow.

The secret is that the citrus fruits or juices should be *fresh or frozen*, not canned—so that their valuable enzymes are still alive and kicking when you drink or eat them. With a small citrus juicer set up and ready to go on your kitchen counter, it takes only a quick three minutes in the morning to make your fresh juice.

Your accelerator health trick is:

Eat citrus fruits or have fresh juice before each meal.

Along with the citrus juices, I've added *cranberry juice* to your regimen. It's a tremendous slimming aid; it flushes toxins and waste from your kidneys, reduces water retention, and gives you a wonderfully clean, lean feeling. For the best results, I suggest using the *pure*, concentrated cranberry juice, as explained in chapter 12. Also, delicious, naturally sweet oranges, apples, pears, and other goodies are great treats for times when you're feeling hungry or in need of something to munch on. To keep within the "code" of proper food combining, the citrus fruits are taken *before* the meal, on an empty stomach, and are best eaten by themselves. That way they are liberated into the bloodstream before you eat other foods.

Slimming Tea

As you read the ingredients for this amazing tea, you will be reminded that your meta-type diet is not only designed to produce weight loss; it is your formula for stronger sex gland and digestive functions, greater energy than ever before, and optimum health. The herbs in this tea are specially designed for the accelerator meta-type and can be found in most health-food or herb stores or ordered from the suppliers listed in appendix 2.

I suggest you drink one to three cups per day of your special tea to stimulate, harmonize, balance, and energize you while you burn off the fat.

To the basic Master Weight-Loss Tea (for the recipe see pages 103–105), you'll need to add those herbs that will stabilize, balance, and support your other endocrine glands that may have been weakened by the hyperactivity of your adrenals or thyroid—namely, the sex glands. Your slimming herbal formula is shown in the accompanying table.

Accelerator Slimming Tea

Basic Formula: One Teaspoon Each
Alisma, poria, rhubarb root, red clover tops, alfalfa leaf, hawthorn berry, radish seed, sargassum, Indian chickweed, evergreen artemesia, astragalus root, fleeceflower root, citrus peel

Accelerator Slimming Formula: Add One Teaspoon Each			
NAME			FUNCTION
Common	Latin	Eastern	
Angelica root—for *women*	*Radix angelicae sinensis*	Dang gui	For the sex glands: supports the ovaries and endocrine system.
Codonopsis root (asiabell root)—for *men*	*Codonopsis pilosula*	Dang shen	For the sex glands: supports the testes and endocrine system.
Safflower	*Carthamus tinctorius*	Hong hua	Opens the pancreas and liver, energizes, balances insulin levels, helps digestion, and burns cholesterol and fats.
Bupleurum root (thorowax root)	*Bupleurum chinense D.C.*	Chai hu	Opens the liver and balances the pancreas.

Note: If you are pregnant, have high blood pressure, or are allergic to grasses or flowers, it's suggested that these teas not be used.

Rules of the Road

Your Eating Schedule

Your adrenal hormones run at a high pitch from approximately 6:00 A.M. to 4:00 P.M. During this time your digestion tends to be underactive, so if you eat heavy foods, they won't digest well. You'll just feel sluggish. Your cortisol level begins to diminish in the late afternoon, which allows your digestive juices to flow once again. This means that it's easier for you to handle heavier meals in the early evening. By then, with your adrenal-produced energy ebbing, you'll need the added energy and nutrients released from foods to get you through the evening and have plenty left for cellular regeneration and repair.

So for you morning is the ideal time to clear out any residual acidic waste from the day before. That makes a light breakfast of fruit perfect. Then a fairly light lunch of nutritious vegetables and grains continues the cleansing and weight-loss program, while a heavier meal at dinnertime supplies the energy and nutrients needed for your body's overnight repairs. Here's your ideal meal balance:

- Light breakfast
- Light lunch
- Plentiful dinner

Late Afternoon—Managing Sinking Energy

As you've learned, your great source of energy wanes when your cortisol production begins to nose-dive in the afternoon, with your adrenal generator grinding slowly to a stop. That's when you grab a sugar fix (such as cake, coffee, or alcohol) or a salt fix (such as peanuts, potato chips, or cheese and crackers). Don't even think about such snacks. They actually send your insulin levels skyrocketing. You'll have a sudden drop in blood sugar, you'll crave starch or sugar, and with those carbohydrates surging, get ready for the roller-coaster ride all over again.

It's fine for you to have a late-afternoon snack to support your waning blood sugar levels, but make it the right kind of snack—from the following list.

> *YOUR LATE-AFTERNOON SNACK*
> Cranberry juice
> Fresh fruit
> Hot green tea

Bedtime Eating—Not a Good Idea

Since you digest your foods quickly but utilize them slowly, if you eat dinner too late, you can bet you'll wake up in a few short hours, triggered by the energy released from your late-night foods. To be sure that you don't end up tossing and turning, or wrestling with gas or heartburn, resist the urge for bedtime snacks.

Accelerator Meals and Menus

Now you've completed the first part of the plan, and here's your reward: the tailor-made diet for your accelerator meta-type. If you've reached this point in the book, you know that losing weight and keeping it off take more than just watching what you eat. And I'm sure you know a lot more about yourself than you did when you picked up *Your Body, Your Diet*.

The meals presented in this section are designed to meet all the needs of your metabolism while giving you the chance to eat a delicious, wide variety of fresh, nutritious foods. The first week may seem like a big adjustment, but by week two, I assure you, you'll be making your juices and tossing together your special meals like a pro.

Eating the Right Foods at the Right Times

It's not just eating the *right kinds of food* but eating at the *right times* that spells success for your weight loss and rejuvenation. As an accelerator, you've learned that eating a lot of acid food will throw you way off balance, making your adrenals explode into hyperactivity and pump out that extra fat.

You require more alkalizing foods—vegetables and fruits—to stabilize your metabolism. You are known as the *strong acid* meta-type, so your natural body pH tends toward 4.5–4. (Chapter 3 provides a detailed explanation of the acid-alkaline aspect of your meta-type.) Meat is high in acidic residue and a perfect food for your meta-opposite, the synthesizers, while leafy green vegetables are a great source of calcium and a perfect food for you accelerators.

This means your diet should consist of foods that are strong alkaline, alkaline, weak alkaline, and weak acid forming ash. Foods that are acid forming should be eaten once or twice per week. Foods that are your own pH tendency—strong acid—should be avoided. Appendix 5 lists the full spectrum of foods and their pH factors.

Here We Go!

To make this adventure of slimming down to a new and healthy you fun, I've taken all the guesswork out of how to shop and prepare your meals. Before you begin, glance through your weekly menus and accelerator elixirs in the accompanying tables and look over the vast array of selections in your Accelerator Food Choices list. At the end of this chapter, you will find your own accelerator shopping list for a week. Then turn to appendix 1 and take a look at the equipment list (which includes all the supplies you'll need to make this as simple as possible), your advance food-preparation suggestions for the week, and your recipes and food-preparation instructions for both men and women.

For any of the foods specified in the weekly menus and recipes, you may substitute comparable foods from the Accelerator Food Choices list.

Eat only the foods that are indicated for you on your individual food choices list. If your favorite isn't there, don't eat it. You can check the "General Food Choices and Their Calorie Content for Each Meta-Type" in appendix 5.

Accelerator Vegetarian Weekly Menus

Alkaline-Based Foods

Larger quantities for men are shown in **boldface**.

WHEN	SATURDAY	SUNDAY	MONDAY	TUESDAY
On rising	Drink the juice of 1 lemon in 4 oz. hot spring water. (Important for your program! The citrus's active enzymes clear out toxic cellular debris, break down fats, alkalize your digestive tract, and are a powerful liver and gallbladder cleanser.)			
Breakfast	Juice of 1 medium grapefruit 2 **(2½)** cups *Dane's Enzyme Fruit Medley* 1 cup herbal tea or Accelerator Slimming Tea	Juice of 1 medium grapefruit 2 **(2½)** cups *Citrus Fruit Salad* 1 cup herbal tea or Accelerator Slimming Tea	Juice of 1 medium grapefruit 2 **(2½)** cups *Dane's Enzyme Fruit Medley* 1 cup herbal tea or Accelerator Slimming Tea	Juice of 1 medium grapefruit 2 **(2½)** cups *Citrus Fruit Salad* 1 cup herbal tea or Accelerator Slimming Tea
Midmorning	1 6-oz. glass cranberry juice (Obtain Knudsen or Ad-Vita cranberry concentrate from your health-food store. Use 2 tbs. concentrate to 6 oz. spring water. Add more water if desired.) 1 cup herbal tea or Accelerator Slimming Tea			
Before lunch	½ grapefruit or 4 oz. grapefruit juice, freshly squeezed. (Try to eat at least ½ hour to 15 minutes before lunch.)			
Lunch	*Health Salad with Quinoa, Fava Beans, Broccoli, Cauliflower, Carrots and Red Onions* 1–2 **(2–3)** cups Accelerator Salad Greens ¼ **(½)** cup Fava Beans ½ **(1)** cup Quinoa 1 **(2)** cup Accelerator Raw Vegetables	*Health Salad with Cottage Cheese and Raw Vegetable Salad* 1–2 **(2–3)** cups Accelerator Salad Greens 1 tbs. Accelerator Salad Dressing 1 **(1½)** cup cottage cheese, low-fat **(1 tbs. Roasted**	*Health Salad with Quinoa, Fava Beans, Broccoli, Cauliflower, Carrots and Red Onions* 1–2 **(2–3)** cups Accelerator Salad Greens ¼ **(½)** cup Fava Beans ½ **(1)** cup Quinoa 1 **(2)** cup Accelerator Raw Vegetables	*Health Salad with Hard-Boiled Eggs and Vegetables* 1–2 **(2–3)** cups Accelerator Salad Greens 2 cups Accelerator Raw Vegetables ⅛ **(¼)** cup Accelerator Salad Dressing 2 sliced Hard-Boiled Eggs **(1 cup cottage**

WHEN	SATURDAY	SUNDAY	MONDAY	TUESDAY
Lunch (cont'd)	1 cup alfalfa sprouts Top with thinly sliced red onion. ⅛ (¼) cup Accelerator Salad Dressing 1 cup herbal tea or Accelerator Slimming Tea	**Hazelnuts)** Sprinkle with paprika and sliced scallions. Add 1 cup Raw Veggie Slaw. 1 cup herbal tea or Accelerator Slimming Tea	1 cup alfalfa sprouts Top with thinly sliced red onion. ⅛ (¼) cup Accelerator Salad Dressing 1 cup herbal tea or Accelerator Slimming Tea	**cheese, low-fat)** 1 cup herbal tea or Accelerator Slimming Tea
Midafternoon	1 6-oz. glass cranberry juice 1 cup herbal tea or Accelerator Slimming Tea			
Before dinner	½ grapefruit (Try to eat at least ½ hour to 15 minutes before dinner.)			
Dinner	*Vege Rejuvenation Dinner* Basmati Brown Rice with Marinated Tofu and Curried Vegetables Health Salad 1 glass Accelerator Elixir 1 cup herbal tea or Accelerator Slimming Tea	*Egg-alicious Dinner* Egg Frittata with Onions, Oregano, and Broccoli Arugula Salad with Goat Cheese, Red Peppers, and Red Onion *½ hour after dinner:* 1 cup mixed berries 1 cup herbal tea or Accelerator Slimming Tea	*Vitality Vegetarian Dinner* Black Bean Soup with Ginger Mexican-Style Brown Rice with Cumin-Flavored Vegetables Jicama Sticks Marinated in Lime Juice *½ hour after dinner:* 1 cup mixed berries 1 cup herbal tea or Accelerator Slimming Tea	*Jump for Joy Carbo Dinner* Roasted Acorn Squash with Mixed Roasted Vegetables (parsnips, beets, carrots, red onions, cauliflower) with Rosemary Spinach Salad 1 glass Accelerator Elixir *½ hour after dinner:* 1 cup Dane's Enzyme Fruit Medley 1 cup herbal tea or Accelerator Slimming Tea

WHEN	WEDNESDAY	THURSDAY	FRIDAY
On rising	Drink the juice of 1 lemon in 4 oz. hot spring water. (Important for your program! The citrus's active enzymes clear out toxic cellular debris, break down fats, alkalize your digestive tract, and are a powerful liver and gallbladder cleanser.)		
Breakfast	Juice of 1 medium grapefruit 2 **(2½)** cups *Dane's Enzyme Fruit Medley* 1 cup herbal tea or Accelerator Slimming Tea	Juice of 1 medium grapefruit 2 **(2½)** cups *Citrus Fruit Salad* 1 cup herbal tea or Accelerator Slimming Tea	Juice of 1 medium grapefruit 2 **(2½)** cups *Dane's Enzyme Fruit Medley* 1 cup herbal tea or Accelerator Slimming Tea
Midmorning	1 6-oz. glass cranberry juice (Obtain Knudsen or Ad-Vita cranberry concentrate from your health-food store. Use 2 tbs. concentrate to 6 oz. spring water. Add more water if desired.) 1 cup herbal tea or Accelerator Slimming Tea		
Before lunch	½ grapefruit or 4 oz. grapefruit juice, freshly squeezed. (Try to eat at least ½ hour to 15 minutes before lunch.)		
Lunch	*Health Salad with Cottage Cheese and Raw Vegetable Salad* 1–2 **(2–3)** cups Accelerator Salad Greens 1 tbs. Accelerator Salad Dressing 1 **(1½)** cup cottage cheese, low-fat **(1 tbs. Roasted Hazelnuts)** Sprinkle with paprika and	*Health Salad with Quinoa, Fava Beans, Broccoli, Cauliflower, Carrots, and Red Onions* 1–2 **(2–3)** cups Accelerator Salad Greens ¼ **(½)** cup Fava Beans ½ **(1)** cup Quinoa 1 **(2)** cup Accelerator Raw Vegetables 1 cup alfalfa sprouts Top with thinly	*Health Salad with Cold Seared Tuna and Mixed Raw Vegetables* 1–2 **(2–3)** cups Accelerator Salad Greens 2 cups Accelerator Raw Vegetables 2 tbs. Salad Dressing **(1 tbs. Roasted Hazelnuts)** *Serve with:* 4 **(6)** oz. cold, sliced seared

WHEN	WEDNESDAY	THURSDAY	FRIDAY
Lunch **(cont'd)**	chopped scallions. 1 cup Raw Veggie Slaw 1 cup herbal tea or Accelerator Slimming Tea	sliced onion. ⅛ (¼) cup Accelerator Salad Dressing 1 cup herbal tea or Accelerator Slimming Tea	tuna (from previous evening) 1 cup herbal tea or Accelerator Slimming Tea
Midafternoon	1 6-oz. glass cranberry juice 1 cup herbal tea or Accelerator Slimming Tea		
Before dinner	½ grapefruit (Try to eat at least ½ hour to 15 minutes before dinner.)		
Dinner	*Hearty Vegetarian Salad Dinner* Wild Rice, Red Beans, Shredded Beets and Carrots, Yellow Squash, And Zucchini 1 glass Accelerator Elixir 1 cup herbal tea or Accelerator Slimming Tea	*Fabulous Fish Dinner* Seared Yellowfin Tuna with Rutabaga Carrot Puree French Green Beans Fennel Salad *½ hour after dinner:* 1 cup mixed berries 1 cup herbal tea or Accelerator Slimming Tea	*Vege-dairian Delight Dinner* Vegetable Lasagna: Layers of cooked Swiss Chard, topped with Scallions, Shredded Carrots, Leeks, and Fennel, mixed with Ricotta Cheese and topped off with Mozzarella cheese Cucumber Yogurt Salad with Dill *½ hour after dinner:* 1 cup Dane's Enzyme Fruit Medley 1 cup herbal tea or Accelerator Slimming Tea

Accelerator Food Choices

Proteins						
FOWL	**FISH**	**DAIRY**	**NUTS**	**SEEDS**	**LEGUMES**	**FRUIT PROTEIN**
Acid Forming	**Acid Forming**	*Note:* If you have allergies, eliminate dairy of any kind.	**Weak Alkaline**	None	**Weak Alkaline**	None
Eggs	Carp		Coconut milk		Soybean curd	
	Yellowtail tuna	**Weak Alkaline Dairy (Use Low-Fat)**		***AVOID***	(tofu)	***AVOID***
AVOID	Hake		**Weak Acid**	**Strong Acid**		**Strong Alkaline**
Strong Acid	Lake perch				**Acid Forming**	
	Bass	Whey	Filberts	Pumpkin seeds		Olives (too salty)
Turkey	Trout	Goat's milk	(hazelnuts)	Sunflower seeds	Lentils	
Goose		Yogurt	Hickory nuts	Squash seeds	Soybeans	**Strong Acid**
Squab		Cow's milk		Safflower seeds	Soy milk	
Chicken	***AVOID***	Cream	**Acid Forming**	Sesame seeds	Adzuki beans	Avocados
Duck	**Strong Acid**	Buttermilk	**(Nonsalted)**	Flaxseeds	Black beans	
Frog legs				Chia seeds	Kidney beans	
Quail	Mackerel	**Cheeses (Use Low-Fat)**	Pecans		Navy beans	
Pheasant	Roe		Pistachios		Pinto beans	
	Halibut	Parmesan	Walnuts		Red beans	
	Red snapper	Limburger	Brazil nuts			
	Sole	Cheddar	Macadamias		***AVOID***	
	Tuna	Brick	Chestnuts		**Strong Acid**	
	Bluefish	Swiss	Almonds			
	Eel				Peanuts	
	Swordfish	**Acid Forming**	***AVOID***			
	Squid (calamari)	Soy milk	**Strong Acid**			
	Cod	(also under				
	Mullet	"Legumes")	Pine nuts			
	Haddock		Water chestnuts			
	Sturgeon	**Weak Acid Cheeses (Use Low-Fat)**	Cashews			
	Ocean perch		Coconut			
	Octopus	Camembert				
	(scungilli)	Brie				
		Edam				
	Purine Forming	Gruyère				
		Cottage				
	Shellfish of any	Farmer				
	kind	Feta				
	Anchovies	Ricotta				
	Caviar	Muenster				
	Herring	Monterey Jack				
	Sardines	Provolone				
	Salmon	Mozzarella				
		Goat				
		Blue				
		Gorgonzola				
		AVOID				
		None				

Carbohydrates

GRAINS	HIGH-STARCH LEGUMES	HIGH-STARCH VEGETABLES	SLIGHTLY STARCHY VEGETABLES	NONSTARCHY VEGETABLES		
Strong Alkaline	**Acid Forming**	**Weak Alkaline**	**Weak Alkaline**	**Alkaline Forming**	**Weak Acid**	**Acid Forming**
Amaranth grain and flakes	Lima Beans Garbanzo beans (chickpeas) Great northern beans Split peas White (fava) beans	Acorn squash **Weak Acid** Butternut squash Hubbard squash Sweet potatoes Pumpkin, canned **Acid Forming** Yams Pumpkin, raw	Carrots Rutabagas **Weak Acid** Beets, cooked Parsnips Jicama **Acid Forming** Beets, raw	Yellow dock, cooked Chicory greens Horseradish Cabbage, cooked Okra, cooked Swiss chard, raw Spinach, cooked Kale, raw Lettuce: cos, romaine, dark green, white Watercress Alfalfa sprouts Dandelion greens Arugula Beet greens, raw	Cauliflower, cooked Eggplant Artichokes Shallots Gingerroot Salsify Soybean sprouts Kohlrabi Chicory Onions Cucumbers Radishes Summer squash, raw	Bamboo shoots Green peas Sugar peas Mungbeans and sprouts Chili peppers Celeriac root Sweet peppers Brussels sprouts Cauliflower, raw Tomatoes
Acid Forming Farina Brown rice Basmati brown rice Wild rice Buckwheat (kasha) Quinoa						**Eliminate If You Have Allergies of Any Kind** Eggplant Tomatoes Peppers
AVOID **Strong Acid** Popcorn Corn grits Rice bran Millet Barley Corn meal Wheat Couscous Bulgur (cracked wheat) Rye Oats Pastas (egg) Sprouted grain bread	*AVOID* **Strong Acid** Black-eyed peas (cowpeas)	*AVOID* **Strong Acid** Field corn Sweet corn Potatoes	*AVOID* None	**Weak Alkaline** Summer squash, cooked Leeks Garden cress Chinese cabbage Snap beans Yellow beans Turnips Scallions Broccoli Lettuce: butter, Boston, iceberg Celery Endive Radicchio Yellow dock, raw Cabbage, raw Spinach, raw Okra, raw Fennel	**Strong Alkaline** Kale, cooked Collards Swiss chard, cooked Parsley Mustard greens, cooked Beet greens, cooked Turnip greens, cooked Lamb's-quarter Mustard spinach **Seaweeds** Agar-agar Irish moss Kelp Dulse Arame	*AVOID* **Strong Acid** Mushrooms Garlic **Purine Forming** Asparagus Mushrooms

FRUIT		OILS	CONDIMENTS	TEAS
Alkaline Forming	**Melons (Eat Alone)**	**Strong Acid (Use Sparingly)**	**Alkaline Forming**	**Black cohosh:** good for your hormones
Loganberries	Watermelon	Avocado	Cane syrup	**Red raspberry:** tonic for hormones
Oranges	Muskmelon	Corn	**Weak Alkaline**	**Dandelion root:** balances your adrenals
Clementines	Cantaloupe	Soybean		
Tangerines	Casaba	Peanut	Pickles	**Lemon balm:** soothes and clears the skin
Kumquats	Crenshaw	Cottonseed	Cane sugar	
Kiwifruits	Honeydew	Olive	**Weak Acid**	**Blue flag:** clears the liver and skin
Weak Alkaline		Safflower	Vinegar	**Passionflower:** calms your adrenals
	Acid Forming	Sunflower	Honey	
Boysenberries	Litchis	Flaxseed	Mustard	**Fennel:** calms and suppresses the appetite
Grapefruit	Passion fruit	Walnut		
Raspberries	Groundberries	Apricot	**Strong Alkaline**	
Strawberries	Pomegranates	Almond	Molasses: blackstrap or light	**Nettle:** stabilizes insulin levels
Plums	Crab apples			
Acerola cherries	Peaches	*AVOID*	Brown sugar	**Chamomile:** soothes and calms (*Careful:* May cause allergies.)
Blueberries		**(Saturated Fats)**	Sorghum	
Nectarines	**Strong Alkaline**	Mayonnaise	Maple syrup	
Gooseberries	Rhubarb	Butter	*AVOID*	**Valerian:** relaxes, calms, and soothes
Pokeberries		Margarine	**Strong Acid**	
Papaya	**Sweet Fruit**		Yeast: all forms	
Grapes: Concord, Thompson	**Alkaline Forming**		**Weak Acid (Salty)**	
Elderberries	Pineapple		Soy sauce	
Sapotes	**Weak Alkaline**			
Cranberries	Figs			
Currants				
Lemons	**Weak Acid**			
Cherries	Apricots, dried			
Blackberries	Raisins			
Limes	Prunes			
Weak Acid	Dates			
Guavas	**Acid Forming**			
Loquats	Persimmons			
Cherimoya	Plantains			
Grapes: muscat, Tokay	Bananas			
Quince	*AVOID*			
Tamarinds	None			
Apples				
Apricots				
Prickly pears				
Pears				
Mangoes				

Accelerator Elixirs for Both Women and Men

Just Plain Sunshine: The "great healer," full of vitamins and minerals—especially vitamins A, D, B, C, E, and K; stabilizes your adrenals.	Carrots: 6 oz. juice (about 6 carrots) Water: 2 oz.
My Favorite: Along with carrot juice, the beet juice builds the blood, increases circulation, and improves the skin, while the coconut milk regenerates the ovaries and testes.	Carrots: 6 oz. juice (about 6 carrots) Beets: 2 oz. juice (about 2 beets) Coconut: 2 oz. milk Water: 2 oz.
Spring Cleanser: A great blood cleanser and cell builder. Alfalfa is full of chlorophyll and cleans out toxic waste, while lettuce is rich in calcium, magnesium, potassium, and iron and stimulates renewed skin and hair growth.	Carrots: 6 oz. juice (about 6 carrots) Lettuce: 4 oz. juice (about 1 head) Alfalfa: 2–3 oz. juice (about 2 boxes) Water: 2 oz.
Adrenal Stabilizer: With carrot juice, parsley is the great adrenal stabilizer and also balances the thyroid gland, cleanses the kidneys, brightens the eyes, and brings oxygen into the body.	Carrots: 6 oz. juice (about 6 carrots) Parsley: 2 oz. juice (about 2 bunches) Water: 2 oz.

You see, it's all done for you, down to the last detail—and my personal promise to you is that this eating plan will keep your accelerator metabolism in perfect balance while helping you achieve a slender, gorgeous physique.

You're on your way to a bright, new, skinny, energetic you. Treat this as a ritual in celebrating your beauty and regeneration.

Your On-Program Cheat Sheet

Naturally there will be days when you just have to cheat. No problem. There's no need to become obsessed with perfection. You can be yourself and still succeed at weight loss on the Your Body, Your Diet plan. Besides, if you try to be flawless, you'll only end up out of balance, in either too much of a yang state or too much of a yin state.

You've still got to forget about chowing down on salt, meats, and coffee, but there are other great-tasting treats that are just ideal for you.

For your accelerator profile, the best snack food is popcorn—and I mean fresh, fragrant, air-popped corn.

Here's a complete list of goodies you can use to put an end to the munchies—fast:

- *Popcorn:* 1 oz. uncooked, with no butter, oil, or salt
- *Raisins:* ¼ cup, or 2 oz.
- *Dates:* ¼ cup pitted, or 2 oz.

- *Prunes:* ½ cup pitted, or 4 oz.
- *Banana:* 1 large
- *Sorbet:* any flavor, 1 cup
- *Fruit ice:* any flavor, 1 cup
- *Frozen yogurt:* any flavor, ½ cup

Looks great, doesn't it? But you have to make a deal with me. In order for you to have these tasty goodies, you need to follow some guidelines. Otherwise, using these cheat foods in the wrong way would sabotage your goal for creating that beautiful body.

CHEAT-FOOD GUIDELINES

- *Eat your cheat foods only at the recommended times.* Cheat foods should be eaten no oftener than once per week, on the weekends (when you're not under stress), and at one meal or one time—only.
- *Eat only the amount suggested.* Your body can handle a small amount of these foods without triggering excessive insulin production. If you eat a large amount, your insulin level will spike and turn your "treat" into a "bad trick" of blubber.
- *Eat only one cheat food at a time.* Don't have several together or you'll wreak havoc with your metabolism and digestion. For instance, raisins *and* popcorn will send you over the top.
- *Never eat your cheat foods when you're under stress.* I guarantee you that's a surefire way to add pounds, not lose them. Only eat cheat foods when you're relaxed—usually on a weekend. Otherwise, your digestion shuts down and your insulin rises, and you become a veritable fat factory.
- *Never eat your cheat foods late at night.* And no bedtime eating in front of the television. You'll end up having a restless night's sleep, and it's mandatory for you to sleep deeply so your body can regenerate itself.

Accelerator Healers and Helpers: Vitamins, Minerals, and Amino Acids

You're ready now to put it all together—a triple-pronged attack plan to restore your healthy body and show quick results. Along with your special tailored diet plan, you can boost the benefits by balancing your foods, juices, and teas with additional vitamins and food supplements. These will help you lose weight even faster and improve your overall health and well-being.

As I discussed in chapter 13, supplementing your diet with extra amino acids, vitamins, or minerals can help restore your master gland's balance while supporting your weaker glands.

For your accelerator meta-type, I suggest a gentle, full-spectrum multiple amino acid, vitamin, and mineral complex containing only those essential nutrients that support your weaker parasympathetic nervous system. This speeds up your weight-loss program, helps tone your muscles, and gives you abundant good health. Your multiple amino acid, vitamin, and mineral complex can be purchased at your local health-food store or ordered from the companies listed in appendix 2.

Remember, since you are an accelerator, your dominant adrenal glands generate the hormones that spark your energy and your digestion, control the way you process those carbs and fats, and do everything from waking you to enabling you to handle stress, play sports, and even display life-saving bursts of strength. By understanding what nourishes and stabilizes your adrenal glands, you can be your own best judge when choosing the right nutrients to support their health.

Don't forget your yin/yang balance. Along with protecting your strong adrenals, you need to build up your weaker opposite parasympathetic endocrine glands: the sex glands (ovaries and testes).

You have learned by now how your adrenal glands, your dominant "speed center," get battle fatigue under your typical accelerator's constant mental and emotional stimulation, both self-induced and from the stress of daily life. The acid-generating foods, the yang types you crave to continue revving your engine, will just guarantee burnout. The job here with your new diet and the vitamin and supplement regimen is to cool down your overheated adrenals, saving their power for more urgent needs. It's like fixing a car accelerator that idles too fast and wastes precious fuel.

The most "famous" of your adrenal hormones you know as adrenaline (or epinephrine), dopamine, and norepinephrine. These are your morning starters and your fight-or-flight stress mobilizers. There are also three hormones synthesized from cholesterol: Cortisol stimulates the thyroid and liver to convert carbohydrates, fats, and protein to energy and metabolizes into cortisone. Aldosterone controls blood pressure and fluid retention by balancing your sodium and potassium levels. Finally, androgens convert into varying degrees of the sex hormones, testosterone and estrogen.

Along with your dominant adrenals, some additional attention must be focused on your weaker, opposite endocrine glands, the sex glands—the male testes and female ovaries.

Under stress and excess weight gain, your body tends to either pump out far too much of the sex hormones or shut down completely. Those hormones—androgens (including testosterone), DHEA (dehydroepiandrosterone), estrogen, and progestins—decrease with age. Your fertility, of course, is at stake here, as well as your sex drive and your secondary sexual characteristics, like breasts, hair, skin and muscle tone, and voice.

The nutrients needed by your adrenal glands are vitamin C and pantothenic acid (B_5). The amino acid tyrosine sparks the regeneration of your adrenals if they've become overworked or exhausted.

Vitamin C is essential for the health of your adrenal glands. That's why you'll see it featured so prominently in your weight-loss program in the form of citrus juices, which are the energizers and scrubbers that start your day and help you better digest your new diet. Vitamin C is water-soluble, which means it isn't stored in the body, so it must be continually taken daily—or sometimes several times a day—to provide adequate amounts needed by your adrenals. This is especially true if your day involves extra demands or you're in a prolonged stress response. Part of its task is to synthesize and metabolize two important amino acids—tyrosine and tryptophan. Tryptophan forms the neurotransmitter serotonin. Serotonin functions as the main regulator for your meta-type's weaker parasympathetic nervous system. Without this you can't chill out, sleep well, or rejuvenate your cells.

Pantothenic acid (B_5), one of the most important substances for your body's metabolism, is vital to healthy adrenals. It's like a railroad signal system, switching your nerve messages. It's responsible for everyday energy and those sudden bursts of energy you need for fight-or-flight stress. It's essential to burn fat, synthesize cholesterol, and restore insulin levels. Pantothenic acid functions as two enzymes—CoA (coenzyme A) and ACP (acyl carrier protein)—building the "good fat" essential for healthy nerves, skin, and cell renewal. It uses PABA (para-aminobenzoic acid) and choline, part of the "Bs" that burn fat for energy, and it burns off the excess fat. With choline it tells you to stop, calm down, and regenerate. Otherwise, you're at risk of becoming a "stress junkie," growing more irritable, anxious, and weary—while packing on more pounds!

Tyrosine is crucial, especially if the adrenals become exhausted. Tyrosine is converted from the amino acid phenylalanine and is essential for your adrenal gland's neurotransmitter production; in turn, it supplies you with your body's energizers, the adrenal hormones—dopamine, epinephrine, and norepinephrine. It's also important for your thyroid gland production, and without it you're almost guaranteed fatigue and depression. A sure sign of a tyrosine shortage is those fierce cravings for bread and sugar.

One word of caution: When taking any of the B vitamins, it's important to know that you shouldn't take an isolated B vitamin—such as pantothenic acid or riboflavin—without taking the whole B-vitamin complement. Otherwise, that solo B will rob your body of the others to activate its energy.

In addition these nutrients are needed for your weaker sex glands:

- *Calcium:* This is not just a bone builder. It helps keep your excitable body calm, toned, and tightened while you're losing weight, generates muscle growth, flushes excess fluids that cause bloating, and helps prevent menstrual cramps or menopausal symptoms.
- *Selenium:* This nutrient affects male ejaculation and prostate problems and also relieves some female menopausal hot flashes.
- *Vitamin E:* This vitamin carries oxygen to strengthen your heart, skin, and sex glands, enhances male potency, and boosts fertility. It stimulates better estrogen production for women and testosterone production for men—so you keep that youthful glow.
- *Essential fatty acids (EFAs):* These nutrients promote ovarian and testicular health, burn fats, and keep your skin moist and radiant.

The Bottom Line

By taking a complete amino acid, vitamin, and mineral combination based on the formulation for your metabolic type, you'll be supplied with the nutrients needed to build up your complementary side, the parasympathetic nervous system. Then you may want to add a few of the vitamins and minerals that we've just discussed, which are also listed in the accompanying table of recommended nutrients.

If you're interested, turn to appendixes 3 and 4 for a more in-depth study of the vitamins, minerals, and amino acids for your meta-type. If you prefer to get all your nutrients from foods, I've listed the foods highest in vitamin, mineral, and amino acid content in the accompanying table.

Accelerator Vitamin, Mineral, and Amino Acid Food Sources

	Adrenals
B complex	<ul><li>B_1: torula yeast, sunflower seeds, rice bran, wheat germ, pine nuts, dried coriander leaf, safflower seeds, soybeans, alfalfa seeds, sesame seeds, and rye flour (dark)</li><li>B_2: almonds, cheese, turnip greens, wheat bran, and soybeans</li><li>B_3 (niacin): fish, nuts, milk, cheese, bran flakes, sesame seeds, and sunflower seeds</li><li>B_6: rice bran, wheat bran, sunflower seeds, avocados, bananas, corn, fish, brown rice, soybeans, and whole grains</li><li>B_{15}: grains, cereals, rice, apricot kernels, and torula yeast</li></ul>

Pantothenic acid (B$_5$)	Cottonseed flour, wheat bran, rice bran, rice polishings, nuts, soybean flour, buckwheat flour, lobster, sunflower seeds, and brown rice *Note:* Avoid lobster (purine food).
Coenzyme Q10	Occurs widely in aerobic organisms (those that utilize air for growth), such as green leafy vegetables and fruits.
Vitamin C (buffered)	Acerola cherries, rose hips, citrus fruit, guavas, hot green peppers, black currants, parsley, turnip greens, poke greens, and mustard greens
Tyrosine	Fish and eggs
Sex Glands	
Vitamin E	Oils (except coconut), alfalfa seeds, nuts, sunflower seed kernels, asparagus, avocados, blackberries, green leafy vegetables, oatmeal, rye, seafood (lobster, shrimp, tuna), and tomatoes *Note:* Avoid seafood and asparagus (too purine for your accelerator metabolism).
Essential fatty acids—vitamin F	• *Oils:* safflower, sunflower, corn, olive, wheat germ, soy, cottonseed, and cod-liver • *Nuts:* walnuts, Brazil nuts, and almonds
Calcium	Cheese, wheat flour, blackstrap molasses, almonds, Brazil nuts, cottonseed flour, dried figs, fish, green leafy vegetables, hazelnuts, milk, oysters, soybean flour, and yogurt *Note:* Avoid oysters (too purine).
Selenium	Brazil nuts, butter, lobster, blackstrap molasses, cider vinegar, clams, crabs, eggs, lamb, mushrooms, oysters, garlic, cinnamon, chili powder, nutmeg, Swiss chard, turnips, wheat bran, and whole grains *Note:* Avoid shellfish and mushrooms (too purine).

There are a few easy things to remember about taking the supplements:

- Try to take amino acids on an empty stomach. (They need adequate amounts of stomach enzymes to be broken down properly.)
- If possible, take enzymes with your meals to aid in your food digestion.
- Take vitamins and minerals after you've eaten, which helps their assimilation.
- The water-soluble vitamins—B complex, vitamin C, and vitamin P (bioflavonoids)—can be taken at any time.
- Your body isn't used to concentrated food substances, so I recommend that you introduce one type of amino acid, vitamin, or mineral into your regimen every few days. Gently and easily is the name of the game.

Accelerator Recommended Nutrients

ENDOCRINE GLAND	NUTRIENT	WOMEN			MEN		
		Number	Strength	Times per Day	Number	Strength	Times per Day
Adrenals	B complex	1	50–75 mg	1	1	100–125 mg	1
	Pantothenic acid	1	250 mg	1–2	1	500 mg	2
	Coenzyme Q10	1	60 mg	2	1	120 mg	2
	Vitamin C (buffered)	1–2	1,000 mg	2–3	1–2	1,000 mg	3
	Tyrosine	1	250 mg	1	1	500 mg	2
Sex glands (ovaries, testes)	Vitamin E	1	400–800 IU	1	1	800 IU	1
	Essential fatty acids	1	300 mg	2–3	2	300 mg	2–3
	Calcium-magnesium	1	500 mg	2–3	2	500 mg	2
	Selenium	0	—	—	1	200 mcg	1

Now taking these extra vitamins, minerals, and supplements will require work—there's no mistaking that. Just as you have to plan meals with the right ingredients, you'll need to organize these. But as your metabolic system moves back into balance, you'll reduce the number of pills you'll need. And along the way, you'll discover that the dividend of glowing good health pays off quickly enough to make Wall Street envious.

Stocking Up

You've now finished reading about the program and are well on your way to a brand-new you. Just wait and see—you'll be slim, sexy, and full of bounce to every ounce. Now to get started, you'll need to stock up and organize. The accompanying list shows all the foods you'll need for the coming week. Double-check this list against your weekly menu and make any adjustments you feel are necessary. Happy regeneration!

Weekly Shopping List for Accelerators

Larger quantities for men are shown in **boldface**.

PRODUCE

Fruit
18 Lemons
14 Grapefruit
2 Limes
3 **(4)** bunches Green grapes
2 Pineapples
2 Papayas
3 **(5)** pt. Strawberries
5 **(6)** Pink grapefruit
5 **(6)** Blood oranges
4 **(5)** Navel oranges
4 **(6)** Clementines
4 **(6)** Tangerines
1 **(7)** pt. Raspberries
2 **(8)** pt. Blueberries
4 Kiwifruits

Vegetables
3 Broccoli
1 **(2)** Cauliflower
5 **(6)** lb. Carrots
3 Red onions
3 bulbs Fennel
1 sm. bulb Jicama
1 **(2)** Yellow squash
2 **(3)** Zucchini
1 Red pepper
3 lb. Yellow (Spanish) onions
1 lb. Ginger
1 Cucumber
1 lg. Turnip/rutabaga
1 bunch Scallions
3 med. Leeks
½ lb. Haricots verts (French green beans)

½ lb. Parsnips
2 lb. Beets
1 sm. **(med.)** Acorn squash
2 bunches Celery
3 bunches Radishes
4 Red peppers

Greens
1 head Romaine lettuce
2 heads Red leaf lettuce
3 heads Boston lettuce
2 lb. Spinach
1 lg. Radicchio
3 heads Belgian endive
1 bunch Arugula
1 bunch Watercress
1 bunch Mint leaves
4 bunches Curly parsley
1 bunch Swiss chard
2 boxes Alfalfa sprouts
2 boxes Radish sprouts

Fresh Herbs
1 bunch Cilantro
1 bunch Rosemary
1 bunch Dill

GROCERIES
1 lb. Fava beans
½ **(1)** lb. Red kidney beans
½ lb. Black beans
½ lb. Quinoa
½ lb. Basmati brown rice
½ lb. Wild rice
2 oz. Hazelnuts (filberts)
1 loaf Sprouted grain bread
2 8-oz. jars Dijon mustard

3 16-oz. jars Pineapple juice
1 8-oz. jar Fat-free mayonnaise
Black pepper
Dried thyme, dried oregano, curry
   powder, turmeric, cinnamon
Herbal teas
Olive/safflower oil

DAIRY
6 Eggs
1 oz. Goat cheese

1 8-oz. Plain yogurt, fat-free
1 8-oz. Ricotta, low-fat
1 4-oz. Mozzarella, low-fat
2 **(3)** 8-oz. Cottage cheese,
   low-fat
1 lb. Tofu, extra firm

FISH
1 6-oz. piece Yellowfin tuna
1 4-oz. piece **(1 7-oz.
   piece)** Yellowfin tuna

15 The Balanced Accelerator Diet

Although you share many characteristics with the accelerator, the subtle differences in your metabolism suggest that you need a diet that's all your own. As the name of your meta-type suggests, you're the most balanced of all the accelerators. You generally manage your weight quite well, unless you fall out of type. If you follow your plan carefully, however, you should be able to kiss those worries good-bye forever. I am going to introduce you to a whole new way of eating, living, and feeling great. Just a few quick words on how your personal balanced accelerator diet works, then on to the menus.

As you read, remember:

- Your dominant gland is the thymus.
- Your weakest gland is the pancreas.
- You're most likely to gain weight in your stomach first, then your hips.

The Science behind Your System

Even though you are the most balanced meta-type in your group, as we discussed briefly in chapter 5, your body chemistry is dominated to a great degree by the activities of the sympathetic nervous system. This means that your metabolism is governed by more nerve stimulation to those glands and organs responsible for energy production—the thymus and the heart, followed by the thyroid gland, adrenals, spleen, and lungs. You start off with a twin bonus—a strong heart and, thanks to your dominant thymus gland, which controls your immune system, a strong natural resistance to illnesses and allergies when you stay in balance.

You have less nerve stimulation to the parasympathetic nervous system–driven organs responsible for digestion, repair, and regeneration of the body: the salivary glands, stomach, pancreas, small intestine, liver, gallbladder, large intestine, kidneys, and bladder.

So your balanced accelerator's primary metabolic focus is to break down carbohydrates and proteins and use them for energy. You're a rather fast metabolizer, similar to the pure accelerator. You break down your foods fairly quickly.

But your unique characteristic is the *way* in which you break down your foods to utilize this energy. Unlike the pure accelerator, you do receive a little more nerve stimulation from your parasympathetic nervous system and therefore produce moderate to low amounts of stomach acid. With a little less nerve stimulation to your energy-producing glands, your digestive ability slows a bit, which means you digest your food in more of an aerobic environment (with more oxygen present). Filled with medium amounts of oxygen, the nutrients reach the cells for transformation into energy and will burn off (oxidize) at a slow to average rate.

So you burn off your blood sugars or energy slightly faster than the pure accelerator. Remember, carbohydrates digest quickly and are the fastest-burning foods. Proteins are slower; fats are slowest. This means that if you eat mostly refined carbohydrates—starches and sugars—they'll tend to break down somewhat quickly, then burn off at an average rate, which gives your body bursts of energy, followed by slower declines. Because of your semifast oxidizing ability and greater production of stomach acid, you can handle some of the slower-burning proteins as well as energy-producing complex carbohydrates to keep your body stable. Fats make your metatype more sluggish.

Since your digestive process takes place in a slightly more oxygenated environment, you have more of an acid-producing chemistry. Also, you retain more of your cell waste products—those aging, disease-prone leftovers—and will need more cell scrubbers, cleansing teas, and juices to keep the rejuvenation process going. So with your fast digestion and fairly fast oxidizing of energy, you'll tend to have:

- Low to moderate production of stomach acid (HCl, or hydrochloric acid)—unless it is completely suppressed by the stress response
- Tissue acidity
- Probable low production of pancreatic enzymes
- Possibly high production of pancreatic insulin

Balance is your key word. You and the pure accelerator have the most abundant energy of all the meta-types. You have a strong creative intellect and powerful intuition and can draw on extra adrenaline readily. So when out of balance, you most easily fall into the adrenal-dominated pure accelerator classification. This makes you susceptible to a constant stress response state, together with adrenal burnout, low blood pressure, irritability, and weight gain.

Metabolically speaking, as a balanced accelerator you require foods of a more alkalinizing nature—such as green, leafy vegetables; fruits; and grains—that support and stimulate your dominant thymus gland. But you also require the slower-burning foods, to keep your blood sugar stable, such as the proteins in fish and chicken. You have *very* low tolerance for refined products such as sugar or alcohol and excess fat. Therefore, your balanced accelerator food formula looks like this:

- Carbohydrates: 50 percent
- Protein: 30 percent
- Fat: 20 percent

Balanced Accelerator Food Choices

After one month on the Your Body, Your Diet plan, you will not only drop excess body fat but also experience a level of vitality and good health that you never dreamed possible. Once you have looked at the basic menus, you will find lists that will show you the wide variety of delicious foods that are best for you. Suggested vitamins, minerals, and supplements for your metabolic makeover are also included, as these can speed up your conversion into perfect balance. The next three subsections give you an overview of the basic principles you'll be following.

What to Avoid

Steer clear of refined carbohydrates, sugar, saturated fats, salt, caffeine, and nicotine. I know this seems like a tough set of restrictions to follow, but making these changes is so important. Your adrenals and thymus get plenty of natural stimulation, so you must eliminate those foods that continue to excite them and give your system a rest. Sugar cravings can be your downfall—and overloading on refined carbohydrates and alcohol, along with those saturated animal fats, can seriously weaken your heart and cardiovascular system as well as give disease-triggering organisms a thriving environment.

Caffeine and nicotine jolt your glands into producing energy with an abrupt crash or into a vicious cycle of continued dependency. Caffeine in any form—tea, coffee, diet drinks, soft drinks, and chocolate—tricks your overworked adrenal and thyroid glands into pumping out their nutrients time and again until they exhaust themselves. The cycle starts with sugar cravings and more insulin production from your pancreas, and fatigue and lethargy set in while the pounds keep piling on. Caffeine's residue is extremely acid and can impair your immune protection.

Nicotine, meanwhile, suffocates the oxygen needed for the immune cells to fend off viruses and infections. Your immune system's fighters need fifty times their size in oxygen to make the lethal juices that kill toxins—a "respiratory burst" that can save you. That's why your meta-type is especially vulnerable to respiratory problems and diseases when you smoke.

Too much salt heightens your meta-type's predisposition to retain water and may cause high blood pressure (later in your life) by stimulating excess aldosterone levels from your adrenals.

Another unwelcome result of saturated fats is free radicals, which can lead to those ugly brown blotches called liver, or age, spots. Since the body temperature is too low to melt these fats, they bond with oxygen and start a chemical chain reaction that destroys good tissue and propels you into the aging process. Remember, if the fat is in a "solid" form, that's the way it stays in your body.

The following table gives you an overview of the foods and other substances that do *not* suit your meta-type.

Your *Never* Foods

REFINED STARCH AND SUGAR	SATURATED FATS	CAFFEINE	NICOTINE	SALT
White sugar	Butter	Coffee	Tobacco in any	MSG (monosodium
White flour	Margarine	Tea	form	glutamate)
Processed syrups	Mayonnaise	Soft drinks		Salty foods
Refined foods	Fatty cheeses	Diet drinks		Olives
Any refined products	Creams	Chocolate		Pretzels
Synthetic additives	Sauces			Potato chips
or sweeteners	Ice cream			Peanuts
Alcohol	Chocolate			Salted nuts
	Fried foods			
	Milk products			

What to Fill Up On

Fish, poultry, grains, selected legumes, and vegetables are your foods of choice. Now you must admit, that's a much fuller list than you expected. You will definitely be able to enjoy a wide variety of delicious foods. You'll just have to lay off the refined carbohydrates. The foods in these groups will help you stabilize your energy, strengthen your weakened pancreas gland, and stop you from putting on excess weight.

The accompanying table lists the foods that best suit your meta-type.

Your *Always* Foods

PROTEINS		CARBOHYDRATES		FATS
Food	Times per Week	Food	Times per Week	
Meat: none (too much saturated fat)	0	Grains: variety	2–3	*Moderate* amount of unsaturated fatty acids—cold-pressed vegetable or nut oils
Fowl: small amount (avoid eggs)	1–2	Legumes: Avoid legumes—except for black-eyed peas (cowpeas).	0	Choose from your food plan
Fish: variety (avoid most shellfish)	2–3	Starchy vegetables: variety	1–2	
Dairy: abundant, nonfat (eliminate if you have allergies; avoid whole-milk products)	2	Slightly starchy vegetables: variety	3–4	
Seeds/nuts: small amount	1–2	Nonstarchy vegetables: abundant	Daily	
Legume protein: abundant tofu (avoid other legumes)	2–3	Fruit: abundant	Daily	

As you've learned, the foods that are required by your specific metabolic type—complex carbohydrates, whole grains, vegetables, seeds, nuts, and fruits—are the ones that feed and support your weaker endocrine gland, the pancreas.

How to Speed Up Weight Loss

Here are a few other tips to stimulate faster weight loss:

• Mix 60 percent grains to 40 percent legumes (beans) or tofu (soybean curd) for a complete protein complement. Tofu is an excellent accompaniment to grains.
• Chew your food slowly and well.
• Try to avoid drinking more than one glass of water or liquid during your meals. Drinking large amounts of liquid during meals dilutes the precious enzymes needed for your digestion.
• Have at least six to eight glasses of water during the day, *not* at mealtimes.

Keeping Your Thymus in Balance

Since you are a balanced accelerator, your dominant thymus gland gives you a powerhouse of health, controlling your immune system and fighting off allergies, viruses, and other illnesses with ease—when you're not out of balance.

Chinese medicine shows how this pyramid-shaped gland in the center of your chest near the heart has a daytime job with your thyroid and adrenal glands. It balances your heart's strong yang activity, oxygenating your blood, feeding your cells, and keeping your immune system flowing under the sympathetic nervous system's domination. At night the parasympathetic system's yin action takes control, restoring and rebuilding your disease- and age-fighting defenses.

When you flip out of balance, your meta-type then has a double risk. You may swing into the accelerator's excessive adrenal activity, putting more stress on your heart and burning out your adrenals and thymus, provoking side effects like weight gain, low libido, excess facial hair, or absence of the menstrual cycle. Or you can tip to the mixed accelerator's burnout damage, with too much or too little thyroid production, developing emotional overreactions, significant weight loss or gain, dry hair or hair loss, fatigue, and, in severe cases of thyroid hyperactivity, protruding eyes.

At the same time, your meta-type's weaker pancreas means that a carbohydrate overload can turn it into an "insulin factory," converting carbohydrates directly to fat. This gland produces two hormones: glucagon, which releases and spends your energy from muscles, and insulin, which saves it as fat. Your meta-type is easily affected by stress, which shuts down your digestion, then stimulates extra insulin to regulate the excess blood sugar. When you overload it with those junk carbs, it gets in the habit of pumping out extra insulin, and you wind up exhausted and carbohydrate-intolerant.

Meanwhile your heart, which works with your thymus on the immune front, is getting overworked. Sugar can weaken your heart muscles as well as your other cells.

Now if your normally strong immune system crashes, you become quite vulnerable to severe allergies, virus or bacteria invasions, or autoimmune illnesses.

Sound alarming? Rest assured that the "balance" in your balanced accelerator system means that you'll respond well to a few basic diet changes, and you'll soon see a major difference.

Your Balanced Accelerator Secret Weapons

Of course everyone, myself included, can find it tough to switch to a whole new way of eating. In addition to willpower, you have to give your body time to adjust to your new lifestyle. So if you find yourself feeling cranky and frustrated, don't worry; it's par for the course. It's just a sign that you're shedding those extra pounds and getting back into balance.

The teas and elixirs in this chapter were created to help you sail through the transition phase of your meta-type diet while making the pounds melt away even faster.

Enzyme-Rich Pineapple and Papaya

For each meta-type there is one food or group of foods that helps to speed up the weight-loss process. For you balanced accelerators, those foods are enzyme-rich fruits.

Your weaker endocrine gland, the pancreas, may be able to supply you with only a small amount of its valuable protein and carbohydrate-splitting enzymes, much less than you need to adequately digest your foods. When foods are incompletely digested, they're more easily stored in your body as fat rather than being completely metabolized and used as nutrients or energy. Remember, all proteins, carbohydrates, and fats—not just fats—will be stored in your body as fat if they're not properly utilized.

If you're repeatedly experiencing the stress response, your pancreatic enzyme production will be further suppressed and your insulin levels may soar, helping turn the carbohydrates you eat into fat.

The key to your weight-loss success is to fortify your diet with enzyme-rich foods that can act as substitutes for your marginal pancreatic enzyme production.

The answer? Fresh *pineapple* and *papaya*. Both pineapple and papaya are enzyme-rich fruits plentiful in *bromelain* and *papain*, whose enzymatic action is similar to the strong digestive activity of the pancreatic enzyme trypsin and the digestive enzyme pepsin. These enzymes easily break down, consume, and wash away those unwanted pounds.

Papaya's papain is a powerful digestive aid, especially beneficial for the digestion and assimilation of proteins. As an assimilator of proteins, papain can even prevent the formation of adhesions as the body heals itself and also help burn off those excess pounds.

Pineapple's bromelain, which also breaks down proteins, is a potent regenerator. Bromelain has the ability to heal and repair your body's cells and tissues. Its duty is to take vitamin C and potassium and bind them with the pineapple's vitamin A content to enhance cellular rejuvenation. This means that as those pounds of fat melt away, bromelain will tone and tighten your skin.

Pineapple and papaya are both rich in vitamins A and C, essential nutrients needed by your overworked immune system. Eating this fertile combination of fruits can invigorate your sluggish glands and organs, especially your liver and gallbladder, stimulating them to efficiently and quickly break down and emulsify your fat. They also act as efficient cleansers, ridding your body of cellular wastes. Remember, fruits are the cleansers, vegetables and grains are the energizers, and proteins are the builders of your body. I've formulated your unique meta-type program to specifically include these nutritious foods to enhance your weight loss. I use a medley of pineapple and papaya with other enzyme-containing fruits for your breakfast and again after lunch and dinner. They'll help you quickly and efficiently break down those excess pounds. To keep within the guidelines of food combining, eat these fruits half an hour after lunch or dinner.

So your balanced accelerator health trick is:

Enjoy pineapple and papaya three times per day.

I've also added *cranberry juice* to your regimen. It's a tremendous slimming aid. It also helps to flush toxins and wastes, reduces water retention, and gives you a wonderfully clean, lean feeling. Remember, this isn't that familiar supermarket-shelf type of cranberry juice; it's pure and concentrated, as explained in chapter 12. Now watch those pounds just melt away.

Slimming Tea

Another important component of your plan is the herbal tea formula I've created to meet the needs of each meta-type. Each tea will harmonize and balance your specific metabolism, facilitating your weight loss. To make yours, you'll need to add a few special ingredients to the basic Master Weight-Loss Tea (see the formula and directions on pages 103–05).

These supplementary herbs should be added in equal proportions to the herbs already in the basic formula. I suggest you drink one to three cups per day of your special tea. The herbs may be purchased at your local health-food store or ordered from the companies listed in appendix 2.

Balanced Accelerator Slimming Tea

Basic Formula: One Teaspoon Each
Alisma, poria, rhubarb root, aloe, red clover tops, alfalfa leaf, hawthorn berry, radish seed, sargassum, Indian chickweed, evergreen artemesia, astragalus root, fleeceflower root, citrus peel

Balanced Accelerator Slimming Formula: Add One Teaspoon Each			
NAME			FUNCTION
Common	Latin	Eastern	
Safflower	Carthamus tinctorius	Hong hua	Opens the pancreas and liver, energizes, balances insulin levels, helps digestion, and burns cholesterol and fats.
Bupleurum root (thorowax root)	Bupleurum chinense D.C.	Chai hu	Opens the liver and balances the pancreas.
Fennel fruit	Foeniculum officinale vulgare	Hui xiang	Excellent for weight loss, opens digestion and liver function, burns fat, and removes waste and mucus.
Dandelion	Taraxacum officinale	Pu gong ying	Reduces water retention and opens the liver and gallbladder to burn fat.

Note: Your thymus gland is already supported by astragalus, and your heart is supported by hawthorn berry, both in the Master Weight-Loss Tea. If you are pregnant, have high blood pressure, or are allergic to grasses or flowers, it's suggested that these teas not be used.

Rules of the Road

Your Eating Schedule

Your energy runs at a high pitch from approximately 6:00 A.M. to 4:00 P.M. During this time your digestion tends to be underactive. If you eat heavy foods, they won't digest well and you'll end up feeling sluggish, even tired or sleepy. You also have a natural tendency to lose energy during the afternoon. Your energy picks up again in early evening and begins to decline around 10:00 or 11:00 P.M.

For balanced accelerators a little food goes a long way. A light breakfast of fruit is the best way for you to start your day. A light to medium lunch will supply you with enough energy to greatly lessen the usual afternoon energy crash. A heavier meal at night supplies you with the energy and nutrients your body needs for its nightly regeneration. Consequently, your eating schedule should be:

- Light breakfast
- Light to medium lunch
- Substantial dinner

Late Afternoon—Living with Low Energy

You've learned that your cortisol level begins to nose-dive in the afternoon. When that happens, most balanced accelerators grab for that sugar fix, such as cake, cookies, bagels, candy, alcohol, or coffee. You might even reach for a fat fix, such as a bagel and cream cheese, cheese and crackers, ice cream, or chocolate. Don't even think of it. These will send your insulin levels skyrocketing, you'll have a sudden drop in blood sugar, you'll start craving more of the starch or sugar, and you'll reach for those carbohydrates—starting the vicious circle all over again. Now you'll be causing your already acid body to become even more acid—especially if you reach for that after-work drink.

It's fine for you to have a late-afternoon snack, to support your waning blood sugar levels, but make it the right kind of snack—from the following types of foods:

YOUR LATE-AFTERNOON SNACK
Cranberry juice
Fresh fruit
Hot green tea

Bedtime Eating—Steering Clear of Snacks

Late-night eating is guaranteed to keep you tossing and turning throughout the night. Even though you digest and break down your foods quickly and tend to burn them more quickly than the pure accelerator, they still burn at a relatively slow rate. This happens as you sleep, so the energy released from the carbohydrates will wake you up or at best give you a restless night's sleep, as well as a lot of gas and even heartburn. So no late dinners or late-night snacks in front of the television.

Balanced Accelerator Meals and Menus

Now you've completed the first part of the plan, and here's your reward: the tailor-made diet for your balanced accelerator meta-type. If you've reached this point in the book, you know that losing weight and keeping it off take more than just watching what you eat.

The meals presented in this section are designed to meet all the needs of your metabolism while giving you the chance to eat a delicious, wide variety of fresh, nutritious foods. The first week may seem like a big adjustment, but by week two, I assure you, you'll be making your juices and tossing together your special meals like a pro.

Eating the Right Foods at the Right Times

Eating the *right kinds of food* at the *right times* is another key to the success of your weight-loss and rejuvenation program. With the acid nature of your balanced accelerator metabolism, you'll find that if you eat a majority of acid foods, it will throw you way out of balance and increase your tissue acidity. Then you'll struggle to regain balance, reach for the wrong foods, feel terrible, and retain that extra fat.

You require the more alkalizing foods to help balance out your body chemistry, just as your counterpart, the balanced synthesizer meta-type, is more alkaline in nature and requires more of the acid forming foods. (Chapter 3 provides a detailed explanation of the acid-alkaline aspect of your meta-type.)

As you've just learned, your metabolism tends to be the most balanced of all the accelerator meta-types, and you require alkaline foods, such as vegetables and fruits, to stabilize your metabolism. You are what is known as the *acid* meta-type, with your natural body pH tending to be 5. You also require some of the weaker acid foods, such as dairy, and can handle some of the more acid-forming foods, such as grains and animal protein, on a "sometimes" basis. You need protein to help maintain the equilibrium of your immune response. Therefore, your diet should consist of foods that are strong alkaline, alkaline, and weak alkaline forming ash. Foods that are weak acid and strong acid can be eaten three times per week. Foods that are your own pH tendency—acid forming—should be avoided. Appendix 5 lists the full spectrum of foods and their pH factors.

Here We Go!

To make this adventure of slimming down to a new and healthy you fun, I've taken all the guesswork out of how to shop and prepare your meals. Before you begin, glance through your weekly menus and balanced accelerator elixirs in the accompanying tables and look over the vast array of selections in your Balanced Accelerator Food Choices list. At the end of this chapter, you will find your own balanced accelerator shopping list for a week. Then turn to appendix 1 and take a look at the equipment list (which includes all the supplies you'll need to make this as simple as possible), your advance food-preparation suggestions for the week, and your recipes and food-preparation instructions for both men and women.

For any of the foods specified in the weekly menus and recipes, you may substitute comparable foods from the Balanced Accelerator Food Choices list.

Eat only the foods that are indicated for you on your individual food choices list. If your favorite isn't there, don't eat it. You can check the "General Food Choices and Their Calorie Content for Each Meta-Type" in appendix 5.

You see, it's all done for you, down to the last detail—and my personal promise to you is that this eating plan will keep your balanced accelerator metabolism in perfect balance while helping you achieve a slender, gorgeous physique.

You're on your way to a bright, new, skinny, energetic you. Treat this as a ritual in celebrating your beauty and regeneration.

Balanced Accelerator Semivegetarian Weekly Menus

Alkaline-Based Foods

Larger quantities for men are shown in **boldface**.

WHEN	SATURDAY	SUNDAY	MONDAY	TUESDAY
On rising	Drink the juice of 1 lemon in 4 oz. hot spring water. (Important for your program! The citrus's active enzymes clear out toxic cellular debris, break down fats, alkalize your digestive tract, and are a powerful liver and gallbladder cleanser.)			
Breakfast	*Dane's Delight* 1 cup herbal tea or Balanced Accelerator Slimming Tea	*Dane's Delight* 1 cup herbal tea or Balanced Accelerator Slimming Tea	*Dane's Delight* 1 cup herbal tea or Balanced Accelerator Slimming Tea	*Dane's Delight* 1 cup herbal tea or Balanced Accelerator Slimming Tea
Midmorning	1 6-oz. glass cranberry juice (Obtain Knudsen or Ad-Vita cranberry concentrate from your health-food store. Use 2 tbs. concentrate to 6 oz. spring water. Add more water if desired.) 1 cup herbal tea or Balanced Accelerator Slimming Tea			
Lunch	*Health Salad with Raw Vegetables and Tofu Scramble* 1 **(2–3)** cup Balanced Accelerator Salad Greens 1 cup broccoli ½ cup diced celery ½ cup shredded red cabbage 2 tsp. Balanced Accelerator Salad Dressing *Serve with:* ½ **(1)** cup Tofu Scramble *½ hour after lunch:* ½ **(1)** cup	*Health Salad with Cold Seared Tuna and Mixed Raw Vegetables* 1 **(2–3)** cup Balanced Accelerator Salad Greens 1 cup broccoli ½ cup diced celery ½ cup shredded red cabbage **(1½ oz. Roasted Hazelnuts)** 2 tsp. Balanced Accelerator Salad Dressing *Serve with:* 2 **(6)** oz. cold seared tuna	*Health Salad with Raw Vegetables, Curried Tofu, and Tabouli* 1 **(2–3)** cup Balanced Accelerator Salad Greens ¼ **(½)** cup carrots ½ **(1)** cup broccoli ¼ cup shredded red cabbage *Serve with:* ½ **(1)** cup Tabouli ¼ **(½)** cup cold Curried Tofu	*Health Salad with Raw Vegetables with Cold Mustard Thyme Chicken* 1 **(2–3)** cup Balanced Accelerator Salad Greens ½ cup carrots 1 cup broccoli ¼ cup diced celery ¼ cup shredded red cabbage **(1½ oz. Roasted Hazelnuts)** 2 tsp. Balanced Accelerator Salad Dressing *Serve with:* 2 **(6)** oz. sliced

WHEN	SATURDAY	SUNDAY	MONDAY	TUESDAY
Lunch (cont'd)	pineapple 1 cup herbal tea or Balanced Accelerator Slimming Tea	(from night before) *½ hour after lunch:* ½ **(1)** cup papaya 1 cup herbal tea or Balanced Accelerator Slimming Tea	*½ hour after lunch:* 1 cup herbal tea or Balanced Accelerator Slimming Tea	mustard thyme chicken *½ hour after lunch:* ½ **(1)** cup pineapple 1 cup herbal tea or Balanced Accelerator Slimming Tea
Midafternoon	1 6-oz. glass cranberry juice 1 cup herbal tea or Balanced Accelerator Slimming Tea			

Dinner	*Fish Fiesta Dinner*
	Seared Yellowfin Tuna with
	  Rutabaga Carrot Puree
	Fiesta Vegetable with
	  Haricots Verts
	
	½ hour after dinner:
	⅓ cup pineapple,
	  papaya, and
	  green grapes
	1 cup herbal tea or
	  Balanced Accelerator
	  Slimming Tea
		Protein Power Dinner
		Baked Chicken Breast with
		  Mustard, Thyme Crust
		Hearty Vegetable Soup
		  Power Salad
		
		½ hour after dinner:
		⅓ cup pineapple,
		  papaya, and
		  blueberries
		1 cup herbal tea or
		  Balanced Accelerator
		  Slimming Tea
			Longevity Dinner
			Amaranth Grain with
			  Roasted Tofu and
			  Vegetables
			Seaweed Health Salad
			1 glass Balanced
			  Accelerator Elixir
			
			½ hour after dinner:
			⅓ cup pineapple
			1 cup herbal tea or
			  Balanced Accelerator
			  Slimming Tea
				*Pasta Party Vegetarian
				  Dinner*
				Egg Pastina with
				  Steamed Artichoke
				Dijon Beets
				Steamed Kale and Tofu
				  with Roasted Onions,
				  Lemon, and Pepper
				Arugula Fennel Salad
				
				½ hour after dinner:
				⅓ cup pineapple, papaya,
				  and strawberries
				1 cup herbal tea or
				  Balanced Accelerator
				  Slimming Tea

WHEN	WEDNESDAY	THURSDAY	FRIDAY
On rising	Drink the juice of 1 lemon in 4 oz. hot spring water. (Important for your program! The citrus's active enzymes clear out toxic cellular debris, break down fats, alkalize your digestive tract, and are a powerful liver and gallbladder cleanser.)		
Breakfast	*Dane's Delight* 1 cup herbal tea or Balanced Accelerator Slimming Tea	*Dane's Delight* 1 cup herbal tea or Balanced Accelerator Slimming Tea	*Dane's Delight* 1 cup herbal tea or Balanced Accelerator Slimming Tea
Midmorning	1 6-oz. glass cranberry juice (Obtain Knudsen or Ad-Vita cranberry concentrate from your health-food store. Use 2 tbs. concentrate to 6 oz. spring water. Add more water if desired.) 1 cup herbal tea or Balanced Accelerator Slimming Tea		
Lunch	*Health Salad with Raw Vegetables, Curried Tofu, and Tabouli* 1 **(2–3)** cup Balanced Accelerator Salad Greens ½ cup carrots 1 cup broccoli ¼ cup shredded red cabbage 2 tsp. Balanced Accelerator Salad Dressing *Serve with:* ½ **(1)** cup Tabouli ¼ **(½)** cup cold Curried Tofu	*Health Salad with Raw Vegetables with Tofu Scramble* 1 **(2–3)** cup Balanced Accelerator Salad Greens 1 cup broccoli ½ cup diced celery ½ cup shredded red cabbage 2 tsp. Balanced Accelerator Salad Dressing *Serve with:* ½ **(1)** cup Tofu Scramble *½ hour after lunch:*	*Health Salad with Ricotta Cheese and Raw Vegetables* 1 **(2–3)** cup Balanced Accelerator Salad Greens ¼ cup carrots 1 cup broccoli ¼ cup diced celery ¼ cup shredded red cabbage 2 tsp. Balanced Accelerator Salad Dressing *Serve with:* 4 **(8)** oz. ricotta cheese, low-fat (Add ¼ cup grated carrots and scallions.

WHEN	WEDNESDAY	THURSDAY	FRIDAY
Lunch **(cont'd)**	½ hour after lunch: 1 cup herbal tea or Balanced Accelerator Slimming Tea	½ **(1)** cup pineapple 1 cup herbal tea or Balanced Accelerator Slimming Tea	Sprinkle with cinnamon, paprika, oregano, or cayenne pepper.)
			½ hour after lunch: ½ **(1)** cup papaya 1 cup herbal tea or Balanced Accelerator Slimming Tea
Midafternoon	1 6-oz. glass cranberry juice 1 cup herbal tea or Balanced Accelerator Slimming Tea		
Dinner	*Calypso Fish Dinner* Calamari Seviche with Lime, Cilantro, and Cayenne Marinated Jicama Sticks Steamed Mixed Vegetables with Cumin Haricots Verts Salad	*Veggie Delight Dinner* Roasted Acorn Squash with Mixed Roasted Vegetables (parsnips, carrots, red onions, fennel, and cauliflower) with Tarragon Spinach and Fennel Salad 1 glass Balanced Accelerator Elixir	*Tofu-Amaranth Vegetarian Dinner* Cold Amaranth Grain, Tofu Salad, Mixed Cold and Cooked Vegetables, with Balanced Accelerator Greens 1 glass Balanced Accelerator Elixir
	½ hour after dinner: ⅓ cup pineapple, papaya, and green grapes 1 cup herbal tea or Balanced Accelerator Slimming Tea	½ hour after dinner: ⅓ cup pineapple, papaya, and raspberries 1 cup herbal tea or Balanced Accelerator Slimming Tea	½ hour after dinner: ½ cup pineapple and papaya 1 cup herbal tea or Balanced Accelerator Slimming Tea

Balanced Accelerator Food Choices

Proteins			
FOWL	**FISH**	**DAIRY**	**NUTS**
Strong Acid	**Strong Acid**	*Note:* If you have allergies, eliminate dairy of any kind.	**Weak Alkaline**
Turkey	Mackerel		Coconut milk
Goose	Roe	**Weak Alkaline**	
Squab	Halibut	**(Use Low-Fat)**	**Weak Acid**
Chicken	Red snapper		Filberts (hazelnuts)
Duck	Sole	Whey	Hickory nuts
Frog legs	Tuna	Goat's milk	
Quail	Bluefish	Yogurt	**Strong Acid**
Pheasant	Eel	Cow's milk	Pine nuts
	Swordfish	Buttermilk	Water chestnuts
AVOID	Squid (calamari)		Cashews
Acid Forming	Cod	**Cheeses (Use Low-Fat)**	Coconut
Eggs	Mullet	Parmesan	
	Haddock	Limburger	**AVOID**
	Ocean perch	Cheddar	**Acid Forming**
	Sturgeon	Brick	Pecans
	Octopus (scungilli)	Swiss	Pistachios
			Walnuts
	Weak Acid	**Weak Acid**	Brazil nuts
	Anchovies	**Cheeses (Use Low-Fat)**	Macadamias
	Caviar	Camembert	Chestnuts
	Herring	Brie	Almonds
	Sardines	Edam	
		Gruyère	
	Shellfish	Cottage	
	Strong Acid	Farmer	
	Abalone	Feta	
		Ricotta	
	Weak Acid	Muenster	
	Oysters	Monterey Jack	
		Provolone	
	AVOID	Mozzarella	
	Acid Forming	Goat	
	Carp	Blue	
	Yellowtail tuna	Gorgonzola	
	Salmon		
	Hake	**AVOID**	
	Lake perch	**Acid Forming**	
	Bass	Soy milk (also under	
	Trout	"Legumes")	
	Crab		
	Lobster	**Saturated Fats**	
	Scallops	Cream	
	Clams and mussels	Buttermilk	
	Shrimp and crayfish		

SEEDS	LEGUMES	FRUIT PROTEIN
Strong Acid	**Weak Alkaline**	**Strong Alkaline**
Pumpkin seeds	Soybean curd (tofu)	Olives
Sunflower seeds		
Squash seeds	**Strong Acid**	**Strong Acid**
Safflower seeds	Peanuts	Avocados
Sesame seeds		
Flaxseeds	*AVOID*	*AVOID*
Chia seeds	**Acid Forming**	
	Lentils	None
AVOID	Soybeans	
None	Soy milk	
	Adzuki beans	
	Black beans	
	Kidney beans	
	Navy beans	
	Pinto beans	
	Red beans	

Carbohydrates

GRAINS		HIGH STARCH LEGUMES	HIGH-STARCH VEGETABLES	
Strong Alkaline	**Eliminate If You Have Any Allergies**	**Strong Acid**	**Weak Alkaline**	**Eliminate If You Have Any Allergies**
Amaranth grain and flakes	Wheat	Black-eyed peas (cowpeas)	Acorn squash	Corn
	Wheat germ			Corn meal
Strong Acid	Rye	*AVOID*	**Strong Acid**	Corn grits
	Barley	**Acid Forming**	Field corn	Potatoes
Popcorn		Lima beans	Sweet corn	
Corn grits	*AVOID*	Garbanzo beans	Potatoes	*AVOID*
Rice bran	**Acid Forming**	(chickpeas)		**Acid Forming**
Millet	Farina	Great northern beans	**Weak Acid**	
Barley	Brown rice	Split peas	Butternut squash	Yams
Corn meal	Basmati brown rice	White (fava) beans	Hubbard squash	Pumpkin, raw
Wheat	Wild rice		Sweet potatoes	
Couscous	Buckwheat (kasha)		Pumpkin, canned	
Bulgur (cracked wheat)	Quinoa			
Rye				
Oats				
Pastinas (egg)				
Sprouted grain bread				

SLIGHTLY STARCHY VEGETABLES		NONSTARCHY VEGETABLES	
Weak Alkaline	Strong Alkaline	Weak Alkaline	Eliminate If You Have *Allergies* of Any Kind
Carrots	Kale, cooked	Summer squash, cooked	Eggplant
Rutabagas	Collards	Leeks	Tomatoes
	Swiss chard, cooked	Garden cress	Peppers
Weak Acid	Parsley	Chinese cabbage	
	Mustard greens, cooked	Snap beans	*AVOID* **Acid Forming**
Beets, cooked	Beet greens, cooked	Yellow beans	
Parsnips	Turnip greens, cooked	Turnips	Bamboo shoots
Jicama	Lamb's-quarter	Scallions	Green peas
	Mustard spinach	Broccoli	Sugar peas
AVOID **Acid Forming**		Lettuce: butter, Boston, iceberg	Mungbeans and sprouts
	Seaweeds	Celery	Chili peppers
Beets, raw		Endive	Asparagus
	Agar-agar	Radicchio	Celeriac root
	Irish moss	Yellow dock, raw	Sweet peppers
	Kelp	Cabbage, raw	Brussels sprouts
	Dulse	Spinach, raw	Cauliflower, raw
	Arame	Okra, raw	Tomatoes
		Fennel	
	Alkaline Forming		
		Weak Acid	
	Yellow dock, cooked		
	Chicory greens	Cauliflower, cooked	
	Horseradish	Eggplant	
	Cabbage, cooked	Artichokes	
	Okra, cooked	Shallots	
	Swiss chard, raw	Gingerroot	
	Spinach, cooked	Salsify	
	Kale, raw	Soybean sprouts	
	Lettuce: cos, romaine, dark green, white	Kohlrabi	
		Chicory	
	Watercress	Onions	
	Alfalfa sprouts	Cucumbers	
	Dandelion greens	Radishes	
	Arugula	Summer squash, raw	
	Beet greens, raw		
	Strong Acid		
	Mushrooms		
	Garlic		

FRUIT		OILS	CONDIMENTS	TEAS
Strong Alkaline	**Weak Acid**	**Strong Acid**	**Strong Alkaline**	**Burdock root:** regulates insulin levels
Rhubarb	Apricots	Avocado	Molasses: blackstrap	**Red raspberry:** tonic for hormones
Alkaline Forming	Prickly pears	Corn	or light	**Dandelion root:**
	Pears	Soybean	Sorghum	regulates blood sugar
Loganberries	Mangoes	Peanut	Maple syrup	**Alfalfa leaf:** cleanses the
Oranges		Cottonseed		blood and clears the
Clementines	**Melons (Eat Alone)**	Olive	**Weak Alkaline**	skin
Tangerines		Safflower	Pickles	**Blue flag:** clears the liver
Kumquats	Watermelon	Sunflower		and skin
Kiwifruits	Muskmelon	Flaxseed	**Weak Acid**	**Passionflower:** calms
	Cantaloupe	Walnut		your adrenals
Weak Alkaline	Casaba	Apricot	Vinegar	**Fennel:** calms and
	Crenshaw	Almond	Honey	suppresses the appetite
Boysenberries	Honeydew		Mustard	**Nettle:** stabilizes insulin
Grapefruit		*AVOID*		levels
Raspberries	**Sweet Fruit**	**(Saturated Fats)**	*AVOID*	**Mint and peppermint:**
Strawberries	**Alkaline Forming**		Yeast—in all forms	calms and relaxes;
Plums	Pineapple	Mayonnaise	Soy sauce	helps digestion
Acerola cherries		Butter	Cane syrup	***Vitex agnus:*** aids
Blueberries	**Weak Alkaline**	Margarine	Cane sugar	hormone balance
Nectarines	Figs		Brown sugar	
Gooseberries				
Pokeberries	**Weak Acid**			
Papaya	Apricots, dried			
Grapes: Concord,	Raisins			
Thompson	Prunes			
Elderberries	Dates			
Sapotes				
Cranberries	*AVOID*			
Currants	**Acid Forming**			
Lemons	Litchis			
Cherries	Passion fruit			
Blackberries	Groundberries			
Limes	Pomegranates			
	Crab apples			
Weak Acid	Peaches			
Guavas	Persimmons			
Loquats	Plantains			
Cherimoya	Bananas			
Grapes: muscat, Tokay				
Quince				
Tamarinds				
Apples				

Balanced Accelerator Elixirs for Both Women and Men

Potassium Powerhouse: Carrot juice leads this potassium-rich formula full of vitamins A, D, B, C, E, and K; celery balances your nerves, stimulates your pancreas, and clears your skin; parsley balances your adrenals; and spinach, full of iron, burns fat.	Carrots: 6 oz. juice (about 6 carrots) Celery: 3 oz. juice (about 1 bunch) Parsley: 2 oz. juice (about 2 bunches) Spinach: 3 oz. juice (about 1 bunch) Water: 2 oz.
Pancreas Balancer: This formula feeds both the pituitary and pancreas glands. Full of vitamins and iron, this juice energizes, nourishes, cleans out, and regenerates your whole endocrine and digestive system—which means cleaning out toxins and fat.	Carrots: 6 oz. juice (about 6 carrots) Spinach: 3 oz. juice (about 1 bunch) Water: 2 oz.
Spring Cleanser: A great blood cleanser and cell builder. Alfalfa is full of chlorophyll and cleans out toxic waste, while lettuce is rich in calcium, magnesium, potassium, and iron and stimulates renewed skin and hair growth.	Carrots: 6 oz. juice (about 6 carrots) Lettuce: 4 oz. juice (about 1 head) Alfalfa Sprouts: 2–3 oz. juice (about 2 to 3 boxes) Water: 2 oz.
Adrenal Stabilizer: With carrot juice, parsley is the great adrenal stabilizer and also balances the thyroid gland, cleanses the kidneys, brightens the eyes, and brings oxygen into the body.	Carrots: 6 oz. juice (about 6 carrots) Parsley: 3 oz. juice (about 3 bunches) Water: 2 oz.

Your On-Program Cheat Sheet

Naturally there will be days when you just have to cheat. No problem. There's no need to become obsessed with perfection. That just causes more tension. You can succeed at weight loss.

For your balanced accelerator profile, the best snack food is crunchy, fragrant, delicious, air-popped popcorn—no butter. Here's a complete list of the goodies you can use to put a stop to the munchies—fast:

SNACKS
- *Popcorn:* 1 oz. uncooked, with no butter or salt
- *Raisins:* ¼ cup, or 2 oz.
- *Dates:* ¼ cup pitted, or 2 oz.
- *Prunes:* ½ cup pitted, or 4 oz.

You'll need to follow some guidelines in order to make these foods work for you. Otherwise, using these cheat foods in the wrong way could sabotage your goal of losing weight.

CHEAT-FOOD GUIDELINES

• *Eat your cheat foods only at the recommended times.* Cheat foods should be eaten only once per week, only on the weekends (when you're not under stress), and just at one meal or one time.

• *Eat only the amount suggested.* Your body can handle a small amount of these foods without triggering excessive insulin production. If you eat a large amount, your insulin level will spike and turn your "treat" into a "bad trick" of fat.

• *Eat only one cheat food at a time.* Don't have several together or you'll wreak havoc with your metabolism. For instance, raisins *and* popcorn or prunes will send you over the top.

• *Never eat your cheat foods when you're under stress.* That's a surefire way to add pounds, not lose them. Only eat them when you're relaxed—usually on a weekend. Otherwise, your digestion will shut down, your insulin level will rise, and you'll become a veritable fat factory.

• *Never eat your cheat foods late at night.* You'll end up having a restless night, and it's important for you to sleep deeply and regenerate your body.

Balanced Accelerator Healers and Helpers: Vitamins, Minerals, and Amino Acids

Now that you're ready to move into high gear, here are some additions to the food plan that will help you lose weight even faster and improve your overall health and well-being. As I discussed in chapter 13, you can enhance the benefits of your meta-type diet with vitamins, minerals, and supplements tailored for you.

For your balanced accelerator meta-type, I suggest that you add a gentle, full-spectrum multiple amino acid, vitamin, and mineral complex containing only those essential nutrients that support your weaker parasympathetic nervous system. This will speed up your weight-loss program, help tone your muscles, and give you abundant good health. Your multiple amino acid, vitamin, and mineral complex can be purchased at your local health-food store or ordered from the companies listed in appendix 2.

If the controlling endocrine gland governed by your dominant nervous system is out of balance, either hyperactive or hypoactive, you may need some additional nutrients in the form of amino acids, vitamins, or minerals besides the full-spectrum amino acid, vitamin, and mineral formula supporting your opposite nervous system. In your case your dominant endocrine gland is the thymus gland and heart.

By learning about what stabilizes your thymus and heart, you can be your own best judge when choosing the nutrients to take for their health. This is particularly true for your meta-type, since the thymus regulates your immune system—pumping out thymosin, a powerful hormone that stimulates those heavy-hitting immune fighters to be on guard against everything from mild food or pollen allergies to life-threatening diseases. Your strong heart keeps the immune system pathways (the lymphatic system) flowing freely.

Of course, fighting major diseases is the thymus's most important role, but the everyday, chronic problems you may face most often when you're not eating right and gaining all that weight are allergies. It's an immune overreaction, as your thymus sends those antibodies to your defense against dust, pollen, drugs, foods, and insect bites, leading to sneezing, hives, and—at its worst—shock that can kill. As you tend to gain weight and burn out your adrenals, you're overloading, and a stress response can trigger an attack. Now you have to resort to antihistamines or cortisone from your doctor or stop the exposure to the offenders.

Along with your thymus gland and heart, some additional attention must be focused on your weaker, opposite endocrine gland, which tends to be the pancreas, with its crucial blood-sugar-regulating hormones, glucagon and insulin. Remember the yin and yang balance. When you experience the stress response and eat improperly, your meta-type is easily pushed into runaway insulin production, converting the excess sugar and fats in your "comfort foods" directly into body bulges, not energy. You're suddenly prone to abrupt blood sugar slumps and fatigue. You also need enough pancreatic enzymes to break down and absorb your food so it won't be stored as ugly fat.

The nutrients needed to gently support your dominant thymus gland are essential fatty acids, vitamin C, vitamin B complex, and zinc.

Essential fatty acids (EFAs) feed your thymus and lymphatic system and encourage a healthy immune response. Fats aren't used just as cushions for your body's organs and as protection from the cold. They're an essential ingredient in your diet. A primary component of all of your body's cell membranes, they're responsible for the manufacture of the adrenal and sex gland steroid hormones from cholesterol. They also act as a major factor in the production of phospholipids, which break down cholesterol and are the "food" for your immune system. Lecithin is a rich source of the phospholipids, as is safflower oil, cranking up your fat furnace. But don't fry them, because heat converts them into the very fats you need to avoid—saturated fats.

Whether animal or plant, the fatty acids are rich in the fat-soluble vitamins A, D, E, and K and are broken down into three groups: triglycerides, which make up 90 percent of the fats and are used to regenerate your body's cells; and phospholipids and cholesterol, the other 10 percent, which are the precursors for the steroid hormones of your adrenal and sex glands.

The phospholipids in polyunsaturated fatty acids are also a basic component of the parasympathetic nervous system's main neurotransmitter, acetylcholine, which you need in order to balance your strong sympathetic side. Acetylcholine also stimulates the production of your immune system's defense cells.

Vitamin C is essential for the health of your immune system. It plays a primary role in almost every part of the body's functioning, from building capillary walls and connective tissue to creating healthy skin and red blood cells to building up the body's resistance to infection and accelerating its healing process. It's crucial for the metabolism of the amino acids needed for the brain's neurotransmitters—tryptophan, which forms the calming, regenerating serotonin for your parasympathetic nervous system; and tyrosine, which forms the adrenal hormones, dopamine, epinephrine, and norepinephrine, used not just for energy but for your allergic responses. Vitamin C is able to control cholesterol because it's necessary in fat and lipid metabolism—it burns off fat. Since it's water soluble, it isn't stored in the body and must be replaced daily.

Vitamin B complex is an organic enzymatic cofactor, meaning that your body's enzymes need the Bs to work properly. This cooperative venture is vital for your immune health as well as for your fat metabolism; it helps you burn off those excess pounds. And the Bs themselves shouldn't be isolated, either. If you take just one, it will rob the body of the other Bs to activate its energy. Vitamins B_2, B_5 (pantothenic acid), B_6, and biotin help form your B cells' antibodies, and B_3 and B_{15} stimulate your immune response. In the fat-burning department, all the Bs work—especially B_3, B_5, and B_{15}, which reduce cholesterol and fatty deposits. Choline and inositol form lecithin, the essential fatty acid needed for your immune system as well as to reduce cholesterol, burn fats, and redistribute body fat. Choline, along with B_5, plays a role in producing acetylcholine, which sends those nerve impulses that signal your body to take a break and restore and repair itself.

Zinc is essential for keeping your immune system strong and balanced. It acts as a traffic officer, directing and overseeing the efficient flow of the body processes, and accelerates the healing time for internal and external wounds. It also has a strong effect on cholesterol and fat reduction.

Protein is the foundation of all the cells and is vitally important for your body's tissue repair. For a balanced accelerator it is especially significant in rebuilding your body's already hardworking immune system. You are constantly producing those disease- and allergy-fighting cells. And the amino acids in protein are responsible for developing your white blood cells, the body's warriors; and for the synthesis of hemoglobin, the oxygen carrier in your red blood cells. They're also essential for your immune system's "respiratory burst" and for the production of the immunoglobulins utilized in the immune antibody response.

I've formulated your diet to include amino acid–rich protein in the form of fish and chicken to provide the appropriate building blocks for your thymus gland and immune function. (The daily intake level of protein should be about 1 gram to 1.5 grams of protein per pound of body weight, depending on the individual's age and circumstances. To convert grams to ounces, multiply the gram figure by .0353.)

The following nutrients are especially good to support your heart:

- *Taurine:* This amino acid relaxes your circulatory system and calms your nervous system. The highest concentration of taurine is in the heart, because it feeds, supports, and stabilizes your heart! It also acts as a "quiet fat buster," stimulating gallbladder bile to burn fats, and helps your metatype's immune system, promoting healing.
- *Carnitine:* This amino acid burns off fat and strengthens the heart by getting rid of excess fat around this essential muscle. It's a vital coenzyme in fat metabolism, and it teams up with vitamins C and E to boost athletic ability and endurance.
- *Vitamin E:* This oil-soluble nutrient from essential fatty acids carries oxygen to cells, boosts your immune system, dissolves blood clots, burns fat, slows cellular aging, promotes healing, and makes your skin glow. If you are prone to high blood pressure, you need to start with only a 200–international unit capsule daily and build up gradually as your blood pressure declines.

Also, the following nutrients support your weaker gland—the pancreas:

- *Alanine:* This is another amino acid from glutamine that stabilizes blood sugar and converts excess blood sugar into energy, not fat. For your meta-type it also stimulates the immune system, along with the amino acid arginine. Both alanine and glycine can be found in your local health-food store, usually in combination with isoleucine in formulas to stabilize blood sugar.
- *Glycine:* This amino acid, known as "food for the brain," also works under the parasympathetic nervous system to regulate the flow of blood

sugar, controlling the release of glucagon. It balances insulin and with taurine helps burn fat by metabolizing bile.

• *Methionine:* The mother of some amino acids (taurine and cystene), methionine breaks down fats and cholesterol, protects the liver and heart, works as an antioxidant to neutralize toxins, and has the extra added attraction of stimulating endorphins, which give pleasure, not pain, in a stress response.

• *Choline and inositol:* These B-complex complements are essential for processing the helpful fats and eliminating the "bad" ones by transporting and breaking down fat. They are also vital for regulating the liver and gallbladder's functions in reducing cholesterol. The combo is a fat buster! They can be found naturally in the form of lecithin or with methionine in capsules called "lipo factors."

• *Chromium:* A "magic-bullet" mineral, chromium is a component of the glucose tolerance factor (produced by your pancreas) that enhances the insulin effect in blood sugar metabolism. It also activates certain pancreatic enzymes in your pancreas to burn fat, utilize cholesterol, and lower blood pressure.

• *Zinc:* Although zinc was listed earlier among the basic supplements, it also helps melt fat by stimulating pancreatic enzymes, helping you utilize proteins, and with chromium it regulates insulin and cholesterol. It's an essential component of all the enzyme systems and a required component in the pancreatic enzyme complex.

The Bottom Line

By taking a complete amino acid, vitamin, and mineral combination based on the formulation for your general metabolic type, you'll be supplied with the nutrients needed to support your complementary side, the parasympathetic nervous system. Then you may want to add a few of the vitamins and minerals we've just discussed. I've provided you with a complete list in the accompanying table.

If you're interested, turn to appendixes 3 and 4 for a more in-depth study of the vitamins, minerals, and amino acids for your meta-type. If you prefer to get all your nutrients from foods, I've listed the foods highest in vitamin, mineral, and amino acid content in the accompanying table.

Balanced Accelerator Vitamin,
Mineral, and Amino Acid Food Sources

Thymus Gland	
Essential fatty acids—vitamin F	• *Oils:* safflower, sunflower, corn, olive, wheat germ, soy, cottonseed, and cod-liver • *Nuts:* walnuts, Brazil nuts, and almonds
Vitamin C (buffered)	Acerola cherries, rose hips, citrus fruit, guavas, hot green peppers, black currants, parsley, turnip greens, poke greens, and mustard greens
B complex	• B_1: torula yeast, sunflower seeds, rice bran, wheat germ, pine nuts, dried coriander leaf, safflower seeds, soybeans, alfalfa seeds, sesame seeds, and rye flour (dark) • B_2: almonds, cheese, turnip greens, wheat bran, and soybeans • B_3 *(niacin):* fish, nuts, milk, cheese, bran flakes, sesame seeds, and sunflower seeds • B_6: rice bran, wheat bran, sunflower seeds, avocados, bananas, corn, fish, brown rice, soybeans, and whole grains • B_{15}: grains, cereals, rice, apricot kernels, and torula yeast
Zinc	Spices, wheat bran, crab, and popcorn
Heart	
Vitamin E	Oils (except coconut), alfalfa seeds, nuts, sunflower seed kernels, asparagus, avocados, blackberries, green leafy vegetables, oatmeal, rye, wheat germ, seafood (lobster, shrimp, tuna), and tomatoes
Amino acids: carnitine and taurine	All animal proteins (fish and fowl) and soy products
Pancreas	
Amino acids: alanine, glycine, and methionine	All animal proteins (fish and fowl) and soy products
Chromium	Blackstrap molasses, cheese, apple peels, bananas, corn meal, vegetable oils, and wheat bran
Zinc, lecithin, *or* choline and inositol (called lipotropic factors)	Listed under "Thymus Gland" • *Choline:* soybeans, cabbage, wheat bran, navy beans, alfalfa leaf meal, rice polishings, rice bran, whole grains, hominy, turnips , and blackstrap molasses • *Inositol:* wheat germ, citrus fruits, blackstrap molasses, fruits, whole grains, bran, nuts, legumes, milk, and vegetables

There are a few easy things to remember about taking the supplements:

• Try to take amino acids on an empty stomach. (They need adequate amounts of stomach enzymes to be broken down properly.)

- If possible, take enzymes with your meals to aid in your food digestion.
- Take vitamins and minerals after you've eaten, which helps their assimilation.
- The water-soluble vitamins—B complex, vitamin C, and vitamin P (bioflavonoids)—can be taken at any time.
- Your body isn't used to concentrated food substances, so I recommend that you introduce one type of amino acid, vitamin, or mineral into your regimen every few days. Gently and easily is the name of the game.

Balanced Accelerator Recommended Nutrients

ENDOCRINE GLAND	NUTRIENT	WOMEN			MEN		
		Number	Strength	Times per Day	Number	Strength	Times per Day
Thymus	Essential fatty	1	300 mg	2	2	300 mg	2
	acids *or* lecithin	1	1,200 mg	1–2	1	1,200 mg	2
	Vitamin C						
	(buffered)	1–2	1,000 mg	2	1–2	1,000 mg	3
	B complex	1–2	50–75 mg	2	1–2	100–125 mg	2
	Zinc	1	30 mg	1	2	30 mg	1
Heart	Taurine	1–2	500 mg	2	1–2	500 mg	3
	Carnitine	1–2	250 mg	2	2	250 mg	2
	Vitamin E	1	200–800 IU	1	1	400–800 IU	1
Pancreas	Alanine	1	500 mg	2	1	500 mg	3
	Glycine	1	500 mg	2	1	500 mg	3
	Methionine	1	500 mg	2	1	500 mg	3
	Chromium	1	100–200 mcg	With meals	1	200 mcg	With meals
	Zinc	See under "Thymus"	—	—	See under "Thymus"	—	—
	Choline and						
	inositol	1	500 mg	1–2	1	1,000 mg	2–3
	Pancreatic						
	enzymes	At your discretion	—	—	At your discretion	—	—

Now taking these extra vitamins, minerals, and supplements will require work—there's no mistaking that. Just as you have to plan meals with the right ingredients, you'll need to organize these. But as your metabolic system moves back into balance, you'll reduce the number of pills you'll need. And along the way, you'll discover that the dividend of glowing good health pays off quickly enough to make Wall Street envious.

Stocking Up

You've now finished reading about the program and are well on your way to a brand-new you. Just wait and see—you'll be slim, sexy, and full of bounce to every ounce. To get started, you'll need to stock up and organize. The accompanying list shows all the foods you'll need for the coming week. Double-check this list against your weekly menu and make any adjustments you feel are necessary. Happy regeneration!

Weekly Shopping List for Balanced Accelerators

Larger quantities for men are shown in **boldface**.

PRODUCE

Fruit
2½ doz. (30) Lemons
3 Limes
2 **(3)** bunches Green grapes
3 **(6)** Pineapples
3 **(6)** lg. Papayas
4 **(6)** pt. Strawberries
1 Blood orange
½ pt. Raspberries
½ pt. Blueberries

Vegetables
3 bunches Broccoli
7 **(8)** lb. Carrots
3 med. Red onions
2 bulbs Fennel
1 sm. **(lg.)** bulb Jicama
3 Yellow squashes
3 Zucchini
3 lb. Yellow (Spanish) onions

½ lb. Ginger
1 lb. Turnip/rutabaga
1 bunch Scallions
4 med. Leeks
½ lb. Haricots verts (French green beans)
2 **(3)** Parsnips
½ **(1)** lb. Beets
1 sm. Acorn squash
2 bunches Celery
3 sm. heads Red cabbage
4 sm. Artichokes
5 bunches Kale
6 **(7)** bulbs Garlic
2 Plum tomatoes (if on diet)

Salad Greens
1 head Romaine lettuce
2 heads Red leaf lettuce
3 heads Boston lettuce
1 **(2)** lb. Spinach
1 sm. **(lg.)** Radicchio

1 **(3)** heads Belgian endive
1 bunch Arugula
1 bunch Watercress
4 bunches Mint leaves
4 bunches Parsley
2 **(3)** boxes Alfalfa sprouts
1 box Radish sprouts

Fresh Herbs
1 bunch Cilantro
1 bunch Rosemary

GROCERIES
½ lb. Amaranth grain
½ lb. Bulgur wheat
1 sm. **(lg.)** loaf Sprouted grain
   bread
½ **(1)** lb. Egg pastina
8-oz. jar Dijon mustard
1 bottle Ad-Vita or Knudsen
   cranberry concentrate

Black pepper
Dried thyme, dried oregano, curry
   powder, turmeric, tarragon,
   cinnamon
Herbal teas
Safflower oil

DAIRY
1 8-oz. Ricotta, low-fat
3 **(5)** lb. Tofu, extra firm

MEAT AND FISH
1 6-oz. **(1 13-oz.)** Chicken breast
   (skin off)
1 5-oz. piece **(2 6-oz. pieces)**
   Yellowfin tuna
1 3-oz. **(1 6-oz.)** Squid (calamari),
   cleaned

16 The Mixed Accelerator Diet

While you share many characteristics with both the balanced accelerator and the accelerator, the differences in your metabolism suggest that you need a diet that's all your own. When out of type, you're more likely to put on weight than either of the other accelerator meta-types. If you follow your plan carefully, however, you can toss those scales in the trash. I am going to introduce you to a whole new way of eating, living, and feeling great. Just a few quick words on how your personal mixed accelerator diet works, then on to the menus.

As you read, remember:

- Your dominant gland is the thyroid.
- Your weakest gland is the pituitary.
- You're most likely to gain weight in your stomach first, then in your hips and thighs.

The Science behind Your System

As with the classic accelerator and balanced accelerator, your body chemistry is generally dominated by the activities of the sympathetic nervous system, but unlike your meta-mates, you receive an almost equal amount of stimulation from the parasympathetic nervous system. This means that your metabolism is fueled by more nerve stimulation to those glands and organs responsible for energy production—the thyroid gland, adrenals, thymus, spleen, lungs, and heart. You have a little less nerve stimulation to the organs responsible for digestion and the repair and regeneration of the body: the salivary glands, stomach, pancreas, small intestine, liver, gallbladder, large intestine, kidneys, and bladder.

Your primary metabolic focus is still for *energetic activity*. Your metabolism tends to be moderately fast but not quite as fast as the other accelerators. In the accelerator category your unique characteristic is the different *way* in which you utilize, or "burn off," your energy.

With good nerve stimulation to your energy-producing glands—albeit less than your meta-mates—you're still able to break down your foods at a somewhat fast pace, but more slowly than either the balanced accelerator or the accelerator. This creates a more oxygenated (that is, aerobic) environment for your food's digestion.

With this type of atmosphere, when the oxygen-rich nutrients reach your body's cells to be turned into energy, they'll burn off somewhat quickly, much faster than with the other two slower-oxidizing accelerators. Remember, "air fans fire." Consequently you tend to break down your foods at a semifast pace and also burn up the energy released by the foods at a semifast pace. Fast in, fast out. (Reread chapter 3 if you need a fuller explanation.)

Unlike the other meta-types in your category, you have strong parasympathetic nerve influence, so you produce an average amount of stomach acid—more than your two meta-mates.

As you've learned, the lighter carbohydrates digest rapidly and are the fastest-burning foods. Proteins are slower; fats are the slowest. So if you eat mostly carbohydrates—*especially* refined starches and sugars—they'll break down rapidly and burn off quickly. You'll experience quick, short spurts of energy, followed by drastic declines in stamina. Your higher level of stomach acid also requires you to eat the heavier and slower-burning proteins.

Since your digestive process takes place in a semioxygenated environment and oxygen burns off the toxic wastes from cells, you tend to retain some cellular toxins.

You have more of a semi–acid-producing chemistry, so with your relatively fast digestion and faster burning off of energy, you'll tend to have:

- Medium production of stomach acid (HCl, or hydrochloric acid)—unless it is completely suppressed by the stress response
- A tendency toward a semiacid body—tissue acidity
- Lower production of pancreatic enzymes
- Probable high production of pancreatic insulin

Metabolically, then, you require foods of a more alkalinizing nature—such as green, leafy vegetables; fruits; and grains—which support your meta-type and stimulate your dominant gland, the thyroid. But with your higher level of stomach acid, you also need an adequate amount of foods that require more time to break down and that burn off more slowly to keep your blood sugar stable, such as the proteins in fish, chicken, and some red meat. Here's where you branch away from your fellow accelerators.

Your *weak acid* metabolism can handle a portion of the strong acid animal protein foods. Your fats should come from a moderate amount of unsaturated oils—not saturated fats—in the form of vegetable oils. There-fore, your mixed accelerator food formula looks like this:

- Carbohydrates: 45 percent
- Protein: 40 percent
- Fat: 15 percent

Mixed Accelerator Food Choices

After one month on the Your Body, Your Diet plan, you will not only drop excess fat but also experience a level of vitality and good health that you never dreamed possible. Once you have looked at the basic menus, you will find lists that will show you the wide variety of delicious foods that are best for you. I've also included suggestions for vitamins, minerals, and supplements to help jump-start your metabolic makeover.

With your energetic balance based between the action-oriented and re-generative nervous systems, you may feel deeply but then intellectualize away those emotions and wind up stuffing them down. It's not just sym-bolic, as you also cram those candy bars or cookies down, too.

Remember that foods, your mind, and your emotions have a direct rela-tionship to your body's health and weight gain. Your meta-type's reactions to emotional stresses, excess mental stimulation, the stress response, or fa-tigue can readily manifest as food cravings if your tired thyroid gland can't answer the call to energetic duty. You'll crave foods that rev it up again, once more resulting in its energetically overproducing or underproducing. Eventually your thyroid will "burn out" and work only at minimal efficiency.

The next three subsections give you an overview of the basic principles you'll be following.

What to Avoid

Steer clear of refined carbohydrates, sugar, caffeine, and nicotine. I know this seems like a tough set of restrictions to follow, but you will adjust. Here's why making these changes is so important. Your thyroid gets plenty of stimulation from your adrenal and thymus glands, so you need to eliminate these things to give your body a rest.

Just remember, "trash, flash, crash." These are all quick-fix ingredients that trick your thyroid into a flash of hormones, followed by a crash—trapping you in a vicious cycle.

Caffeine, perhaps the world's favorite stimulant these days, is deceptive. It's not just lattes and soft drinks that cost you. Black coffee and diet sodas still pull that trigger, because as your thyroid and adrenal hormones surge and slump, you'll crave those deadly sweets and breads. Your pancreas pumps out extra insulin to try to stabilize your blood sugar, and your energy plunges. That leaves you facing two more problems: The insulin stores the blood sugar not as energy in the muscles but as fats, those unwanted bulges. Then your overloaded pancreas leaves you carbohydrate-intolerant. Even a bit of bread or pasta turns to fat. Caffeine also makes your body more acid—which not only triggers those sugar cravings but causes your body to hold on to the cellular wastes that leave you puffy and dry.

Nicotine, drugs, and alcohol—stimulants and depressants—reduce your oxygen supply and, with your lesser pituitary output, leave you weary and fuzzy-thinking. Alcohol and nicotine trick the adrenals into producing energy hormones and cancel out your body's natural calming influences, so they wind up making you more anxious. That's why the minute you start to come "down," you feel compelled to reach for another cigarette, drink, or drug to spike your high.

The following table gives you an overview of the foods and other substances that do *not* suit your meta-type.

Your *Never* Foods

REFINED CARBOHYDRATES	SUGAR	WHITE-FLOUR PRODUCTS	CAFFEINE	NICOTINE, DRUGS
All packaged foods	White sugar	White pasta	Coffee	Tobacco in any form
Synthetic additives	Cane sugar	White bread	Tea	
Sweeteners	Brown sugar	Cakes	Soft drinks	Drugs
Cakes	Maple syrup	Doughnuts	Diet drinks	**FATS**
Cookies	Honey	Cookies		Butter
Doughnuts	Processed syrup	Muffins		Margarine
	Alcohol			Mayonnaise

What to Fill Up On

Fish, poultry, some red meat, low-fat dairy, selected legumes, and vegetables are your foods of choice.

Now you must admit, that's a much fuller list than you expected. You will definitely be able to enjoy a wide variety of delicious foods. You'll just have to lay off the refined carbohydrates mentioned in the table. The recommended foods will help you stabilize your energy, strengthen your overworked thyroid gland, and avoid putting on excess weight.

The accompanying table lists the foods that best suit your meta-type.

Your *Always* Foods

PROTEINS		CARBOHYDRATES		FATS
Food	Times per Week	Food	Times per Week	
Meat: variety	2–3 per *month*	Grains: abundant	2–3 per week	*Moderate* amount of
Fowl: abundant	2–3 per week	Legumes: small		unsaturated fatty
Eggs	2 per week	amount	1–2 per week	acids—cold-pressed
Fish: abundant	2–3 per week	Starchy vegetables:		vegetable or nut oils
Shellfish	1 per week	variety	1–2 per week	Choose from your food
Dairy: small amount		Slightly starchy		plan.
(stimulates pituitary		vegetables: small		
function)	3–4 per week	amount	1–2 per week	
Nuts: some	1 per week	Nonstarchy		
Seeds: variety	1–2 per week	vegetables: abundant	Daily	
Legume protein:		Fruit: variety	Daily	
variety	1–2 per week			

The foods that are required by your specific metabolic type—light dairy foods, complex carbohydrates, and proteins—are also ones that feed and support your weaker endocrine gland, the pituitary.

One reason for light dairy is to stimulate your weaker pituitary. Milk's hormone, prolactin, is known to boost a nursing mother's milk production as well as infants' brain development, the functioning of the pituitary gland, and intellectual growth.

How to Speed Up Weight Loss

Here are a few other tips to stimulate faster weight loss:

• Mix 60 percent grains to 40 percent legumes (beans) or tofu (soybean curd) for a complete protein complement. Tofu is an excellent accompaniment to grains.

• Chew your food slowly and well.

• Try to avoid drinking more than one glass of water or liquid during your meals. Drinking large amounts of liquid during meals dilutes the precious enzymes needed for your digestion.

• Have at least six to eight glasses of water during the day, *not* at mealtimes.

Keeping Your Thyroid in Balance

Although the other meta-types will definitely experience problems when their dominant gland is out of balance, your dominant gland, the thyroid, can wreak all types of havoc if it is not in balance. The thyroid plays a critical role in weight maintenance and good health. Since your thyroid is the bridge between your two major nervous systems, it can easily get pulled out of its metabolic profile if it is the least bit weak from overwork.

You have another bridge, too—the bridge between the accelerator and synthesizer meta-types—and your dominant thyroid is a "crossover" gland: a powerful trigger for energy and regeneration. It's like a diamond necklace, draped at the front of your neck, two lobes surrounding the larynx, with four "pearls," the parathyroids. Your thyroid's potent hormones are triggered by the pituitary and adrenal glands—with megaspurts throughout the day.

Those short "pulsatile" bursts don't provide you with sustained energy. If you're eating only refined carbohydrates, they'll stimulate your thyroid to secrete its hormone, thyroxine, and both the thyroxine and the carbohydrates will give you a double dose of *quick flashes of energy*, followed by *dramatic energy crashes*.

Constant overuse weakens your thyroid, robbing you of the all-important cell-repair function overnight and thwarting your hopes of stopping the energy drain.

On the flip side of this coin, deeply buried emotions suddenly needing to erupt can just as easily pull you into your complementary parasympathetic system. Unlike your two meta-type partners, who easily intellectualize and bury their feelings, you have deep feelings that lie very near the surface, and when they abruptly erupt, you're into an emotional stress response, triggering the adrenals and thyroid into overdrive—followed by the crash.

This is important for you to recognize. In the whole spectrum of meta-types, your meta-type can most easily split into *hyperactivity* or *hypoactivity*—each requiring a different diet and healing protocol.

A *hyperactive thyroid* reaction can result either from an overactive adrenal or pituitary response or from low parathyroid function. (The parathyroid glands produce a hormone that equalizes your thyroid's function.)

When your thyroid's overproduction has been stimulated by an out-of-balance pituitary function or low parathyroid function, you will have an abnormally fast metabolism. You'll digest and burn off your foods rapidly, resulting in either too much weight loss or an inability to hold on to any weight. You'll begin to eat excessively, and in some cases nodules can erupt on your thyroid gland due to its higher hormone production. Untreated, this condition can produce very severe health problems.

If your hyperactive thyroid is due to an out-of-balance pituitary or low parathyroid performance, then a more calming general diet is needed, with the emphasis on building up weight, not losing it.

If, however, your hyperactive thyroid is due to overactive adrenal production resulting in excess weight gain, then the more calming accelerator diet can generally be followed. (But you'll eliminate all fish, because that extra iodine content in fish stimulates thyroid function.)

Since this is a book about weight loss, we'll concentrate on the type of thyroid problem that leads to overweight problems—the *hypoactive thyroid* profile.

Hypoactive problems are generally the result of either a tired thyroid gland's being constantly overused or a lowered pituitary function. Since your weaker gland tends to be the pituitary, more often than not hypoactive conditions are seen in mixed accelerators when they've flipped out of balance and into the mixed synthesizer type.

Extreme symptoms of a hypoactive thyroid include dry, lusterless hair; dry skin; low blood pressure drops; and a slow pulse.

To help you determine the condition of your thyroid, use the simple self-test in the accompanying box, which was developed by Broda Barnes, M.D.

Your basal temperature reflects the heat your body produces when it is at complete rest. This heat is generated by the way your energy or blood glucose is burned off, or utilized, in every cell of your body. The rate of these reactions generally determines the amount of heat or energy you

How to Assess Your Thyroid Function

Obtain a "basal thermometer," available at most pharmacies. Before you go to sleep, shake the thermometer down and place it near your bed. Next morning, *immediately* upon waking, place the mercury end of the thermometer in the middle of your bare armpit, pressing your arm gently against your body. Leave it there for ten minutes. Take it out, read it, and record your results below. The most important thing is to be *very still*. Women are advised to record their temperature during the first two weeks of their menstrual cycle for an accurate reading. It's advisable to take your reading every morning for one week. If you generally have a reading below the *normal range* of 97.8 to 98.2, you may indeed have a low thyroid function. If your reading is above the normal range, you may have an overactive thyroid gland, or you could be harboring some infection.

Date _____ Temperature _____

Date _____ Temperature _____

Date _____ Temperature _____

Date _____ Temperature _____

Date _____ Temperature _____

Date _____ Temperature _____

Date _____ Temperature _____

generate. The hormones your thyroid gland secretes control this rate at which energy is burned, so your thyroid influences your basal temperature and literally acts as a "thermostat." When the thermostat is set at "high," fuel is burned at a rapid rate, resulting in a high temperature (hyperthyroid). When the thermostat is on "low," fuel consumption is slow and a cooler temperature results, indicating that you may have an underactive (hypoactive) thyroid gland. You can determine how your thyroid is functioning by taking your own basal temperature.

Before we move on, let's look again at supporting your weaker endocrine gland, your pituitary. In partnership with the hypothalamus, it governs all your body's hormones, from the morning wake-up call to the intense danger signals of "fight or flight"; it also determines whether you're a "lark" or a "night owl" and controls your cell-repair systems. One of its growth hormones is even responsible for the redistribution of fat in your body.

When your body goes into overdrive from a continued stress response or when you persist in eating foods that are wrong for your metabolism, your pituitary suffers. It will automatically *try* to keep up with the constant demands but won't be able to sustain it. Your energy-producing glands rage, but when the pituitary signals fade, those once-strong thyroid, adrenal, and sex glands shut down.

Your Mixed Accelerator Secret Weapons

Now I know—from firsthand experience—just how tough it can be to switch to a whole new way of eating. In addition to having to apply lots of willpower, you have to give your body time to adjust to your new lifestyle. If you find yourself feeling cranky and frustrated, relax; it's par for the course. It's just a sign that you're shedding those extra pounds and getting back into balance.

The teas and elixirs in this chapter were created to help you sail through the transition phase of your meta-type diet while making the pounds melt away even faster.

Savory Sea Greens

For each meta-type there is one food or group of foods that helps to speed up the weight-loss process. For you those foods are ocean plants. Reaping the benefits of sea vegetables, by the way, is a beauty secret that's been with us for ages. The ancient Eastern sages knew that one of the ways to possess a youthful, slim body and achieve longevity was the abundant use of ocean plants. But the most important news about sea vegetables for you is the fact that they are a treasure-house of minerals, the most abundant of which is *iodine*—the mineral needed most by your weakened thyroid gland.

Would you believe that two-thirds of the body's iodine reserve is used by your thyroid gland to make its hormone, thyroxine? That's right. Without iodine your thyroid isn't able to control the way your body uses energy and how you metabolize food. The second magical ingredient in ocean plants is mannitol, a natural sugar (no, it won't make you fat or increase your blood sugar). It helps your body make thyroxine and is then used by your thyroid to help send hormones into your bloodstream to keep your fat-burning mechanisms working smoothly.

Four basic kinds of sea greens are generally available to us (although others can be found at your health-food store). The first is *seaweed*—originating from Japan—in the form of thin sheets called *nori*. You can crumble it and sprinkle it on foods or salads. It's also delicious toasted. Then there is *kelp*, which grows along the Pacific and Atlantic coasts. It usually comes in powdered form and is my favorite. It's a prime source of iodine that's especially potent in regulating thyroxine production. You can sprinkle it over salads, grains, vegetables, or protein dishes. It has a wonderfully rich taste. A third type, *Irish moss* (also known as carrageen), is full of vitamins and minerals. The fourth, *blue-green algae,* is a powerhouse of vitamins A and D as well as the mineral zinc, which is highly concentrated in the thyroid. Blue-green algae with its zinc component may well ignite thyroxine production. Use it also as a seasoning agent or even as a flavoring. I use these savory sea greens in a powerful drink I developed just for your meta-type.

Miraculous Thin and Trim Cocktail

The following weight-loss secret comes in the form of a delicious beverage full of all the nutrients needed to properly feed your thyroid gland so it can naturally keep pumping out its hormones.

You know that your thyroid gland needs iodine and zinc. It also needs the amino acid tyrosine, which acts as the building block of your thyroid's fat-burning hormone, thyroxine. Your thyroid needs other important nutrients, too, such as manganese, iron, and several B-complex vitamins—B_1 (thiamine), B_2 (riboflavin), and B_3 (niacin). All of these nutrients are present in a tasty drink I've designed just for you—the Miraculous Thin and Trim Cocktail.

The basis for this cocktail is *pineapple juice*. It just happens to be full of the enzyme bromelain, which stimulates thyroid and pituitary function and literally helps dissolve those unwanted pounds of fat and flab.

My first choice, of course, is fresh pineapple juice. If that's not available, then use unsweetened pure pineapple juice from a bottle—not a can. (You can substitute fresh grapefruit juice for the pineapple juice if you're in a pinch, but the results won't be as wonderful as with the pineapple juice.)

This cocktail also contains *wheat germ* (rich in manganese), *black-strap molasses* (which has abundant iron and B-complex vitamins), and *kelp* or *blue-green algae* (loaded with iodine and zinc).

A final, optional ingredient is *cod-liver oil*, a great source of iodine and unsaturated fatty acids.

Mixing all these ingredients together and drinking this marvelous energizer before breakfast will allow you to say good-bye to nervousness, weight gain, depression, irritability, low energy, a cold body, and bad memory and welcome a great body, vibrant energy, gorgeous skin and hair, a youthful appearance, and a razor-sharp mind. (For the recipe, see Miraculous Thin and Trim Cocktail, on page 394.)

Slimming Tea

Another important component of your plan is the herbal tea formula I've created to meet the needs of each meta-type. Each tea will harmonize and balance your specific metabolism, facilitating your weight loss. To make yours, you'll need to add a few special ingredients to the basic Master Weight-Loss Tea (see the formula and directions on pages 103–05).

These supplementary herbs should be added in equal proportions to the herbs already in the basic formula. I suggest you drink one to three cups per day of your special tea. The herbs may be purchased at your local health-food store or ordered from the companies listed in appendix 2.

Mixed Accelerator Slimming Tea

Basic Formula: One Teaspoon Each			
Alisma, poria, rhubarb root, red clover tops, alfalfa leaf, hawthorn berry, radish seed, sargassum, Indian chickweed, evergreen artemesia, astragalus root, fleeceflower root, citrus peel			
Mixed Accelerator Slimming Formula: Add One Teaspoon Each			
NAME			FUNCTION
Common	Latin	Eastern	
Licorice root	*Radix glycyrrhizae*	Gan cao	Great for supporting and stimulating the adrenals and providing energy
Burdock root	*Arctium lappa*	Nui bang zi	Soothes the hypothalamus and stimulates the pituitary gland to release its hormones; also helps to metabolize carbohydrates.
Safflower	*Carthamus tinctorius*	Hong hua	Opens the pancreas and liver, energizes, balances insulin levels, helps digestion, and burns cholesterol and fats.
Angelica root—for women	*Radix angelicae sinensis*	Dang gui	Supports the ovaries and endocrine system.
Codonopsis root (Asiabell root)—for men	*Codonopsis pilosula*	Dang shen	Supports the testes and endocrine system.

Note: If you are pregnant, have high blood pressure, or are allergic to grasses or flowers, it's suggested that these teas not be used. Licorice should not be used if you have high blood pressure.

Rules of the Road

Your Eating Schedule

In the morning you require abundant stimulation to create the essential energy for your body's activity. But you must rely on your weaker pituitary gland to activate your adrenals, which, in turn, stimulate your dominant thyroid gland's hormonal production. Since the pituitary is your weaker gland, it must rely on glucose, oxygen, amino acids, unsaturated fatty acids, and calcium—not itself—to have enough energy and strength to manufacture its own hormones. Therefore, you must supply the nutrients needed to stimulate your pituitary's function. Then your thyroid will produce its hormones in stable—not erratic—bursts throughout the day, giving you a steady energy supply.

A light to medium breakfast composed of fresh fruits (for glucose) or proteins (for amino acids and calcium) works best, along with your morning Thin and Trim Cocktail. They're the answer to meeting your pituitary's requirements and keeping yourself filled with abundant energy.

With your adrenals' cortisol level diminishing in the early to late afternoon, a medium lunch is necessary to activate your thyroid hormones again. Remember, foods also stimulate thyroid production. This helps you avoid that late-afternoon crash, keeps your thyroid hormones pumping out in stable bursts, and carries you over the energetic gap until your parasympathetic nervous system takes over at night.

As evening approaches, you'll receive hormonal impulses from your parasympathetic nervous system through your pituitary, now properly fed from the day's food intake. Your energy returns, so you'll need only a medium dinner to supply enough nutrients for the stimulus required for your cellular repair and the actual regeneration of your body that takes place overnight. Consequently, your eating schedule should be:

- Light to medium breakfast
- Medium lunch
- Medium dinner

Late Afternoon—Keeping Your Energy High

You've learned that your adrenal cortisol level begins to nose-dive in the afternoon, and you'll feel that more strongly than either the balanced accelerator or the accelerator. Most mixed accelerators grab for that sugar fix—cake, cookies, candy, alcohol, or coffee. You might also reach for the baked goods—bagels or crackers. Don't even think of it. These foods will send your insulin levels skyrocketing, you'll have a sudden drop in blood sugar, you'll start craving more of the starch or sugar, and the vicious circle starts all over again. You'll be causing your already acid body to become even more acid—especially if you reach for that after-work drink.

It's fine for you to have a late-afternoon snack to support your waning blood sugar levels, but it has to be the right kind of snack, from the following list:

YOUR LATE-AFTERNOON SNACK
Raw vegetables or fruit, 1 cup
Hot herbal tea or green tea

Bedtime—Laying Off Late-Evening Snacks

As you've learned, you tend to digest your foods fairly quickly but *utilize* them in your cells more quickly than the balanced accelerator and accelerator. That means that if you eat dinner very late or eat before you go to sleep, you'll wake in a few short hours, triggered by the energy released from your late-night eating. You'll end up tossing and turning and may even have a lot of gas or get heartburn. So no late dinners or late-night snacks in front of the television.

Mixed Accelerator Meals and Menus

Now you've completed the first part of the plan, and here's your reward: the tailor-made, one-month diet for your mixed accelerator metatype. If you've reached this point in the book, you know that losing weight and keeping it off takes more than just watching what you eat.

The meals presented in this section are designed to meet all the needs of your metabolism while giving you the chance to eat a delicious, wide variety of fresh, nutritious foods. The first week may seem like a big adjustment, but by week two, I assure you, you'll be making your juices and tossing together your special meals like a pro.

Eating the Right Foods at the Right Times

Eating the *right kinds of food* at the *right times* is another key to the success of your weight-loss and rejuvenation program. With the semiacid nature of your mixed accelerator metabolism, if you eat a majority of acid foods, it will throw you out of balance and increase your tissue acidity. Then you'll try to balance yourself by reaching for the wrong foods, which

The following meal—consisting of meat, vegetables, and salad—can be enjoyed two times per *month*:

Skinny-Minnie Regeneration Dinner

Meat: 4 **(6)** oz., from the meats on your Mixed Accelerator Food Choices list (bake, broil, or grill—lean, no fat) with
Vegetables: 2 cups, from the nonstarchy vegetables on your list and
Salad: as much as desired, from the nonstarchy vegetables on your list (for example, spinach, fennel, radicchio, and assorted sprouts, mixed with 1 tsp. Mixed Accelerator Salad Dressing)
1 cup herbal tea, from the teas on your list, or Mixed Accelerator Slimming Tea

will cause you to retain that extra fat and feel terrible physically and emotionally. You require the more alkalizing foods to balance your body chemistry, just as your counterpart, the mixed synthesizer, is more semialkaline in nature and requires more of the acid forming foods.

Your metabolism tends to be the least acid of all the accelerator meta-types, which bridges to the more alkaline parasympathetic system. You require alkaline foods, such as vegetables and fruits, to stabilize your metabolism as well as acid forming foods, such as grains and animal protein. You need protein to keep the equilibrium of your pituitary and hypothalamus. You are known as the *weak acid* meta-type, with your natural body pH tending to be 6.2. (Chapter 3 provides a detailed explanation of the acid-alkaline aspect of your meta-type.) This means that your diet should consist of the foods that are strong alkaline, alkaline, and strong acid forming ash. Foods that are acid forming and weak alkaline can be eaten three to four times per week. Foods that are the same as your own pH tendency—weak acid forming—should be avoided. Appendix 5 lists the full spectrum of foods and their pH factors.

Your mixed meta-type gives you more flexibility than your counterparts, so you'll find yourself adapting with ease.

Here We Go!

To make this adventure of slimming down to a new and healthy you fun, I've taken all the guesswork out of how to shop and prepare your meals. Before you begin, glance through your weekly menus and mixed

Mixed Accelerator Semiomnivore Weekly Menus

Alkaline to Acid-Based Foods

Larger quantities for men are shown in **boldface.**

WHEN	SATURDAY	SUNDAY	MONDAY	TUESDAY
On rising	Miraculous Thin and Trim Cocktail			
Breakfast	Mushroom and Egg Fritatta with Scallions and Basil 1 cup herbal tea or Mixed Accelerator Slimming Tea	Spinach and Egg Surprise 1 cup herbal tea or Mixed Accelerator Slimming Tea	Sunrise Special Orange, tangerine, kiwi, strawberries, and raspberries with lemon and mint 1 cup herbal tea or Mixed Accelerator Slimming Tea	Power Punch Morning Drink Low-fat milk and protein powder with almond or vanilla 1 cup herbal tea or Mixed Accelerator Slimming Tea
Midmorning	1 orange 1 cup herbal tea or Mixed Accelerator Slimming Tea	1 peach 1 cup herbal tea or Mixed Accelerator Slimming Tea	4 oz. plain yogurt, low-fat 1 cup herbal tea or Mixed Accelerator Slimming Tea	1 orange 1 cup herbal tea or Mixed Accelerator Slimming Tea
Lunch	Health Salad with Raw Vegetables, Tabouli, and Curried Tofu 1 **(2–3)** cup Mixed Accelerator Salad Greens ½ cup carrots ¼ cup sliced mushrooms ¼ cup scallions 2 tsp. Mixed Accelerator Salad Dressing Serve with: ½ **(¾)** cup cooked tabouli ½ **(¾)** cup	Health Salad with Raw Vegetables and Cold Seared Tuna 1 **(2–3)** cup Mixed Accelerator Salad Greens 1 cup carrots ½ cup sliced mushrooms ½ cup scallions 2 tsp. Mixed Accelerator Salad Dressing Serve with: 4 **(6)** oz. cold sliced tuna (from previous	Health Salad with Raw Vegetables and Cold Mustard Thyme Chicken 1 **(2–3)** cup Mixed Accelerator Salad Greens ½ **(1)** cup carrots ¼ **(½)** cup sliced mushrooms ¼ **(½)** cup scallions 2 tsp. Mixed Accelerator Salad Dressing Serve with: 4 oz. cold sliced chicken (from previous	Health Salad with Raw Vegetables and Tofu Scramble 1 **(2–3)** cup Mixed Accelerator Salad Greens 1 cup carrots ½ cup sliced mushrooms ½ cup scallions 2 tsp. Mixed Accelerator Salad Dressing Serve with: ¾ **(1)** cup Tofu Scramble ½ slice toasted

WHEN	SATURDAY	SUNDAY	MONDAY	TUESDAY
Lunch (cont'd)	Curried Tofu 1 cup herbal tea or Mixed Accelerator Slimming Tea	evening) 1 cup herbal tea or Mixed Accelerator Slimming Tea	evening) 1 cup herbal tea or Mixed Accelerator Slimming Tea	sprouted grain bread cut into croutons 1 cup herbal tea or Mixed Accelerator Slimming Tea
Midafternoon	½ cup each: carrot and fennel sticks 1 cup herbal tea or Mixed Accelerator Slimming Tea	½ cup each: carrot sticks and raw mushrooms 1 cup herbal tea or Mixed Accelerator Slimming Tea	½ cup each: carrot and celery sticks 1 cup herbal tea or Mixed Accelerator Slimming Tea	½ cup each: carrot and fennel sticks 1 cup herbal tea or Mixed Accelerator Slimming Tea
Dinner	*Thin Fin Dinner* Seared Yellowfin Tuna Carrot Rutabaga Puree Steamed Asparagus Salad *½ hour after dinner:* ⅓ cup each: pineapple, papaya, and green grapes 1 cup herbal tea or Mixed Accelerator Slimming Tea	*Chicken Surprise* Hearty Vegetable Soup Mustard, Thyme, and Roasted Garlic Chicken Healthy Salad with Watercress *½ hour after dinner:* ⅓ cup each: pineapple, papaya, and raspberries 1 cup herbal tea or Mixed Accelerator Slimming Tea	*Couscous Supreme* Couscous and Roasted Peanuts with Curried Vegetables Carrots, Rutabagas, Zucchini, Yellow Squash and Tomatoes Savory Salad with Seaweed 1 glass Mixed Accelerator Elixir *½ hour after dinner:* ½ cup fresh pineapple 1 cup herbal tea or Mixed Accelerator Slimming Tea	*Carrot and Rutabaga* *Pasta Delight* Egg Pastina with Roasted Garlic and Fresh Basil Mixed Roasted Vegetables and Tofu Carrots, Rutabagas and Mushrooms with Rosemary Radicchio and Fennel Salad *½ hour after dinner:* 1 cup herbal tea or Mixed Accelerator Slimming Tea

WHEN	WEDNESDAY	THURSDAY	FRIDAY
On rising	*Miraculous Thin and Trim Cocktail*		
Breakfast	*Tropical Delight* Orange, tangerine, kiwi, papaya, and green grapes, with lemon and mint 1 cup herbal tea or Mixed Accelerator Slimming Tea	*Power Punch Morning Drink* Low-fat milk and protein powder with almond or vanilla 1 cup herbal tea or Mixed Accelerator Slimming Tea	*Fruit Frolic* Orange, tangerine, kiwi, blueberries, and nectarine, with lemon and mint 1 cup herbal tea or Mixed Accelerator Slimming Tea
Midmorning	4 oz. plain yogurt, low-fat 1 cup herbal tea or Mixed Accelerator Slimming Tea	1 peach 1 cup herbal tea or Mixed Accelerator Slimming Tea	1 cup strawberries 1 cup herbal tea or Mixed Accelerator Slimming Tea
Lunch	*Health Salad with Raw Vegetables and Cold Seared Tuna* 1 **(2–3)** cup Mixed Accelerator Salad Greens 1 cup carrots ½ cup sliced mushrooms ½ cup scallions 2 tsp. Mixed Accelerator Salad Dressing *Serve with:* 4 **(6)** oz. cold seared tuna (from Saturday's dinner)	*Health Salad with Raw Vegetables and Tofu Scramble* 1 **(2–3)** cup Mixed Accelerator Salad Greens 1 cup carrots ½ cup sliced mushrooms ½ cup scallions 2 tsp. Mixed Accelerator Salad Dressing *Serve with:* ¾ **(1)** cup Tofu Scramble ½ slice toasted sprouted grain	*Health Salad with Raw Vegetables, Cottage Cheese and Scallions* 1 **(2–3)** cup Mixed Accelerator Salad Greens ½ cup carrots ½ cup sliced mushrooms ½ cup scallions 2 tsp. Mixed Accelerator Salad Dressing *Serve with:* 1 **(1½)** cup low-fat cottage cheese ½ cup grated carrots

WHEN	WEDNESDAY	THURSDAY	FRIDAY
Lunch **(cont'd)**	1 cup herbal tea or Mixed Accelerator Slimming Tea	bread cut into croutons 1 cup herbal tea or Mixed Accelerator Slimming Tea	¼ cup chopped scallions 1 cup herbal tea or Mixed Accelerator Slimming Tea
Midafternoon	½ cup each: carrot and celery sticks 1 cup herbal tea or Mixed Accelerator Slimming Tea	½ cup each: carrot and fennel sticks 1 cup herbal tea or Mixed Accelerator Slimming Tea	½ cup each: carrot sticks and raw mushrooms 1 cup herbal tea or Mixed Accelerator Slimming Tea
Dinner	*Simply Veggies* Roast Acorn Squash Lemon Pepper Kale Tarragon Carrots Spinach Salad 1 glass Mixed Accelerator Elixir *½ hour after dinner:* ⅓ cup each: peaches, oranges, and raspberries 1 cup herbal tea or Mixed Accelerator Slimming Tea	*Seafood Supreme* Scallops Seviche with Lime and Cilantro Mixed Steamed Vegetables Carrots, Rutabagas, Yellow Beans, and Red Pepper, with cumin Watercress Salad *½ hour after dinner:* ⅓ cup each: pineapple, papaya, and green grapes 1 cup herbal tea or Mixed Accelerator Slimming Tea	*Tabouli, Tofu, and Veggie Health Salad* Mixed Salad Greens with Grated Carrots, with Tabouli Steamed Kale with Garlic and Tofu 1 glass Mixed Accelerator Elixir *½ hour after dinner:* 1 cup fresh strawberries 1 cup herbal tea or Mixed Accelerator Slimming Tea

Mixed Accelerator Food Choices

Proteins								
MEAT	**FOWL**	**FISH**		**DAIRY**	**NUTS**	**SEEDS**	**LEGUMES**	**FRUIT PROTEIN**
Strong Acid	Strong Acid	Strong Acid	Shellfish Strong Acid	*Note:* If you have allergies, eliminate dairy of any kind.	Strong Acid	Strong Acid	Strong Acid	Strong Alkaline
Venison	Turkey	Mackerel	Abalone	**Weak Alkaline (Use Low-Fat)**	Pine nuts	Pumpkin seeds	Peanuts	Olives
Veal	Goose	Roe			Water chestnuts	Sunflower seeds	**Weak Alkaline**	**Strong Acid**
Beef, lean	Squab	Halibut	**Acid Forming**	Whey	Cashews	Squash seeds		Avocados
Lamb, lean	Chicken	Red snapper		Goat's milk		Safflower seeds	Soybean curd (tofu)	
Rabbit	Duck	Sole	Crab	Yogurt	Coconut	Sesame seeds		**AVOID**
Organ meats	Frog legs	Tuna	Lobster	Cow's milk	**Weak Alkaline**		**Acid Forming**	None
	Quail	Bluefish	Scallops	Cream		Flaxseeds		
AVOID	Pheasant	Eel	Clams and mussels	Buttermilk	Coconut milk	Chia seeds	Lentils	
Pork (ham, bacon, roast)	**Acid Forming**	Swordfish	Shrimp and crayfish	**Cheeses (Use Low-Fat)**	**Acid Forming**	**AVOID**	Soybeans	
		Squid (calamari)				None	Soy milk	
	Eggs	Cod	**AVOID**	Cottage	Pecans		Adzuki beans	
		Mullet	**Weak Acid**	Parmesan	Pistachios		Black beans	
	AVOID	Haddock		Limburger	Walnuts		Kidney beans	
	None	Ocean perch	Anchovies	Cheddar	Brazil nuts		Navy beans	
		Sturgeon	Caviar	Brick	Macadamias		Pinto beans	
		Octopus (scungilli)	Herring	Swiss	Chestnuts		Red beans	
			Sardines		Almonds			
		Acid Forming	Oysters	**Acid Forming**			**AVOID**	
					AVOID		None	
		Carp		Soy milk (also under "Legumes")	**Weak Acid**			
		Yellowtail tuna			Filberts (hazelnuts)			
		Salmon		**AVOID**				
		Hake		**Weak Acid Cheeses**	Hickory nuts			
		Lake perch						
		Bass		Camembert				
		Trout		Brie				
				Edam				
				Gruyère				
				Farmer				
				Feta				
				Ricotta				
				Muenster				
				Monterey Jack				
				Provolone				
				Mozzarella				
				Goat				
				Blue				
				Gorgonzola				

				Carbohydrates		
GRAINS	**HIGH-STARCH LEGUMES**	**HIGH-STARCH VEGETABLES**	**SLIGHTLY STARCHY VEGETABLES**	**NONSTARCHY VEGETABLES**		
Strong Alkaline	Strong Acid	Strong Acid	Weak Alkaline	Strong Alkaline	Weak Alkaline	Eliminate If You Have Allergies of Any Kind
Amaranth grain and flakes	Black-eyed peas (cowpeas)	Field corn Sweet corn Potatoes	Carrots Rutabagas	Kale, cooked Collards Swiss chard, cooked	Summer squash, cooked	Eggplant Tomatoes
Strong Acid	**Acid Forming**	**Weak Alkaline**	**Acid Forming**	Parsley Mustard greens, cooked	Leeks Garden cress Snap beans	Peppers
Popcorn Corn grits	Lima beans Garbanzo beans (chickpeas)	Acorn squash	Beets, raw	Beet greens, cooked	Yellow beans Turnips	**AVOID** **Cabbage Family**
Rice bran Millet Barley	Great northern beans Split peas	**Acid Forming** Yams	**AVOID** **Weak Acid**	Turnip greens, cooked Lamb's-quarter	Scallions Lettuce: butter, Boston,	Broccoli Chinese cabbage Cabbage
Corn meal Wheat Couscous	White (fava) beans	Pumpkin, raw **Eliminate If You Have**	Beets, cooked Parsnips Jicama	Mustard spinach **Seaweeds**	iceberg Celery Endive	Brussels sprouts Cauliflower
Bulgur (cracked wheat) Rye	**AVOID** None	**Any Allergies** Corn		Agar-agar Irish moss Kelp	Radicchio Yellow dock, raw	**Weak Acid** Eggplant
Oats Pastinas (egg) Sprouted grain bread		Corn meal Corn grits Potatoes		Dulse Arame	Okra, raw Spinach, raw Fennel	Artichokes Shallots Gingerroot Salsify
Acid Forming		**AVOID** **Weak Acid**		**Alkaline Forming**	**Acid Forming**	Soybean sprouts Kohlrabi
Farina Brown rice Basmati brown rice		Butternut squash Hubbard squash Sweet potatoes		Yellow dock, cooked Chicory greens Horseradish	Bamboo shoots Green peas Sugar peas	Chicory Onions Cucumbers Radishes
Wild rice Buckwheat (kasha) Quinoa		Pumpkin, canned		Okra, cooked Swiss chard, raw Spinach, cooked	Mungbeans and sprouts Chili peppers	Summer squash, raw
Eliminate If You Have Any Allergies				Kale, raw Lettuce: cos, romaine, dark green, white	Asparagus Celeriac root Sweet peppers Tomatoes	
Wheat Wheat germ Rye Barley				Watercress Alfalfa sprouts Dandelion greens	**Strong Acid** Mushrooms Garlic	
AVOID None				Arugula Beet greens, raw		

FRUIT		OILS	CONDIMENTS	TEAS (CATEGORY 17)
Strong Alkaline	**Acid Forming (Eat Alone)**	**Strong Acid**	**Strong Alkaline**	Licorice root: strengthens the adrenals (Don't use if you have high blood pressure.)
Rhubarb	Watermelon	Avocado	Molasses: blackstrap or light	Red raspberry: hormone tonic
Alkaline Forming	Muskmelon	Corn	Sorghum	Black cohosh: balances your hormones
Loganberries	Cantaloupe	Soybean		
Oranges	Casaba	Peanut	**Weak Alkaline**	Alfalfa leaf: cleanses the blood, clears the skin, and "alkalizes" your body
Clementines	Crenshaw	Cottonseed	Pickles	
Tangerines	Honeydew	Olive		Blue flag: raises your metabolism and clears the liver and skin
Kumquats		Safflower	**AVOID Weak Acid**	
Kiwifruits	**Sweet Fruit Alkaline Forming**	Sunflower	Vinegar	Ginger: aids your digestion
	Pineapple	Flaxseed	Honey	
Weak Alkaline		Walnut	Mustard	Cinnamon: invigorates
Boysenberries	**Weak Alkaline**	Apricot	Yeast—in all forms	Lemon grass: reduces fluid retention
Grapefruit	Figs	Almond	Soy sauce	
Raspberries			Cane syrup	White oak bark: high in calcium
Strawberries	**Acid Forming**	**AVOID (Saturated Fats)**	Cane sugar	
Plums	Persimmons	Mayonnaise	Brown sugar	Vitex agnus: aids hormone balance
Acerola cherries	Plantains	Butter	Maple syrup	
Blueberries	Bananas	Margarine		
Nectarines				
Gooseberries	**AVOID Weak Acid**			
Pokeberries	Guavas			
Papaya	Loquats			
Grapes: Concord, Thompson	Cherimoya			
Elderberries	Grapes: muscat, Tokay			
Sapotes	Quince			
Cranberries	Tamarinds			
Currants	Apples			
Lemons	Apricots			
Cherries	Prickly pears			
Blackberries	Pears			
Limes	Mangoes			
Acid Forming	**Weak Acid**			
Litchis	Apricots, dried			
Passion fruit	Raisins			
Groundberries	Prunes			
Pomegranates	Dates			
Crab apples				
Peaches				

Mixed Accelerator Elixirs for Both Women and Men

Potassium Powerhouse: Carrot juice—the "great healer," full of vitamins and minerals—leads this potassium-rich formula full of vitamins A, D, B, C, E, and K; celery balances your nerves and clears your skin; parsley balances your thyroid and adrenals; and spinach, full of iron, burns fat. This formula supplies the full spectrum of minerals needed by your thyroid gland.

Carrots: 6 oz. juice (about 6 carrots)
Celery: 3 oz. juice (about 1 bunch)
Parsley: 2 oz. juice (about 2 bunches)
Spinach: 3 oz. juice (about 1 bunch)
Water: 2 oz.

Energizer: Vitamin-filled carrots and iron-rich spinach energize, clean out, and regenerate your whole digestive system—which means cleaning out toxins and fat. Spinach supplies the iron needed by your thyroid gland.

Carrots: 6 oz. juice (about 6 carrots)
Spinach: 3 oz. juice (about 1 bunch)
Water: 2 oz.

Pituitary Power: Calcium-rich carrot juice is exactly what your pituitary needs, coupled with magnesium-rich celery juice, also high in iron, furnishing a balance of these minerals in perfect ratio. Parsley acts as a stabilizer of both the adrenals and the thyroid, equalizing pituitary function.

Carrots: 6 oz. juice (about 6 carrots)
Celery: 3 oz. juice (about 1 bunch)
Parsley: 2 oz. juice (about 2 bunches)
Water: 2 oz.

Adrenal Stabilizer: With carrot juice, parsley is the great adrenal stabilizer and also balances the thyroid gland, cleanses the kidneys, brightens the eyes, and brings oxygen into the body.

Carrots: 6 oz. juice (about 6 carrots)
Parsley: 3 oz. juice (about 3 bunches)
Water: 2 oz.

accelerator elixirs and look over the vast array of selections in your Mixed Accelerator Food Choices list. At the end of this chapter, you will find your own mixed accelerator shopping list for a week. Then turn to appendix 1 and take a look at the equipment list (which includes all the supplies you'll need to make this as simple as possible), your advance food-preparation suggestions for the week, and your recipes and food-preparation instructions for both men and women.

For any of the foods specified in the weekly menus and recipes, you may substitute comparable foods from the Mixed Accelerator Food Choices list.

Eat only the foods that are indicated for you on your individual food choices list. If your favorite isn't there, don't eat it. You can check the "General Food Choices and Their Calorie Content for Each Meta-Type" in appendix 5.

You see, it's all done for you, down to the last detail—and my personal promise to you is that this eating plan will keep your mixed accelerator metabolism in perfect balance while helping you achieve a slender, gorgeous physique.

You're on your way to a bright, new, skinny, energetic you. Treat this as a ritual in celebrating your beauty and regeneration.

Your On-Program Cheat Sheet

Naturally there will be days when you just have to cheat. No problem. There's no need to become obsessed with perfection. You can still succeed at weight loss on the Your Body, Your Diet plan. Besides, if you try to be flawless, you'll only end up out of balance, in either too much of a yang state or too much of a yin state.

For your mixed accelerator profile, your cheat food of choice is popcorn (air popped with no butter), followed by chocolate, figs, and fruit ices. Did I say chocolate? Yes. It's packed with the amino acid arginine and the mineral magnesium—which are great to stimulate your weaker pituitary function.

Here's a complete list of goodies you can use to beat the munchies:

- *Popcorn:* 1 oz. uncooked, with no butter or salt
- *Chocolate:* 2 oz. only
- *Figs, dried:* ¼ cup pitted, or 2 oz.
- *Fruit ice:* any flavor, 1 cup

The list looks pretty good, right? But you have to make a deal with me: you need to follow some guidelines so that you can have these great goodies and really enjoy them. Eating these cheat foods at random would sabotage your goal for creating that beautiful body.

CHEAT-FOOD GUIDELINES
- *Eat your cheat foods only at the recommended times.* Cheat foods should be eaten once per week, on the weekends (when you're not under stress), and at one meal or one time—only.
- *Eat only the amount suggested.* Your body can handle a small amount of these foods without triggering excessive insulin production. If you eat a large amount, your insulin level will spike and turn your "treat" into a "bad trick" of blubber.
- *Eat only one cheat food at a time.* Don't have several together or you'll wreak havoc with your metabolism and digestion. For instance, chocolate *and* popcorn will send you over the top.
- *Never eat your cheat foods when you're under stress.* I guarantee you that's a surefire way to add pounds, not lose them. Only eat cheat foods

when you're relaxed—usually on a weekend. Otherwise, your digestion shuts down and your insulin rises, and you become a veritable fat factory.

• *Never eat your cheat foods late at night.* And no bedtime eating in front of the television. You'll end up having a restless night's sleep, and it's mandatory for you to sleep deeply so your body can regenerate itself.

Mixed Accelerator Helpers and Healers: Vitamins, Minerals, and Amino Acids

This section of your program is dedicated to the additions to the food plan that can help facilitate your weight loss and improve your overall well-being: vitamins, minerals, and supplements.

For your mixed accelerator meta-type, I recommend a gentle, full-spectrum multiple amino acid, vitamin, and mineral complex containing *only* those essential nutrients that support your opposite parasympathetic nervous system. This will speed up your weight-loss program, help tone your muscles, and give you abundant good health. The multiple amino acid, vitamin, and mineral complex for your meta-type can be purchased at your local health-food store or ordered from the companies listed in appendix 2.

If the controlling endocrine gland governed by your dominant nervous system is out of balance, either *hyperactive* or *hypoactive*, you may need some additional nutrients in the form of amino acids, vitamins, or minerals besides the full-spectrum amino acid, vitamin, and mineral formula supporting your opposite nervous system.

The following information should help you understand just what role each vitamin and mineral in your supplement program plays in helping regulate your dominant thyroid and weaker pituitary functions. This knowledge will enable you to be your own best judge when choosing which nutrients to take to support their health.

You'll also need to focus on your weaker opposite parasympathetic endocrine gland—the pituitary—the one at the opposite end of the "energetic strength" of your thyroid gland. Your whole body must be working at optimal speed and balance to guarantee you a rapid weight-loss and health-building program.

Your thyroid produces three major hormones, the most important of which is *thyroxine (T4)*, which increases the rate of energy being burned from the release of carbohydrates and increases the rate of protein synthesis, or how amino acids are "assembled" for cellular repair. It also stimulates the breakdown and mobilization of lipids, or "fats," needed for cellular repair, to bolster immune function, and to act as insulation for your body or provide energy needed for current use or store energy for later use. And finally it stimulates the activity in your nervous system and is heightened in the stress response.

Triiodothyronine (T3) is five times more potent than T4 and accounts for 95 percent of the circulating thyroid hormone. Its main function is to be stimulated in the stress response, giving an added boost to energy production.

Calcitonin ensures the strength of your bones and is an essential component of the stress response. It regulates your body's calcium and phosphate ion levels by *inhibiting* the rate with which calcium and phosphorus leave the bones, thereby *reducing* the calming effect in the body and maintaining your strong bones. It's released in great quantities during the stress response and helps to maintain the stimulatory effect of the "fight or flight" reaction.

As I mentioned earlier, entwined with your thyroid gland is a balancing set of four parathyroid glands, which serve as the "bridge keeper" to the thyroid and discharge the parathyroid hormone (PTH).

It's important to maintain a balance between the thyroid and parathyroid functions. If the blood calcium level falls too low (from overproduction of thyroid hormones) or there's not enough calcium in the body, PTH releases calcium *back* from the bones into the bloodstream as a negative-feedback system to regulate the action of the thyroid's hormones. It can also cause absorption of calcium from the intestines by influencing the metabolism of vitamin D. Its action is to release more calcium into the blood and to stabilize the stimulatory effect of the stress response.

This is how you gain weight from constant stress. If the parathyroids are constantly overworking, calming the body down from stress, your thyroid activity slows to a halt; calcitonin, thyroxine, and T3 are suppressed and you become fatigued and depressed and gain weight. PHT also causes your kidneys to conserve blood calcium and stimulates the excretion of phosphates (phosphoric acid salts), which maintain the acid-base balance of your body, increasing the danger of kidney stones. Stress is dangerous.

Your thyroid gland is activated in three ways. Early in the day, when your thyroid gland is under the domination of the sympathetic nervous system (usually between the hours of 7:00 A.M. and 4:00 P.M.), your hypothalamus signals the pituitary with its hormone, corticotropin-releasing hormone (CRH), to get your body ready to wake up for the day's activity according to your own "inner clock." Your pituitary responds by releasing its hormone, adrenocorticotropic hormone (ACTH), which speeds not to your thyroid gland but to your adrenal glands. Your adrenals then activate their hormones, norepinephrine and epinephrine, which stimulate cortisol production from the adrenal cortex. The adrenal's cortisol *then* activates your thyroid's hormone production—stimulating carbohydrate and glucose metabolism by signaling the liver through the pancreas to release its stored energy and transform fats and proteins into energy.

The second way your thyroid gland is stimulated is by the stress response, triggered by a call from your adrenals. The third way it's activated is by eating, especially complex carbohydrates.

The nutrients needed to gently support your dominant thyroid gland are the amino acid tyrosine; the B-complex vitamins and vitamins C and A; the minerals calcium, zinc, manganese, and iodine; and unsaturated fatty acids (essential fatty acids).

Tyrosine, synthesized from the dominant amino acid of the sympathetic nervous system, phenylalanine, is the major amino acid that produces your thyroid gland's hormone, thyroxine. Tyrosine is also the elemental ingredient for your adrenal glands' neurotransmitter production of dopamine, norepinephrine, and epinephrine (adrenaline), which fuel your sympathetic nervous system and provide you with energy. With a sluggish thyroid, the one thing you do need is plenty of the building material for your own hormone production.

Without ample amounts of this crucial amino acid, fatigue and depression may become a way of life. Tyrosine is almost gobbled up by the body in high adrenal activity or in the stress response. So if your adrenals have been making your thyroid work double time, your tyrosine levels may be low—one of the culprits responsible for those uncontrollable sugar or bread cravings. Remember, tyrosine is the main amino acid for both your adrenal and thyroid hormones and can be depleted quickly. Now it's abundant in proteins, but to facilitate your weight loss, a nutritional supplement of tyrosine might be a good idea.

The B-complex vitamins—B_1, B_2, and niacin (B_3)—are of vital importance in supporting your thyroid's hormone production, as I mentioned in describing your morning Miraculous Thin and Trim Cocktail. Two other members of the B-complex family are also essential: vitamin B_{12} and folic acid are needed for your thyroid's proper functioning.

When taking any of the B vitamins, it is important to remember that *you should not take an isolated B*—for instance, B_1 or B_2—without taking the whole B-vitamin complement. Otherwise, to activate its energy, the lone B would rob your body of the other B vitamins.

Vitamin C helps to conserve the iodine in your body and is essential for the metabolism of tyrosine. It plays a primary role in almost every part of your body's functioning, from building blood capillary walls and forming connective tissue to creating healthy skin and red blood cells, building resistance to infection, and accelerating the healing process. Another major function of vitamin C is its ability to control cholesterol, because it's required for fat and lipid metabolism. It burns off fat. Vitamin C is water-soluble and not stored in the body, so it must be taken on a daily basis—and sometimes several times a day if you're in a continued stress response. As you might imagine, it's used more rapidly when you're under stress.

Vitamin A is also necessary for thyroxine production. There should be ample amounts of this sunshine vitamin, along with vitamin D, in your Thin and Trim Cocktail.

Calcium, as you've already discovered, is important to keep a steady balance between your thyroid and parathyroids. Keeping your blood calcium levels high and in equilibrium will quiet the parathyroids, calm your body if you're experiencing the stress response, and stimulate your thyroid. Calcium and phosphorus work together for healthy bones and teeth; calcium and magnesium work together for nerves and cardiovascular health. It's commonly recommended to have a two-to-one relationship between calcium and magnesium or phosphorus.

Zinc is a magic mineral for you. It's a major component in your thyroid gland itself, and it also helps to stimulate your pancreatic enzyme production, for digestion—and that's important to speed up your weight loss by burning off fat and cholesterol. It's essential for the synthesis and metabolism of proteins and nucleic acids and for your pancreas's insulin-producing function. Zinc also acts as a "traffic officer"—directing and overseeing the efficient flow of the body processes. And if all that weren't enough, it accelerates the healing time for internal and external wounds as well.

Iodine has already been discussed (see page 184).

Unsaturated fatty acids (essential fatty acids) in the form of vegetable oils also stimulate your body's glandular action, especially that of your thyroid. They're a primary component of all of your body's cell membranes, and they manufacture your adrenal and sex gland steroid hormones from cholesterol. They also act as a major factor in the production of phospholipids, the "good guys" that break down cholesterol, help to clear away cholesterol deposits from your artery walls, and provide a concentrated source of energy. Both lecithin and safflower oil are rich sources of phospholipids and will help to burn off those excess pounds rapidly. Here's an important thing to remember: don't cook or fry with these oils. Heat can change the chemical composition of the fats, from unsaturated fatty acids to damaging saturated fat.

As you've now learned, your weaker pituitary needs support. It is tucked into the base of your brain, alongside the hypothalamus, that link between body and mind and regulator for our inner clocks. It works nonstop and should be strong and actively balanced in releasing the growth hormones, thyroid-stimulating hormones, and sex-stimulating hormones, which activate the repair and regeneration of your body. Without full support, you'll age quickly, lose that youthful sexual interest, and see your precious energy vanish.

For your weaker pituitary gland, the best daily supplements are:

• *Glucose* and *oxygen:* Both of these are essential for your proper brain function, especially for your weaker hypothalamus and pituitary. I've given you glucose from the pineapple juice in your Miraculous Thin and Trim Cocktail and the fruits for breakfast. Do a lot of deep breathing in good, clean air to oxygenate your lungs and bloodstream. Don't smoke. It robs the body of oxygen.

The following amino acids also support the pituitary:

• *Phenylalanine:* A precursor to tyrosine, phenylalanine affects the "exciters," your adrenal and thyroid hormones. It also supplies your pituitary with the basics to make ACTH, the pituitary hormone that gives your adrenal glands their morning wake-up call.

• *5-hydroxytryptophan (5-HTP):* This amino acid affects the "soothers," such as serotonin, and all the regenerative hormones, such as the pituitary's growth hormone.

• *GABA (gamma-aminobutyric acid):* Known as a "natural Valium," GABA helps relieve anxiety and depression. It's synthesized from glutamic acid and glutamine. It also can calm a hyperactive appestat (appetite-adjustment function) in your pituitary.

• *Glycine:* Synthesized from glutathione and creatinine, glycine helps regenerate cells, fights fat, and calms. It's essential for the strength of your pituitary's function.

• *Arginine* and *ornithine:* These twin regenerators boost production of the growth hormone that regulates insulin, burns fat, builds muscle, detoxifies your liver, and boosts your immune system. They also boost sperm production. (One exception: if you have any tendency to herpes outbreak, skip the arginine.)

Here are the other nutrients that support your pituitary:

• *B complex:* For your meta-type the B-complex vitamins help stabilize your emotions, reducing irritability, anxiety, and depression. B_1, B_3, B_5,

B_6, and B_{12} perform those functions, while B_5 stimulates cells in the glands, heart, and other muscles.

• *Choline* and *inositol:* These vitamins, which are part of the B complex, work both to break down fat and to soothe nerves. Both occur naturally in the form of lecithin.

• *Vitamin C:* With respect to the pituitary, vitamin C's role is to synthesize amino acids needed to transmit those essential pituitary hormones.

• *Unsaturated fatty acids* (essential fatty acids): These are needed for producing energy, stimulating growth, preventing cholesterol deposits, and burning fat, as well as for stimulating the function of all glands, especially your pituitary. You'll get plenty of the unsaturated fatty acids in your Miraculous Thin and Trim Cocktail in the form of the cod-liver oil or in the oils in your diet. If you feel you might have very weak pituitary function, you may want to take some additional unsaturated fatty acids in the form of capsules.

• *Calcium:* This mineral feeds and strengthens your pituitary gland, working with magnesium for healthy nerves and cardiovascular system, and working with phosphorus for healthy bones and teeth. It's commonly felt that it's best to have two parts calcium to one part phosphorus or magnesium.

• *Magnesium:* This mineral also helps to energize the pituitary to receive and transmit nerve and muscle impulses, stabilizes emotions, balances hormone production, maintains the acid-alkaline balance of your body, and regulates your blood sugar metabolism and protein synthesis. It's essential for growth and repair.

The Bottom Line

By taking a complete amino acid, vitamin, and mineral combination based on the formulation for your general metabolic type, you'll be supplied with the nutrients needed to support your complementary side, the parasympathetic nervous system. Then you may want to add a few of the vitamins and minerals that we've just discussed, which are also listed in the accompanying table of recommended nutrients.

If you're interested, turn to appendixes 3 and 4 for a more in-depth study of the vitamins, minerals, and amino acids for your meta-type. If you prefer to get all your nutrients from foods, I've listed the foods highest in vitamins, minerals, and amino acid content in the accompanying table.

Mixed Accelerator Vitamin, Mineral, and Amino Acid Food Sources

Thyroid Gland	
Tyrosine B complex	All animal proteins (meat, fowl, and fish) and soy products • B_1: torula yeast, sunflower seeds, rice bran, wheat germ, pine nuts, dried coriander leaf, safflower seeds, soybeans, alfalfa seeds, sesame seeds, and rye flour (dark) • B_2: almonds, cheese, turnip greens, wheat bran, and soybeans • B_3: (niacin): fish, nuts, milk, cheese, bran flakes, sesame seeds, and sunflower seeds • B_6: rice bran, wheat bran, sunflower seeds, avocados, bananas, corn, fish, brown rice, soybeans, and whole grains • B_{15}: grains, cereals, rice, apricot kernels, and torula yeast
Vitamin C	Acerola cherries, rose hips, citrus fruit, guavas, hot green peppers, black currants, parsley, turnip greens, poke greens, and mustard greens
Vitamin A	Carrots, cod-liver oil, liver, dark green leafy vegetables (spinach, dandelion greens, chard, kale, etc.), yellow foods (pumpkins, sweet potatoes, etc.), and some seafood (oysters, salmon, and swordfish)
Calcium	Cheese, wheat flour, blackstrap molasses, almonds, dried figs, fish with soft edible bones, green leafy vegetables, milk, oysters, soybean flour, and yogurt
Zinc	Spices, wheat bran, crab, and popcorn
Essential fatty acids—vitamin F	• Oils: safflower, sunflower, corn, olive, wheat germ, soy, cottonseed, and cod-liver • Nuts: walnuts, Brazil nuts, and almonds
Pituitary	
Amino acids B complex Lecithin or choline and inositol (called lipotropic factors)	All animal proteins (meat, fish, and fowl) and soy products As listed under "Thyroid Gland" • Choline: soybeans, wheat bran, navy beans, alfalfa leaf meal, rice polishings, rice bran, whole grains, hominy, turnips, and blackstrap molasses. Note: avoid cabbage. • Inositol: wheat germ, citrus fruits, blackstrap molasses, fruits, whole grains, bran, nuts, legumes, milk, and vegetables
Vitamin C	As listed under "Thyroid Gland"
Essential fatty acids	As listed under "Thyroid Gland"
Calcium	As listed under "Thyroid Gland"
Magnesium	Cottonseed, peanut, and soybean flour, sesame seeds, wheat bran and germ, blackstrap molasses, nuts, peanut butter, whole grains, and torula yeast

There are a few easy things to remember about taking the supplements:

• Try to take amino acids on an empty stomach. (They need adequate amounts of stomach enzymes to be broken down properly.)
• If possible, take enzymes with your meals to aid in your food digestion.

Mixed Accelerator Recommended Nutrients

ENDOCRINE GLAND	NUTRIENT	WOMEN			MEN		
		Number	Strength	Times per Day	Number	Strength	Times per Day
Thyroid	Tyrosine	1	500 mg	1	1	500 mg	2
	B complex	1	50–75 mg	2	1	100–125 mg	2
	Vitamin C (buffered)	1	1,000 mg	2–3	1–2	1,000 mg	3
	Calcium and magnesium	1	500 mg	3	1–2	500 mg	3
	Zinc	1	30 mg	1	1	60 mg	1
	Essential fatty acids	1	300 mg	2	2	300 mg	2
	or lecithin	1	1,200 mg	1–2	1	1,200 mg	2
Pituitary	Phenylalanine	1	500 mg	Morning	2	500 mg	Morning
	5-hydroxytrytophan	1	50 mg	Dinner	2	50 mg	Dinner
	GABA	1	500 mg	2	1–2	500 mg	2
	Glycine	1	500 mg	2	1–2	500 mg	2
	Arginine and ornithine	1	500 mg	2	2	500 mg	2
	B complex	See under "Thyroid"	—	—	See under "Thyroid"	—	—
	Choline and inositol	1–2	500 mg	1–2	1–2	1,000	2
	Vitamin C (buffered)	See under "Thyroid"	—	—	See under "Thyroid"	—	—
	Essential fatty acids	See under "Thyroid"	—	—	See under "Thyroid"	—	—
	Calcium	See under "Thyroid"	—	—	See under "Thyroid"	—	—
	Magnesium	See under "Thyroid"	—	—	See under "Thyroid"	—	—

Note: Do not take arginine or ornithine if you are susceptible to herpes simplex outbreaks.

- Take vitamins and minerals after you've eaten, which helps their assimilation.
- The water-soluble vitamins—B complex, vitamin C, and vitamin P (bioflavonoids)—can be taken at any time.
- Your body isn't used to concentrated food substances, so I recommend that you introduce one type of amino acid, vitamin, or mineral into your regimen every few days. Gently and easily is the name of the game.

Taking these extra vitamins, minerals, and supplements will require work—there's no mistaking that. Just as you have to plan meals with the right ingredients, you'll need to organize these. But as your metabolic system moves back into balance, you'll reduce the number of pills you'll need. And along the way, you'll discover that the dividend of glowing good health pays off quickly enough to make Wall Street envious.

Stocking Up

You've now finished reading about the program and are well on your way to a brand-new you. Just wait and see—you'll be slim, sexy, and full of bounce to every ounce. Now to get started, you'll need to stock up and organize. The accompanying list shows all the foods you'll need for the coming week. Double-check this list against your weekly menu and make any adjustments you feel are necessary. Happy regeneration!

Weekly Shopping List for Mixed Accelerators

Larger quantities for men are shown in **boldface**.

PRODUCE

Fruit
4 Lemons
1 Lime
1 med. bunch Green grapes
2 Pineapples
2 lg. Papayas
2 pt. Strawberries
1 pt. Raspberries
½ pt. Blueberries
9 **(12)** Oranges

7 **(10)** Tangerines
3 **(6)** Kiwifruits
2 Nectarines
1 Peach

Vegetables
10 **(11)** lb. Carrots
2 bulbs Fennel
1 med. Yellow squash
1 med. Zucchini
2 **(3)** lb. Rutabaga
2 bunches Scallions

2 med. Leeks
1 lb. Yellow beans
1 med. Acorn squash
3 bunches Celery
1 lg. bunch Kale
4 8-oz. Mushrooms
3 bulbs Garlic
6 Plum tomatoes (if on diet)
1 Red pepper

Salad Greens
1 **(2)** head Romaine lettuce
1 **(2)** head Red leaf lettuce
4   lb. Spinach
1 med. Radicchio
2 bunches Arugula
3 bunches Watercress
4 bunches Mint leaves
11 bunches Parsley
1 box Alfalfa sprouts
1 **(2)** head Chicory
1 **(2)** head Green leaf lettuce

Fresh Herbs
1 bunch Cilantro
1 bunch Rosemary
1 bunch Basil

GROCERIES
1 container Whey protein powder
½ lb. Couscous
½ lb. Bulgur wheat

1 loaf Sprouted grain bread
1 lb. Egg pastina
1 8-oz. jar Dijon mustard
4 **(6)** oz. Peanuts
1 qt. Pineapple juice (in glass)
Black pepper
Dried thyme, dried oregano, curry
    powder, turmeric, tarragon,
    cinnamon
Herbal teas
Safflower oil
Blackstrap molasses
Wheat germ
Cod-liver oil
Blue-green algae

DAIRY
6 Eggs
1 **(3)** 8-oz. Cottage cheese,
    low-fat
1 pt. Milk, low-fat
4 **(6)** 8-oz. Plain yogurt, fat-free
3 lb. Tofu, extra firm

MEAT AND FISH
1 8-oz. **(11-oz.)** piece Chicken
    breast (skin off)
2 pieces: 1 8-oz., 1 3-oz.
    **(2 pieces: 1 12-oz.,
    1 6-oz.)** Yellowfin tuna
4 **(6)** oz. Scallops (sea or bay)

17 The Synthesizer Diet

As a synthesizer, you have probably spent a lot of time fighting your own battle of the bulge. Well, get ready to celebrate your victory over that excess weight once and for all. When you master your personal diet plan, your constant worries about those excess pounds will be a thing of the past. I am going to introduce you to a whole new way of eating, living, and feeling great. Just a few quick words on how your synthesizer diet works, then on to the menus.

As you read, remember:

- Your dominant gland is the pituitary.
- Your weakest gland is the thyroid.
- You're most likely to gain weight fairly evenly over your body.

The Science behind Your System

You are the most sensitive of all the synthesizer meta-types and are primarily dominated by the yin forces of the parasympathetic nervous system, with little influence from the yang sympathetic nervous system.

Your dominant pituitary gland is the "master gland" of the body, which controls and directs how your body will function energetically *and* regenerate itself under the directions from the pituitary's partner, the hypothalamus. Within the hypothalamus are housed your individual circadian rhythms, your "inner time clock" created by the specific programming in your DNA pattern. Based on these rhythms, your pituitary sends out its hormones at the appointed times to keep your body running smoothly.

Your natural energy and metabolism are driven by abundant nerve stimulation to those glands and organs responsible for the regeneration, repair, and growth of your body: your pituitary gland, salivary glands, stomach, pancreas, liver, gallbladder, small and large intestines, kidneys, and bladder. Much less nerve stimulation goes to the organs that produce energy: your adrenal, thymus, and thyroid glands and your spleen, lungs, and heart.

This simply means that you need to eat regularly—and right—to draw energy from your foods instead of automatically producing energy through the sympathetic nervous system as the accelerator meta-types do.

While accelerators need to reach for the veggies for balance, synthesizers will learn to load up on proteins, especially meats. You've probably had some success—temporarily—on those high-protein diets. But you'll soon see why balance is essential for your meta-type, too—and why those rich, creamy pastas and double lattes you love are your downfall.

Since your primary metabolic focus is to break down and utilize carbohydrates and proteins for cell repair, growth, and the regeneration of your body, you tend to be a *very slow metabolizer*. Although you produce ample stomach acid needed for those heavier protein foods, without that extra energy burst from your weaker adrenals and thyroid glands, your foods take a long time to break down. This digestion takes place in what is called an aerobic environment (that is, in the presence of oxygen).

Since your foods require plenty of time to break down in your stomach, they mix with more oxygen (aerobic environment) before passing into the small intestine for further digestion. Finally, when those oxygen-rich nutrients arrive in your cells to be converted to energy, they'll burn off in a flash.

You know from the energy rush of a candy bar, cola, or even fruit that carbohydrates break down quickly and are the fastest-burning foods, while proteins break down and burn off more slowly. Fats are the slowest to break down and burn off. That's why those refined carbohydrates give your meta-type quick bursts of energy followed by rapid declines, providing no sustaining energy or endurance. You'll feel like a Ping-Pong ball, bouncing from abrupt flashes of energy to dramatic plunges into fatigue.

This means you need a diet with slower-burning proteins and fats, as well as some of the energy-producing *complex* carbohydrates, to provide you with more level, sustained energy.

With your tendency to have a strong alkaline body chemistry, coupled with a slow digesting and fast oxidizing capacity, you'll tend to have:

- Ample production of stomach acid (HCl, or hydrochloric acid)—although there can be much less if production is suppressed by the stress response
- Strong tissue alkalinity
- Good production of pancreatic enzymes—if you are not under stress
- Balanced production of pancreatic insulin—if you are not experiencing the stress response

Luckily for your metabolism, you're inclined to have lower levels of toxic cellular waste. Your oxygen-rich nutrients help to rid your cells of poisonous debris.

Metabolically speaking, you require foods of an acid nature—such as proteins like meat, fowl, fish, seeds, and nuts. You also require some of those foods that supply you with energy—the complex carbohydrates in vegetables, fruits, and some grains. Your fats should come from a moderate amount of unsaturated oil—*not* saturated fat—in the form of vegetable oils (unsaturated fatty acids). You can't tolerate refined carbohydrates (sugars and starches), packaged and refined products (too much sugar), or dairy products. Therefore, your synthesizer food formula looks like this:

- Protein: 55 percent
- Carbohydrates: 30 percent
- Fat: 15 percent

Synthesizer Food Choices

After one month on the Your Body, Your Diet plan, you will not only drop excess fat but also experience a level of vitality and good health that you never dreamed possible. Once you have looked at the basic menus, you can turn to lists that will show you the wide variety of delicious foods that are best for you. Suggested vitamin and mineral supplements are also included. The next three subsections give you an overview of the basic principles you'll be following.

What to Avoid

Steer clear of dairy products, chocolate, sugar, refined carbohydrates, nicotine, and alcohol. These restrictions may seem stringent, but they are an important part of jump-starting your weight-loss program.

Here's why: Since you are a synthesizer, the minute you eat refined (or even some complex) carbohydrates, your weaker thyroid won't be able to sustain the demand for long. As it gives up and your energy wanes, you reach for another "fix." Your pancreas floods your system with extra insulin, not converting those "carbs" to energy and sleek muscles but escorting them directly to your fat tissues. You end up tired, irritable, and probably depressed, overweight, and carbohydrate-intolerant. So less and less makes you grow more and more.

Dairy and chocolate both overstimulate your active pituitary gland while blocking absorption of its most-needed mineral, magnesium. Even though chocolate mimics a "love" drug—triggering hormones to stimulate sexuality and sensuality—you synthesizers already get enough pituitary stimulation. On you it just goes directly into extra weight. Chocolate contains large quantities of theobromine, a powerful stimulant that can dilate heart muscles and blood vessels and fuels your pituitary gland. Dairy products are also dangerous for you. The prolactin in milk, a boon for babies' brain and pituitary gland growth, is also believed to overstimulate your already revved-up pituitary.

Nicotine, drugs, and alcohol (stimulants and depressants) have a devastating effect on your meta-type—far more dangerous than for most others. By overloading your pituitary gland and depriving you of oxygen, they trigger the hangover that keeps you repeating the cycle and depresses you easily. Alcohol interferes with your brain's signals to relax, and instead your pituitary jolts its weaker partners, your adrenal and thyroid glands. You'll keep reaching for that next cigarette, drink, or drug to spike your "high." Your pituitary begins working overtime pumping out those growth hormones that make you bigger and bigger; when it's exhausted, your whole endocrine system screeches to a halt.

You'll be amazed at how much better you look and feel without these foods literally weighing you down.

The following table gives you an overview of the foods and other substances that do *not* suit your meta-type.

Your *Never* Foods

DAIRY PRODUCTS	REFINED CARBOHYDRATES	SUGAR	CHOCOLATE	NICOTINE, DRUGS
All milk products	All packaged foods	White sugar	Cocoa	Tobacco in any form
Cream	Synthetic additives	Cane sugar	Chocolate in any form	Drugs
Sour cream	Sweeteners	Brown sugar	(semisweet, bittersweet,	
Buttermilk	Cakes	Processed syrup	Dutch, milk)	**FATS**
Milk	Cookies	Alcohol	Cola drinks (from	
Ice cream	Doughnuts		cocoa bean/leaf)	Butter
Cheese	Pastry			Margarine
Yogurt	Muffins			Mayonnaise
Whey	Bagels			
	White pasta			
	White bread			

What to Fill Up On

Proteins (poultry, lean meats, and fish) and a limited amount of vegetables, fruits, and grains are your foods of choice. You must admit, this is a
pretty impressive list. There are lots of delicious foods on your eating plan,
perfect for your synthesizer meta-type. These foods stimulate and sustain
your energy while keeping you balanced. They keep your blood sugar stable while melting off extra pounds. Proteins ground your parasympathetic
system's intense emotional energy while stimulating your sympathetic system's intellectual and physical energy. They also help strengthen your relatively weak adrenal glands while supporting your thyroid's production of
thyroxine, the hormone that keeps your metabolic rate high. After looking
over the complete list of recommended foods in the accompanying table,
you'll see that you will have plenty of opportunities to enjoy great-tasting
meals while watching your excess weight disappear.

The foods required by your specific metabolic type—complex carbohydrates (grains, vegetables, and fruits) and the amino acids in proteins
(meat, fish, fowl, seeds, and nuts)—are those that feed and support your
weaker endocrine gland, the thyroid.

Your *Always* Foods

PROTEINS		CARBOHYDRATES		FATS
Food	Times per Week	Food	Times per Week	
Meat: abundant	2–3	Grains: variety	1	*Moderate* amount of
Fowl: abundant	2	Legumes: variety	1	unsaturated fatty
Fish: abundant	2	Starchy vegetables: variety	1–2	acids—cold-pressed
Dairy: none	0	Slightly starchy vegetables:		vegetable or nut oils
		variety	2–3	Choose from your
Seeds/nuts: abundant	2–3	Nonstarchy vegetables: variety	Daily	food plan.
Legume protein: variety	1	Fruit: some	Daily	

How to Speed Up Weight Loss

Here are a few other tips to stimulate faster weight loss:

- Chew your food slowly and well.
- Try to avoid drinking more than one glass of water or liquid during your meals. Drinking large amounts of liquid during meals dilutes the precious enzymes needed for your digestion.
- Have at least six to eight glasses of water during the day, *not* at mealtimes.

Keeping Your Pituitary in Balance

Your dominant pituitary gland is a tiny but powerful organ tucked in the brain, in a protected hollow just behind the bridge of your nose. It is the control center for the body, from your wake-up and sleep cycle to the hormones crucial for growth, sex and fertility, cell repair, and—when it's in balance—mobilizing fat into energy and sleek muscles, not unsightly bulges. Out of balance, you become at risk for diabetes or its opposite, hypoglycemia.

Your pituitary works with your hypothalamus as your inner time clock, relaying messages between your mind, body, and emotions, twenty-four hours a day. The hypothalamus regulates both the parasympathetic and sympathetic nervous systems, determining which hormones to release—and at what time—for overnight repairs or your daily energy.

Your supergland acts as a kind of "relay station" between your intellectual mind (cerebrum) and emotional mind (limbic system, located in the temporal lobe of your brain), connecting them to your physical body by sending hormones and nerve impulses to all of your cells. These hormones are based on your bodily cycles or a need for either an emotional or an intellectual response from your body.

It's why your meta-type—when in balance—is so good at healing and age-defying regeneration. The growth hormone you produce also promotes bone growth and mobilizes fat for energy. Sounds great? Sure, since it redistributes fat in your body.

But if your power gland becomes overstimulated, then the extra blood sugar from the refined carbohydrates and fats can often cause hyperglycemia or diabetes, especially if you've been bingeing on sugars and starches to maintain that "pituitary high." Also, the continued overproduction of the growth hormone will just prod the body to keep re-creating itself—turning you into a "fat factory" while you sleep.

When you've been hooked on a pituitary high and come crashing down, you'll start craving those foods that restimulate your tired pituitary as your pituitary has now been trained to overproduce its hormones. The result is that you keep gaining weight.

This master gland of your body gets *plenty* of its own natural stimulation from your thoughts, self-induced stress, and emotional reactions. While your deep emotions can be your strength, they also mean you're most vulnerable to stress and depression—and the eating binges that go with them. Sugar triggers those emotional slumps and depressions, while proteins provide the amino acids needed to feed your weaker energy-producing glands and your intellectual side.

On the flip side, your pituitary also produces thyroid-stimulating hormone (TSH), which stimulates your weakest gland, the thyroid. Unfortunately, it's all on the wrong schedule for you, so you're sluggish in the morning, have bursts of energy at night, and then are restless overnight.

When you need energy in the mornings, or when you need it during the day for your daily activity and burning off those pounds, your weaker thyroid gland gets its only stimulation from your weaker adrenal gland, not the strong stimulation from the pituitary.

Your pituitary also produces certain sex hormones that trigger the production of testosterone in the male's testes, which in turn produce strong sperm, and estrogen in the female's ovaries, stimulating egg production. Although they are obviously important for fertility, they are also essential for your sex drive and mental and emotional acuity. If the pituitary goes into overload, however, women can begin producing testosterone (manufactured in the ovaries or in the adrenals as androgens), leading to disrupted menstrual cycles, mood swings, excess body or facial hair, and fatigue. In men overload would bring excess body or facial hair, or baldness. And in both sexes it can produce nervousness, restlessness, depression, anger, and diminished or dormant libido. No fun for you—or those around you.

You also need to build up your weaker gland, your thyroid, the engine that produces its hormone, thyroxine, to burn fat fast all day and at night convert energy to repair your cells.

Your weaker thymus gland may make you vulnerable to colds, the flu, or infections. Your weaker adrenals make you susceptible to fatigue, allergies, and depression.

Sugar and refined carbohydrates, which are *exactly* the foods loved by bacteria and viruses, will further weaken your thymus as well as cause your adrenals to burn out quickly! Moreover, your thymus gland and your whole immune response are automatically shut down in a prolonged stress response. So with your vulnerability to intense emotionality and susceptibility to stress, you're a prime target for all kinds of imbalanced immune responses, especially allergies or asthma.

Your Synthesizer Secret Weapons

Now I know—from firsthand experience—just how tough it can be to switch to a whole new way of eating. In addition to having to apply a lot of willpower, you have to give your body time to adjust to your new lifestyle. If you find yourself feeling cranky and frustrated, relax; it's par for the course. It's just a sign that you're shedding those extra pounds and getting back into balance.

The teas and elixirs in this chapter were created to help you sail through the transition phase of your meta-type diet while making the pounds melt away even faster.

Call-to-Arms Weight-Buster Morning Drink

You need to give your pituitary a wake-up call so it can begin releasing its hormone, adrenocorticotropic hormone. ACTH will in turn activate your adrenal glands so that they will release their hormones, setting in motion the liberation of your stored blood sugar—*energy*. The released blood sugar then acts as the fuel to wake you up and get you going. This energy should run from about 6:00 A.M. to 3:00 P.M. The inner clock in your hypothalamus is set to trigger your pituitary's activation at a later time, so you need to help jump-start it in the morning.

I've designed a drink for synthesizers that wakes them right up: the

Call-to-Arms Weight-Buster Morning Drink. It contains all the essential ingredients needed by your pituitary gland to release ample amounts of ACTH, alerting your adrenals to swing into action—ginger, capsicum, flaxseed oil, apple cider vinegar, kelp, and honey in a base of fresh spring water.

Ginger is an excellent herb for your digestion, stimulating your pituitary and building up your immune system. It's also a superior herb to boost your digestive activity and speed up your weight loss. It's highly beneficial for your meta-type because it's rich in magnesium, the mineral needed to give your pituitary gland a wake-up call. Ginger also contains vitamins A, C, and B-complex factors as well as calcium, phosphorus, iron, sodium, and potassium.

Capsicum, known as cayenne pepper, is one of the best morning stimulants for the pituitary and thyroid glands. This fantastic herb helps raise your metabolic rate—the secret to burning off those excess pounds.

Apple cider vinegar has long been known as a remedy for weight problems, but it must be the cider vinegar made from apples that still contain their valuable minerals: phosphorus, chlorine, potassium, sodium, magnesium, calcium, sulfur, iron, fluorine, silicon, and many trace minerals.

Apple cider vinegar's secret is that it raises your metabolic rate—speeds up the way you burn fat. How? It allows your bloodstream to be filled with much more oxygen than is normal, which in turn raises the rate at which your cells burn off fat.

Apple cider vinegar also helps to stimulate your mental clarity, improves your memory, and helps to clear the toxins from your liver.

Honey is the perfect morning food for your meta-type because it's rich in two simple sugars, levulose (fruit sugar) and dextrose (grape sugar), and much lower in sucrose (cane sugar). Levulose is a high-powered energy producer—higher and better than even dextrose and especially sucrose. Now honey normally is already predigested, and with these sugars it's able to go right into your bloodstream, giving you the immediate energy needed to raise your blood sugar levels in order to activate your brain, your pituitary, and consequently your adrenals and thyroid gland.

Honey is also rich in the vitamins and minerals necessary to feed your slower-waking pituitary.

The best is dark honey, such as buckwheat and heather, because of its higher mineral content. *Tupelo honey* has the highest content of levulose and is a powerful energizer. Honey is a perfect food for your meta-type, but *only* in the morning before your dominant glands kick in.

Kelp or *blue-green algae* contains abundant iodine—the important mineral required by your thyroid gland. Two-thirds of your body's iodine reserve is used by your thyroid gland to make its potent hormone, thyroxine, which is responsible for activating the way your body burns off or uses energy. It influences your mental, physical, and hormonal growth; metabolizes all of your nutrients; stimulates your energy; and regulates the way you oxidize, or burn off, fat.

Another ingredient in kelp is mannitol—a natural sugar essential to the composition of thyroxine. Mannitol is also an energizer that helps your weaker endocrine glands produce their hormones, which in turn activate all the organs and glands of your body—so you burn fat. Kelp is also rich in calcium, a mineral that is crucial in providing a stable equilibrium between your thyroid and parathyroid glands, helping build your bones, stabilizing your nerves, and enlivening your skin and hair.

Blue-green algae is a powerhouse of vitamins A and D as well as the mineral zinc, which is highly concentrated in your thyroid gland. Blue-green algae with its zinc component may well ignite your weaker thyroid's thyroxine production. It can also be used as a seasoning agent or flavoring.

Flaxseed oil or *unsaturated fatty acids* in the form of oils will be the most powerful tonic for your pituitary gland. These unsaturated fatty acids lubricate and activate your pituitary into releasing its hormones in a steady rhythm throughout the morning and early-afternoon hours. This in turn helps your thyroid and adrenals supply a continuous flow of hormones, keeping metabolic harmony in your body.

Mixing all of these ingredients together and taking this drink *before breakfast* will wake you right up, energize you, and literally set your body in motion to melt away those excess pounds. (For the recipe, see Call-to-Arms Weight-Buster Morning Drink, on page 400.)

Seeds

The second important part of your weight-loss food plan is keeping your appetite under control.

Eating a small amount of raw unsalted seeds and nuts at dinnertime—when your pituitary can become hyperactive—keeps that rambunctious synthesizer appetite happy. The nuts and seeds are rich sources of essential fatty acids and amino acids and are alive with enzymes that help to keep your blood sugar stable and those pounds melting away.

SYNTHESIZER'S APPETITE-CONTROL SNACK
Seeds or nuts: 1 oz., at dinnertime (Choose from pine nuts, cashews, peanuts, pecans, pistachio nuts, walnuts, almonds, filberts, pumpkin seeds, sunflower seeds, sesame seeds, or flaxseeds.)

Burdock, Sassafras, and Hops Relaxer

Most experts agree that when you gain weight quickly, especially all over the body, your pituitary gland is out of whack due to low levels of the mineral magnesium in the body. To correct this, I have developed a tea that contains three essential herbs rich in magnesium: burdock, sassafras, and hops. When I give this tea to my synthesizer clients, they calm down quickly and lose weight consistently, and their pituitary gland becomes balanced.

Burdock, a rich source of magnesium, will aid your pituitary gland in adjusting its hormonal output. When mixed with sassafras, it becomes a soother to your hypothalamus. It also contains anywhere from 27 to 45 percent of an insulin-like substance that helps the metabolism of carbohydrates and is one of the herbal kingdom's best blood purifiers, promoting kidney function and clearing toxic debris from the blood. Burdock also contains a lot of vitamins: C (good for your adrenals), A, P (bioflavonoids), and E; the B-complex vitamins (especially para-aminobenzoic acid, or PABA); and small amounts of sulfur, silicon, copper, iodine, and zinc.

Sassafras, along with burdock, is excellent when used as an appetite-control tonic to quiet your busy hypothalamus and pituitary glands. Sassafras also stimulates the action of your liver, keeping your blood clean, and has a wonderful spicy odor.

Hops is one of the best nerve tonics known to herbalists. Rich in magnesium, it is very strong yet very safe to use. It also contains properties that calm your active nighttime hunger pains by relaxing the stimulation to the gastric nerves. Its main uses are to alleviate nervous eating and promote a good night's sleep. Perhaps that explains beer's universal appeal from ancient times.

One to two cups taken in the evening or along with your seeds and nuts will immediately help stabilize your pituitary's energy. (For the recipe, see Burdock, Sassafras, and Hops Relaxer, on page 403.)

Cranberry Juice

I've also added cranberry juice to your regimen. It's a tremendous slimming aid that also helps flush toxins and waste from your kidneys. It reduces extra water retention and gives you a wonderfully clean and lean feeling. Check chapter 12 to find out what kind to buy and the ways to make this delicious juice.

Slimming Teas

Another important component of your plan is the herbal tea formula I've created to meet the needs of each meta-type. Each tea will harmonize and balance your specific metabolism, facilitating your weight loss. To make yours, you'll need to add a few special ingredients to the basic Master Weight-Loss Tea (see the formula and directions on pages 103–05).

Synthesizer Slimming Tea

Basic Formula: One Teaspoon Each			
Alisma, poria, rhubarb root, red clover tops, alfalfa leaf, hawthorn berry, radish seed, sargassum, Indian chickweed, evergreen artemesia, astragalus root, fleeceflower root, citrus peel			
Synthesizer Slimming Formula: Add One Teaspoon Each			
NAME			FUNCTION
Common	Latin	Eastern	
Licorice root	*Radix glycyrrhizae*	Gan cao	Great for supporting and stimulating the adrenals and thyroid—an energizer for your body.
Laminaria	*Lamineria japonica aresh*	Kun bu	Stimulates the thyroid gland, speeding up your metabolism; reduces fat.
White atractylodes	*Atractylodes macrocephala*	Bai zhu	Powerful immune stimulant; also helps to reduce water retention.
Safflower	*Carthamus tinctorius*	Hong hua	Opens the pancreas and liver, energizes, balances insulin levels, helps digestion, burns cholesterol, and stimulates the adrenals.
Burdock root	*Arctium lappa*	Nui bang zi	Soothes the hypothalamus and stimulates the pituitary gland to balance its hormone release; also helps to metabolize carbohydrates.
Fennel fruit	*Foeniculum officinale vulgare*	Hui xiang	Excellent for weight loss, opens digestion and liver function, burns fat, and removes waste and mucus.

Note: If you are pregnant, have high blood pressure, or are allergic to grasses or flowers, it's suggested that these teas not be used. Licorice root should not be used if you have high blood pressure.

These supplementary herbs should be added in equal proportions to the herbs already in the basic formula. I suggest you drink one to three cups per day of your special tea. The herbs may be purchased at your local health-food store or ordered from the companies listed in appendix 2.

Rules of the Road

Your Eating Schedule

Since your body clock is guided by the parasympathetic nervous system—which works hardest during the nighttime, from about 4:00 P.M. to 6:00 A.M.—this is the time your body regenerates itself and redistributes fat.

With your energy highest in the late afternoon and evening, dinner is the time when your meals should be the lightest and focused on protein. This helps stabilize your blood sugar levels and supplies you with the amino acids for your cellular repair and regeneration.

Your less energetic time is likely to be in the morning, when you're under the complete domination of your opposite sympathetic nervous system with your weaker energy-producing glands, the thyroid and adrenals. Your thyroid and adrenals try to rise to the energetic occasion and create enough energy for your daily activities. But since they're your weaker opposite glands, they'll be having a hard time supplying you with enough of their hormones to get you up and about.

That's why they require support and stimulation from the foods you eat in the morning. Remember, you need to eat to get your energy. A good protein breakfast and lunch stimulate your thyroid and adrenals, stabilizing your blood sugar levels, reducing your insulin levels, and melting those pounds away. Your blood sugar level can then remain stable during the approaching cortisol crash in the late afternoon. The bonus: it keeps you away from those energy-killers—starches, sugars, and dairy products. The key to your eating schedule is:

- Medium to substantial breakfast
- Substantial lunch
- Light dinner

Late Afternoon—Battling Low Energy

While your least energetic time is in the morning, you also experience a less energetic period in the late afternoon—just as the cortisol levels from your adrenals begin to plummet and your dominant parasympathetic system begins to take over. Without a substantial lunch, you'll feel your blood sugar drop. You'll experience fatigue, sleepiness, headaches, and irritability. If you're not able to get that kind of lunch, you can help stave off that adrenal cortisol drop with a late-afternoon protein snack of seeds or nuts. That will help stabilize your blood sugar and curb your appetite.

> *YOUR LATE-AFTERNOON SNACK*
> Protein snack of seeds or nuts, 1 oz. (*only* if you haven't eaten a substantial lunch)
> Cranberry juice
> Hot herbal tea or green tea

Bedtime Eating—A Good Bet

If you're following your proper diet, you shouldn't need to eat before bed. But if you'd like a snack, stick to protein. If you want to save your afternoon snack and have it before you go to bed, okay. But no more than that. You can handle proteins, since they are digested slowly and are the foods that facilitate cellular regeneration. They won't wake you up by their conversion to energy. But stay away from carbohydrates. No cookies, candy, bread, fruit, ice cream, and so forth. They break right down into glucose or blood sugar—energy—and you don't want that extra blood sugar liberated into your bloodstream. It will wake you up and turn immediately to fat.

Synthesizer Meals and Menus

Now you've completed the first part of the plan, and here's your reward: the tailor-made diet for your synthesizer meta-type. If you've reached this point in the book, you know that losing weight and keeping it off take more than just watching what you eat.

The meals presented in this section are designed to meet all the needs of your metabolism while giving you the chance to eat a delicious, wide variety of fresh, nutritious foods. The first week may seem like a big adjustment, but by week two, I assure you, you'll be making your juices and tossing together your special meals like a pro.

Eating the Right Foods at the Right Times

Eating the *right kinds of food* at the *right times* is another key to the success of your weight-loss and rejuvenation program. With the very alkaline nature of your synthesizer metabolism, if you eat a majority of strong alkaline foods, it will throw you far out of balance. Then, instinctively struggling to balance yourself, you'll reach for the wrong type of acid foods—sugars and starches—that will cause you to retain that extra fat, and you'll wind up feeling terrible.

You require the right kind of acid foods to balance your body chemistry, just as your counterpart, the accelerator meta-type, is more acid in nature and requires more of the alkaline forming foods.

Your metabolism tends to be the most alkaline of all the synthesizer meta-types, so you require the most acid foods, such as animal proteins and grains, to help stabilize your metabolism. You also need some of the more weak alkaline and alkaline foods, such as vegetables and fruits, to balance out your equilibrium. You are known as the *strong alkaline* meta-type, with your natural body pH tending to be 8–7.5. (Chapter 3 has a detailed explanation of the acid-alkaline aspect of your meta-type.) Therefore, your diet should consist of foods that are strong acid, acid forming, and weak acid. Foods that are alkaline and weak alkaline forming can be eaten one to three times per week. Foods that are the same as your own pH tendency—strong alkaline forming—should be avoided. Appendix 5 lists the full spectrum of foods and their pH factors.

Here We Go!

To make this adventure of slimming down to a new and healthy you fun, I've taken all the guesswork out of how to shop and prepare your meals. Before you begin, glance through your weekly menus and synthesizer elixirs in the accompanying tables and look over the vast array of food selections in your Synthesizer Food Choices list. At the end of this chapter, you will find your own synthesizer shopping list for a week. Then turn to appendix 1 and take a look at the equipment list (which includes all the supplies you'll need to make this as simple as possible), your advance food-preparation suggestions for the week, and your recipes and food-preparation instructions for both men and women.

For any of the foods specified in the weekly menus and recipes, you may substitute comparable foods from the Synthesizer Food Choices list.

Eat only the foods that are indicated for you on your individual food choices list. If your favorite isn't there, don't eat it. You can check the "General Food Choices and Their Calorie Content for Each Meta-Type" in appendix 5.

You see, it's all done for you, down to the last detail—and my personal promise to you is that this eating plan will keep your synthesizer metabolism in perfect balance while helping you achieve a slender, gorgeous physique.

You're on your way to a bright, new, skinny, energetic you. Treat this as a ritual in celebrating your beauty and regeneration.

Synthesizer Carnivore Weekly Menus

Acid-Based Foods

Larger quantities for men are shown in **boldface**.

WHEN	SATURDAY	SUNDAY	MONDAY	TUESDAY
On rising	Call-to-Arms Weight-Buster Morning Drink			
Breakfast	Salmon Surprise Poached Eggs Florentine with Salmon and Sesame Seeds 1 cup herbal tea or Synthesizer Slimming Tea	Protein Power Breakfast Steak and Scrambled Eggs with Steamed Asparagus and Sesame Seeds 1 cup herbal tea or Synthesizer Slimming Tea	Quick and Easy Slim and Thin Protein Drink 1 cup herbal tea or Synthesizer Slimming Tea	Spanish Supreme Egg Fritatta with Tomatoes, Peppers, Mushrooms, Onions, Basil, and Pinoli Nuts 1 cup herbal tea or Synthesizer Slimming Tea
Midmorning	1 6-oz. glass cranberry juice (Obtain Knudsen or Ad-Vita cranberry concentrate from your health-food store. Use 2 tbs. concentrate to 6 oz. spring water. Add more water if desired.) 1 cup herbal tea or Synthesizer Slimming Tea			
Lunch	Skinny-Minnie Regeneration Lunch Filet of Beef Super Salad with Raw Zucchini, Yellow Squash, Tomatoes, Carrots, Mushrooms, and Cashews 1 cup herbal tea or Synthesizer Slimming Tea	Moroccan Makeover Couscous Moroccan-Style Vegetables Tomato, Summer Squash, Mushrooms, Eggplant, and Chickpeas, with Seaweed Red Onion and Sprout Salad 1 glass Synthesizer Elixir 1 cup herbal tea or Synthesizer Slimming Tea	Egg-a-licious Lunch Vegetable Omelet with Onions, Peppers, Mushrooms, and Peas Roasted Garlic Mashed Potatoes Fennel and Carrot Salad 1 cup herbal tea or Synthesizer Slimming Tea	Chicken Dijon Dijon Mustard and Thyme Roasted Chicken Roasted Garlic Mashed Potatoes Sunshine Salad with Raw Zucchini, Yellow Squash, Carrots, and Mushrooms 1 cup herbal tea or Synthesizer Slimming Tea
Midafternoon	1 6-oz. glass cranberry juice 1 cup herbal tea or Synthesizer Slimming Tea			
Dinner	Combine ¼ **(½)** cup each: peaches, pears, apricots, and grapes Top with 1 **(2)** oz.	Combine ¼ **(½)** cup each: Balsamic Strawberries, blueberries, apricots, and	Great Grapefruit 1 cup Burdock, Sassafras, and Hops Relaxer Tea	Combine ¼ **(½)** cup each: peaches, pears, apricots, and grapes Top with 1 **(2)** oz.

WHEN	SATURDAY	SUNDAY	MONDAY	TUESDAY
Dinner (cont'd)	cashews 1 cup Burdock, Sassafras, and Hops Relaxer Tea	mangoes Top with 1 **(2)** oz. pecans 1 cup Burdock, Sassafras, and Hops Relaxer Tea		cashews or pecans 1 cup Burdock, Sassafras, and Hops Relaxer Tea

WHEN	WEDNESDAY	THURSDAY	FRIDAY
On rising	Call-to-Arms Weight-Buster Morning Drink		
Breakfast	*Quick and Easy Slim and Thin Protein Drink* 1 cup herbal tea or Synthesizer Slimming Tea	*Chicken Delight* Chicken and Scrambled Eggs with Mushrooms, Peas, Fennel, Red Onions, and Pignoli Nuts 1 cup herbal tea or Synthesizer Slimming Tea	*Quick and Easy Slim and Thin Protein Drink* 1 cup herbal tea or Synthesizer Slimming Tea
Midmorning	1 6-oz. glass cranberry juice (Obtain Knudsen or Ad-Vita cranberry concentrate from your health-food store. Use 2 tbs. concentrate to 6 oz. spring water. Add more water if desired.) 1 cup herbal tea or Synthesizer Slimming Tea		
Lunch	*Hearty Vegetarian Salad* Couscous Moroccan-Style Vegetables with Red Onions, Sprouts, and Synthesizer Salad Greens 1 glass Synthesizer Elixir 1 cup herbal tea or Synthesizer Slimming Tea	*Fabulous Fish Fiesta* Ginger Soy Salmon Steamed Sugar Snap Peas, Onions, Carrots, and Corn Cucumber Salad 1 cup herbal tea or Synthesizer Slimming Tea	*Outrageous Omelet* Shrimp-Filled Omelet Steamed Green Beans Tomato and Onion Salad 1 cup herbal tea or Synthesizer Slimming Tea
Midafternoon	1 6-oz. glass cranberry juice 1 cup herbal tea or Synthesizer Slimming Tea		
Dinner	Great Grapefruit 1 cup Burdock, Sassafras, and Hops Relaxer Tea	Combine ¼ **(½)** cup each: peaches, pears, apricots, and grapes Top with 1 **(2)** oz. cashews 1 cup Burdock,	Combine ¼ **(½)** cup each: Balsamic Strawberries, blueberries, apricots, and mangoes

WHEN	WEDNESDAY	THURSDAY	FRIDAY
Dinner (cont'd)		Sassafras, and Hops Relaxer Tea	Top with 1 **(2)** oz. pecans 1 cup Burdock, Sassafras, and Hops Relaxer Tea

Synthesizer Elixirs for Both Women and Men

Thyroid Energizer: Stimulating both your thyroid and adrenal glands, the carrot juice along with the beet juice builds your blood; provides the nutrients needed by your thyroid gland to produce its hormone, thyroxine; increases your circulation; balances your hormonal levels; and literally rebuilds your skin.

Carrots: 6 oz. juice (about 6 carrots)
Beets: 3 oz. juice (about 2 beets)
Cucumber: 3 oz. juice (about 1 cucumber)
Water: 2 oz.

Adrenal Stabilizer: With carrot juice, parsley is the great adrenal stabilizer and also balances the thyroid gland, cleanses the kidneys, brightens the eyes, and brings oxygen into the body.

Carrots: 6 oz. juice (about 6 carrots)
Parsley: 3 oz. juice (about 3 bunches)
Water: 2 oz.

Immune Energizer: Full of vitamins and iron, this juice energizes, nourishes, and regenerates your whole immune system. Spinach builds iron-rich blood, which nourishes your immune warriors, cleans out toxins, and burns up excess fat. It also supplies the iron needed by your thyroid gland. Dandelion greens clear out a toxic liver and support your thymus gland.

Carrots: 6 oz. juice (about 6 carrots)
Spinach: 3 oz. (about 1 bunch)
Dandelion greens: 2 oz. (about 1 large bunch) (optional)
Water: 2 oz.

Pituitary Balancer: The "great healer," carrot juice, is full of the vitamins and minerals most needed by your pituitary: the vitamins A, D, B, C, E, and K and especially the minerals calcium and magnesium. Celery juice calms your nerves and balances your pituitary gland. Parsley is the great adrenal stabilizer.

Carrots: 6 oz. juice (about 6 carrots)
Celery: 3 oz. juice (about 1 bunch)
Parsley: 2 oz. juice (about 2 bunches)
Water: 2 oz.

Synthesizer Food Choices

				Proteins				
MEAT	**FOWL**	**FISH**		**DAIRY**	**NUTS**	**SEEDS**	**LEGUMES**	**FRUIT PROTEIN**
Strong Acid	Strong Acid	Strong Acid	Weak Acid	Acid Forming	Strong Acid	Strong Acid	Strong Acid	Strong Acid
Venison	Turkey	Mackerel	Anchovies	Soy milk	Pine nuts	Pumpkin	Peanuts	Avocados
Veal	Goose	Roe	Caviar	(also under	Water	seeds		
Beef, lean	Squab	Halibut	Herring	"Legumes")	chestnuts	Sunflower	Acid	AVOID
Lamb,	Chicken	Red snapper	Sardines		Cashews	seeds	Forming	Strong
lean	Duck	Sole		AVOID	Coconut	Squash seeds		Alkaline
Rabbit	Frog legs	Tuna	Shellfish			Safflower	Lentils	
Organ	Quail	Bluefish	Strong Acid	All dairy	Weak	seeds	Soybeans	Olives
meats	Pheasant	Eel			Alkaline	Sesame	Soy milk	
Pork		Swordfish	Abalone			seeds	Adzuki beans	
(ham,	Acid	Squid			Coconut milk	Flaxseeds	Black beans	
bacon,	Forming	(calamari)	Acid			Chia seeds	Kidney beans	
roast)		Cod	Forming		Acid		Navy beans	
	Eggs	Mullet			Forming	AVOID	Pinto beans	
AVOID		Haddock	Crab		(Nonsalted)		Red beans	
	AVOID	Ocean perch	Lobster			None		
None		Sturgeon	Scallops		Pecans		Weak	
	None	Octopus	Clams and		Pistachios		Alkaline	
		(scungilli)	mussels		Walnuts			
			Shrimp and		Brazil nuts		Soybean curd	
		Acid	crayfish		Macadamias		(tofu)	
		Forming			Chestnuts			
			Weak Acid		Almonds		AVOID	
		Carp						
		Yellowtail	Oysters		Weak Acid		None	
		tuna						
		Salmon	AVOID		Filberts			
		Hake			(hazelnuts)			
		Lake perch	None		Hickory nuts			
		Bass						
		Trout			AVOID			
					None			

Carbohydrates						
GRAINS	HIGH-STARCH LEGUMES	HIGH-STARCH VEGETABLES	SLIGHTLY STARCHY VEGETABLES	NONSTARCHY VEGETABLES		
Strong Acid	**Strong Acid**	**Strong Acid**	**Weak Acid**	**Strong Acid**	**Weak Acid**	**Alkaline Forming**
Popcorn	Black-eyed peas (cowpeas)	Field corn	Beets, cooked	Mushrooms	Chicory	Swiss chard, raw
Corn grits		Sweet corn	Parsnips	Garlic	Onions	Spinach, cooked
Rice bran	**Acid Forming**	Potatoes	Jicama		Cucumbers	Kale, raw
Millet				**Acid Forming**	Radishes	Lettuce: cos,
Barley	Lima beans	**Weak Alkaline**	**Weak Alkaline**		Summer squash,	romaine, dark
Corn meal	Garbanzo beans			Bamboo shoots	raw	green, white
Wheat	(chickpeas)	Acorn squash	Carrots	Green peas		Watercress
Couscous	Great northern		Rutabagas	Sugar peas	**Weak Alkaline**	Alfalfa sprouts
Bulgur	beans	**Acid Forming**		Mungbeans and		Dandelion greens
(cracked	Split peas		**Acid Forming**	sprouts	Summer squash,	Arugula
wheat)	White (fava)	Yams		Chili peppers	cooked	Beet greens, raw
Rye	beans	Pumpkin, raw	Beets, raw	Asparagus	Leeks	
Oats				Celeriac root	Garden cress	**Strong Alkaline**
Pastinas	**AVOID**	**Weak Acid**	**AVOID**	Sweet peppers	Chinese cabbage	
(egg)				Brussels sprouts	Snap beans	Parsley
Sprouted grain	None	Butternut squash	None	Cauliflower, raw	Yellow beans	
bread		Hubbard squash		Tomatoes	Turnips	**Eliminate If You**
		Sweet potatoes			Scallions	**Have Allergies**
Acid Forming		Pumpkin, canned		**Seaweeds**	Broccoli	**of Any Kind**
Farina		**Eliminate If**		Strong alkaline	Lettuce: butter,	Eggplant
Brown rice		**You Have**		seaweeds are	Boston, iceberg	Tomatoes
Basmati brown		**Any Allergies**		permissible due	Celery	Peppers
rice				to possible low	Endive	
Wild rice		Corn		thyroid function.	Radicchio	**AVOID**
Buckwheat		Corn meal		Agar-agar	Yellow dock, raw	**Strong Alkaline**
(kasha)		Corn grits		Kelp	Cabbage, raw	
Quinoa		Potatoes		Irish moss	Okra, raw	Kale, cooked
				Dulse	Spinach, raw	Collards
Eliminate If		**AVOID**		Arame	Fennel	Swiss chard,
You Have Any						cooked
Allergies		None		**Weak Acid**	**Alkaline**	Mustard greens,
Wheat				Cauliflower,	**Forming**	cooked
Wheat germ				cooked		Beet greens,
Rye				Eggplant	Yellow dock,	cooked
Barley				Artichokes	cooked	Turnip greens,
				Shallots	Chicory greens	cooked
AVOID				Gingerroot	Horseradish	Lamb's-quarter
Strong Alkaline				Salsify	Cabbage, cooked	Mustard spinach
Amaranth				Soybean sprouts	Okra, cooked	
grain and				Kohlrabi		
flakes						

FRUIT		OILS	CONDIMENTS	TEAS
Acid Forming	**Weak Alkaline**	**Strong Acid**	**Weak Acid**	**Licorice root:** strengthens the adrenals (Don't use if you have high blood pressure.)
Litchis	Elderberries	Avocado	Vinegar	
Passion fruit	Sapotes	Corn	Honey	**Black cohosh:** balances your hormones
Groundberries	Cranberries	Soybean	Mustard	
Pomegranates	Currants	Peanut		**Alfalfa leaf:** blood cleanser and immune builder
Crab apples	Lemons	Cottonseed	**Weak Alkaline**	
Peaches	Cherries	Olive	Pickles	**Bayberry:** stimulates the adrenals and thyroid
Weak Acid	Blackberries	Safflower		
	Limes	Sunflower	**Weak Acid**	**Dandelion root:** metabolizes cholesterol
Guavas		Flaxseed	Soy sauce	
Loquats	**Melons (Eat Alone)**	Walnut		**Burdock root:** regulates insulin levels
Cherimoya	Watermelon	Apricot	*AVOID*	
Grapes: muscat, Tokay	Muskmelon	Almond	Yeast—in all forms	**Juniper berry:** strengthens your adrenals and kidneys
Quince	Cantaloupe		Cane syrup	
Tamarinds	Casaba	*AVOID*	Cane sugar	**Fennel:** curbs your appetite and aids digestion
Apples	Crenshaw	*(Saturated Fats)*	Brown sugar	
Apricots	Honeydew	Mayonnaise	Molasses: blackstrap or light	**White oak bark:** strengthens the thyroid gland
Prickly pears		Butter		
Pears	**Sweet Fruit**	Margarine	Sorghum	**Gota kula:** high in magnesium; stimulates the thyroid
Mangoes	**Acid Forming**		Maple syrup	
Alkaline Forming	Persimmons			**Comfrey:** feeds and soothes the pituitary
	Plantains			
Loganberries	Bananas			**Chamomile:** high in magnesium; feeds the pituitary; soothes and calms (*Careful:* May cause allergies.)
Oranges				
Clementines	**Weak Acid**			
Tangerines	Apricots, dried			
Kumquats	Raisins			
Kiwifruits	Prunes			
	Dates			
Weak Alkaline				
	Weak Alkaline			
Boysenberries	Figs			
Grapefruit				
Raspberries	**Alkaline Forming**			
Strawberries	Pineapple			
Plums				
Acerola cherries	*AVOID*			
Blueberries	**Strong Alkaline**			
Nectarines	Rhubarb			
Gooseberries				
Pokeberries				
Papaya				
Grapes: Concord, Thompson				

Your On-Program Cheat Sheet

Naturally there will be days when you just have to cheat. No problem. There's room in the Your Body, Your Diet plan for you to indulge yourself a little and still take off weight. Besides, if you try to change everything about how you eat at once and never give yourself a break, you're bound to end up frustrated.

For your synthesizer profile, pretzels are the cheat food of choice. Raisins, dates, and other fruits are also just perfect for your meta-type. The best pretzels for you are sourdough, without salt (try Snyder's of Hanover)— and baked, not fried.

Here's a complete list of snacks to help you beat the munchies—fast:

- *Hard pretzel:* 1 unsalted
- *Raisins:* ¼ cup, or 2 oz.
- *Dates:* ¼ cup pitted, or 2 oz.
- *Prunes:* ½ cup pitted, or 4 oz.
- *Apricots, dried:* ½ cup pitted, or 4 oz.
- *Banana:* 1

You'll need to follow some guidelines in order to make these foods work for you. Otherwise, using these cheat foods in the wrong way could undermine your goal of losing weight.

CHEAT-FOOD GUIDELINES
- *Eat your cheat foods only at the recommended times.* Cheat foods should be eaten no oftener than once per week, on the weekends (when you're not under stress), and at one meal or one time—only.
- *Eat only the amount suggested.* Your body can handle a small amount of these foods without triggering excessive insulin production. If you eat a large amount, your insulin level will spike and turn your "treat" into a "bad trick" of blubber.
- *Eat only one cheat food at a time.* Don't have several together or you'll wreak havoc with your metabolism and digestion. For instance, raisins *and* pretzels will send you over the top.
- *Never eat your cheat foods when you're under stress.* I guarantee you that's a surefire way to add pounds, not lose them. Eat cheat foods only when you're relaxed—usually on a weekend. Otherwise, your digestion shuts down and your insulin rises, and you become a veritable fat factory.
- *Never eat your cheat foods late at night.* You'll end up having a rest-

less night's sleep, and it's mandatory for you to sleep deeply so your body can regenerate itself.

Synthesizer Healers and Helpers: Vitamins, Minerals, and Amino Acids

This section of your program is dedicated to the additions to the food plan that will help you lose weight even faster and improve your overall health and well-being. As I discussed in chapter 13, you can enhance the benefits of your meta-type diet with vitamins, minerals, and supplements tailored for you.

For synthesizers I recommend a gentle, full-spectrum multiple amino acid vitamin and mineral complex containing only those essential nutrients that support the sympathetic nervous system. This will speed up your weight-loss program, help tone your muscles, and give you abundant good health. The nutrients recommended here can be purchased at your local health-food store or ordered from the companies listed in appendix 2.

If the controlling endocrine gland governed by your dominant nervous system is out of balance, either hyperactive or hypoactive, you may need some additional nutrients in the form of amino acids, vitamins, or minerals besides the full-spectrum amino acid, vitamin, and mineral formula supporting your opposite nervous system. In your case your dominant endocrine gland is the pituitary.

As you learned earlier, this tiny gland in the brain delivers powerful hormones that control everything from your wake-up alertness to nighttime rest and recuperation. It governs the growth hormone that can trigger not only how you repair cells but how you fight aging. It also musters fat and the sex hormones that determine not only your fertility but your libido as well.

Your pituitary's daytime routine is to crank out the jolt of electricity under the hypothalamus's influence to get your adrenals and thyroid working. We'll talk more in a moment about your weaker thyroid and adrenals, which need more support to finish the job.

Your pituitary's nighttime role provides you with plenty of regenerating growth hormone and the sex hormones, testosterone and estrogen, which rule your sex drive and fertility. When you're in balance, your abundant and powerful growth hormone (GH) lets you keep that age-defying glow. Its thyroid-stimulating hormone (TSH) stimulates your thyroid hormones to burn carbohydrates and break down fats to rebuild those cells and rid yourself of toxic wastes.

Along with the focus on your pituitary gland, some additional attention must be given to your weaker opposite sympathetic endocrine gland, your thyroid. This energy-producing gland, when out of balance, produces too little of the hormones essential to boost your metabolic generator and burn off those excess pounds. Its hormone, thyroxine, not only has that daylong task of governing the production of energy, but at night it switches signals to rest and repair your worn cells. Your other energy-producing glands—the adrenals and the thymus, which also controls your immune protection—are on the weaker side, too, and need support.

Your meta-type's adrenal glands, the dominant glands of the yang sympathetic nervous system, aren't very strong in the mornings—even when you're in metabolic balance—and you are susceptible to the stress response, fatigue, allergies, and depression. Your weaker thymus gland also can make your immune system falter, leaving you vulnerable to colds, flu, or infections.

You won't want to get out of bed in the mornings, you'll feel fatigued during the day, and you'll have spurts of energy at night. Along with packing on the pounds, these glandular weaknesses may trigger hair loss, irregular menstrual periods, or low sex drive.

Sugar and refined carbohydrates—which, as I mentioned earlier, are exactly the foods loved by bacteria and viruses—will further weaken your thymus and also cause your adrenals to burn out quickly.

The nutrients needed to gently balance your pituitary gland are glucose and oxygen; the amino acids phenylalanine, tryptophan, gamma-aminobutyric acid (GABA), and glycine; vitamin B complex and choline; vitamin C; unsaturated fatty acids (vitamin F); and the mineral magnesium.

Glucose is provided by the honey in the Call-to-Arms Weight-Buster Morning Drink, which will give your blood sugar a morning jump start.

For *oxygen* do lots of deep breathing, sending that oxygenated blood to the brain quickly.

Amino acids (proteins)—phenylalanine, tryptophan, GABA, and glycine—are the building blocks most effective for gently boosting your meta-type. Since your diet is so high in all the amino acids in meat, fish, fowl, seeds, and nuts, I don't recommend the addition of any *extras*, but I do want you to be aware of how important the amino acids are to your meta-type so you will understand why protein is critical in your diet. Phenylalanine is essential to excite your yang sympathetic nervous system and is a precursor to tyrosine, which regulates all your energizing and fat-burning adrenal and thyroid hormones. Tryptophan works similarly on the yin parasympathetic nervous system for the soothing neurotransmitters serotonin and tryptamine, and the pituitary's growth hormone. GABA, known as the natural Valium, helps ease anxiety and depression, while glycine, similar to GABA, helps calm anxiety and is also essential to regeneration and fighting fat.

The standard daily intake level of protein should be about 1 gram to 1.5 grams per pound of body weight. To convert grams to ounces, multiply the gram figure by .0353.

I suggest you take a full complement of the *B-complex vitamins* to feed your pituitary. B_1 nourishes your pituitary and helps to stabilize your brain's emotional messages; B_3 helps to eliminate negative emotional shifts and reduces irritability, anxiety, and depression; B_5 also reduces irritability, restlessness, and mental depression; B_6 calms your hypothalamus and central nervous system; B_{12} reduces irritability, feeds your pituitary, and alleviates anxiety, depression, apathy, and nervousness. Choline along with B_5 produces the other neurotransmitter of your parasympathetic nervous system, acetylcholine, which stimulates all glandular cells as well as skeletal, cardiac, and smooth muscle cells and is used in all the neuromuscular junctions in your parasympathetic system. Choline works together with inositol as a fat-buster duo that transports and breaks down fat while soothing nerves. They occur naturally in the form of lecithin.

Vitamin C supports your pituitary by utilizing the key amino acids that produce your parasympathetic and sympathetic nerve messengers, tryptophan and tyrosine.

Magnesium, the pituitary's magic mineral, energizes your pituitary to receive messages from the hypothalamus and transmit them throughout the body. It regulates your other hormones, maintains the acid-alkaline balance of your body, and is critical in regulating the metabolism of blood sugar, digesting proteins, and utilizing calcium and vitamin C.

Unsaturated fatty acids are needed for producing energy, stimulating growth, preventing cholesterol deposits, burning fat, and stimulating the function of all glands, especially your pituitary. But you should be getting plenty of unsaturated fatty acids in your Call-to-Arms Weight-Buster Morning Drink in the form of the flaxseed oil or in the oils taken in your diet.

The following supplements support your weaker thyroid gland:

• *Tyrosine,* an amino acid, sparks your thyroid's energizing hormone, thyroxine. Your new eating strategy with plenty of proteins should be sufficient, but if you experience sugar and bread cravings, this is a signal that you may be low and a supplement may be in order.

• *Vitamin B complex:* For thyroid support the B_{12} and folic acid in the vitamin B complex are important. The other Bs have already been discussed.

• *Vitamin C:* Its role here is to help conserve iodine in your body and metabolize tyrosine, which are crucial to building blood capillaries, healthy skin, and the healing process—as well as burning fat.

• *Zinc:* This is another magic mineral for you. It stimulates the pancreatic enzymes and insulin production, reducing cholesterol. It's a major factor as you front-load your diet with proteins to recapture its meta-balance.

The Bottom Line

By taking a complete amino acid, vitamin, and mineral combination based on the formulation for your general metabolic type, you'll be supplied with the nutrients needed to support your complementary side, the sympathetic nervous system. Then you may want to add a few of the vitamins and minerals we've just discussed, which are also listed in the accompanying table of recommended nutrients. If you're interested, turn to appendix 3 for a more in-depth study of the vitamins, minerals, and amino acids for your meta-type. If you prefer to get all your nutrients from foods, I've listed the foods highest in vitamin, mineral, and amino acid content in the accompanying table.

Synthesizer Vitamin, Mineral, and Amino Acid Food Sources

Pituitary	
Amino acids B complex	All animal proteins (meat, fish, and fowl) and soy products • B_1: torula yeast, sunflower seeds, rice bran, wheat germ, pine nuts, dried coriander leaf, safflower seeds, soybeans, alfalfa seeds, sesame seeds, and rye flour (dark) • B_2: almonds, turnip greens, wheat bran, and soybeans • B_3 *(niacin):* fish, nuts, bran flakes, sesame seeds, and sunflower seeds • B_6: rice bran, wheat bran, sunflower seeds, avocados, bananas, corn, fish, brown rice, soybeans, and whole grains • B_{15}: grains, cereals, rice, apricot kernels, and torula yeast
Lecithin *or* choline and inositol (called lipotropic factors)	• *Choline:* soybeans, cabbage, wheat bran, navy beans, alfalfa leaf meal, rice polishings, rice bran, whole grains, hominy, turnips, and blackstrap molasses • *Inositol:* wheat germ, citrus fruits, blackstrap molasses, fruits, whole grains, bran, nuts, legumes, and vegetables

Vitamin C	Acerola cherries, rose hips, citrus fruit, gauvas, hot green peppers, black currants, parsley, turnip greens, poke greens, and mustard greens
Essential fatty acids—vitamin F	• *Oils:* safflower, sunflower, corn, olive, wheat germ, soy, cottonseed, and cod-liver • *Nuts:* walnuts, Brazil nuts, and almonds
Magnesium	Cottonseed, peanut, and soybean flour; sesame seeds; wheat bran and germ; blackstrap molasses; nuts; peanut butter; whole grains; and torula yeast
Thyroid Gland	
Tyrosine	All animal proteins (meat, fowl, and fish) and soy products
B complex	As listed under "Pituitary"
Vitamin C	As listed under "Pituitary"
Zinc	Spices, wheat bran, crab, and popcorn
Essential fatty acids—vitamin F	As listed under "Pituitary"

There are a few easy things to remember about taking the supplements:

• If you are taking amino acids, try to take them on an empty stomach. (They need adequate amounts of stomach enzymes to be broken down properly.)
• If possible, take enzymes with your meals to aid in your food digestion.
• Take vitamins and minerals after you've eaten, which helps their assimilation.
• The water-soluble vitamins—B complex, vitamin C, and vitamin P (bioflavonoids)—can be taken at any time.
• Your body isn't used to concentrated food substances, so I recommend that you introduce one type of vitamin or mineral into your regimen every few days. Gently and easily is the name of the game.

Taking these extra vitamins, minerals, and supplements will require work—there's no mistaking that. Just as you have to plan meals with the right ingredients, you'll need to organize these. But as your metabolic system moves back into balance, you'll reduce the number of pills you'll need. And along the way, you'll discover that the dividend of glowing good health pays off quickly enough to make Wall Street envious.

Synthesizer Recommended Nutrients

ENDOCRINE GLAND	NUTRIENT	WOMEN			MEN		
		Number	Strength	Times per Day	Number	Strength	Times per Day
Pituitary	B complex	1–2	50–75 mg	2	1–2	100–125 mg	2
	Choline and						
	inositol	1	500 mg	1–2	2	500 mg	1–2
	Vitamin C (buffered)	1–2	1,000 mg	2–3	1–3	1,000 mg	3
	Magnesium	1	250 mg	1–2	1	500 mg	2
Thyroid	Tyrosine	1	500 mg	2–3	2	500 mg	3
	B complex	See under "Pituitary"	—	—	See under "Pituitary"	—	—
	Vitamin C (buffered)	See under "Pituitary"	—	—	See under "Pituitary"	—	—
	Zinc	1	30 mg	1	2	30 mg	1
	Essential fatty						
	acids	1	300 mg	2	2	300 mg	2–3
	or lecithin	1	1,200 mg	1–2	1	1,200 mg	2–3

Stocking Up

You've now finished reading about the program and are well on your way to a brand-new you. Just wait and see—you'll be slim, sexy, and full of bounce to every ounce. Now to get started, you'll need to stock up and organize. The accompanying list shows all the foods you'll need for the coming week. Double-check this list against your weekly menu and make any adjustments you feel are necessary. Happy regeneration!

Weekly Shopping List for Synthesizers

Larger quantities for men are shown in **boldface**.

PRODUCE

Fruit
1 Grapefruit
3 Apricots
1 pt. Strawberries
1 pt. Blueberries
2 Pears
1 lg. Mango
2 Peaches
1 sm. bunch Green grapes
6 Lemons

Vegetables
1 lb. Ginger, fresh
1 lb. Yellow (Spanish) onions
5 lb. Carrots
2 Cucumbers
4 lb. Spinach
1 bunch Celery
1 bunch Dandelion greens
   (optional)
1 lg. Yellow squash
1 lg. Zucchini
2 10-oz. Mushrooms
2 bulbs Garlic
8 Plum tomatoes
1 Red onion
1 sm. Japanese eggplant
1 lb. Asparagus
2 Red peppers
2 **(3)** Beets
1 sm. **(lg.)** ear Sweet corn
1 sm. bulb Fennel
1 sm. bunch Radishes
¼ lb. (or 10 oz. frozen) Peas
3 Yukon gold potatoes

¼ lb. Sugar snap peas
¼ lb. Green or yellow beans
1 bunch Basil, fresh
5 bunches Parsley

Salad Greens
2 heads Boston lettuce
1 head Red leaf lettuce
1 Chicory
1 Escarole
1 Radicchio
1 box Radish sprouts

GROCERIES
8 oz. Pecans
11 **(19½)** oz. Cashews
3 oz. Pine nuts
2 **(6)** oz. Sesame seeds
1 16-oz can Chickpeas
½ lb. Couscous
1 8-oz. jar Dijon mustard
1 bottle Apple cider vinegar
1 bottle Balsamic vinegar
1 bottle Rice vinegar
1 16-oz. jar Dark or Tupelo
   honey
2 qt. Soy milk
1 container Soy-based protein
   powder
1 container Kelp powder or blue-
   green algae
1 package Seaweed of choice
1 bottle Almond extract
1 bottle Ad-Vita or Knudsen
   cranberry juice concentrate
1 tube Harissa (Moroccan spice)
Saffron, dried thyme, cinnamon,

nutmeg, cardamom seed,
turmeric, cayenne pepper
Soy sauce
Herbal teas (include the
ingredients for Burdock,
Sassafras, and Hops Relaxer.)
Safflower oil
Flaxseed oil

DAIRY

18 Eggs

MEAT AND FISH

2 pieces: 1 4-oz, 1 10-oz. **(1 6-oz.,
1 1-lb.)** cutlet Chicken breast
(no skin)
2 pieces: 1 4-oz., 1 6-oz. **(1 6-oz.,
1 8-oz.)** filet Salmon
4 oz. (peeled weight) Shrimp
1 9-oz **(15-oz.)** filet Beef (filet
mignon)

18 The Balanced Synthesizer Diet

If you are a true balanced synthesizer, you have probably fought—and lost—the battle to keep your weight under control quite a few times. Well, you can relax. Once you master your personal diet plan, your worries about your weight will be a thing of the past. I am going to introduce you to a whole new way of eating, living, and feeling great. Just a few quick words on how your personal balanced synthesizer diet works, then on to the menus. As you read, remember:

- Your dominant gland is the pancreas.
- Your weakest gland is the thymus.
- You're most likely to gain weight in your hips and thighs.

The Science behind Your System

You are the most balanced of all the synthesizers. You'll *naturally* receive a greater proportion of nerve stimulation to those endocrine glands and organs responsible for the growth, repair, and regeneration of your body—primarily your pancreas gland, with its powerful enzymes and master hormones, glucagon and insulin, which spell the difference between a body that feels like a "fat factory" and one that feels like a sleek, energy-efficient machine.

In turn, your pancreas is supported by your parasympathetic meta-type partners, the pituitary and sex glands, along with your dominant organs of digestion—the salivary glands, stomach, liver, gallbladder, small intestine, large intestine, kidneys, and bladder. Unlike the pure synthesizer, who receives little stimulation from the sympathetic nervous system, you have somewhat more stimulation to your sympathetic energy-producing glands—the thyroid, adrenals, thymus, spleen, heart, and lungs.

Your body, like that of your fellow synthesizers, is *mainly* focused on its repair and regeneration, but you have more of a balancing influence as well, from the process of generating energy and stabilizing it during the day.

With this low nerve stimulation to your energy-producing glands, you tend to be a slow metabolizer, and—again like the pure synthesizer—you produce a fair amount of stomach acid. Consequently, you break down your foods slowly, so digestion takes place in an aerobic environment (with oxygen present) as your food mixes with your HCl (hydrochloric acid—that is, stomach acid) and oxygen. (Refer to chapter 3 for a more in-depth discussion.)

This oxygen-filled digestion results in your burning off energy or sugar instantly in your cells (remember, "air fans fire"). Like the pure synthesizer, you require the heavier and slower-burning proteins; but unlike your meta-mate, you can handle more of the *complex* carbohydrates, since the action of your adrenals and thyroid is stronger than that of the synthesizer.

But *refined* carbohydrates and sugars already are quick-burning. So you need to eat a combination of slow-burning proteins and slower-burning, energy-producing complex carbohydrates to keep your energy levels balanced. Quick-burning refined breads, sugars, and carbohydrates are your downfall, giving you that Ping-Pong effect of energy highs and lows. The slower-burning proteins are your lifesavers.

With a predisposition toward an *alkaline body chemistry* and its slower digesting and fast oxidizing capacity, you'll tend to have:

- Good to generous production of stomach acid—although there can be less if production is suppressed by the stress response
- Tissue alkalinity
- Good production of pancreatic enzymes
- Balanced production of pancreatic insulin—if you are not under stress

You'll also incline toward low levels of cellular toxic waste. When the oxygen-rich nutrients reach your cells for transformation into energy or to feed them, they help to clear out any unwanted debris.

Balance is important for you, since your emotional side is strong—with feelings first, intellectual sorting-out later. If you're not balanced with the proper foods to boost your thinking processes, you tend to be pulled further into the emotional side.

Metabolically speaking, the ideal diet for you includes acid and slower-oxidizing proteins, in the form of meat, fowl, fish, and dairy products, along with slower-burning *complex* carbohydrates found in grains, legumes, and some vegetables and fruits.

As I mentioned, you need to avoid refined carbohydrates (sugars and starches) as well as packaged and refined products that have too much sugar. Excess saturated fat slows you down and clogs your arteries. Your balanced synthesizer food formula will look like this:

- Protein: 50 percent
- Carbohydrates: 30 percent
- Fat: 20 percent

Balanced Synthesizer Food Choices

After one month on the Your Body, Your Diet plan, you will not only drop excess fat but also be introduced to a level of vitality and good health that you never dreamed possible. Once you have looked at the basic menus, you will see food lists that will show you the wide variety of delicious foods that are best for you. Suggested vitamins, minerals, and other supplements are also included. The next three subsections give you an overview of the basic principles you'll be following.

What to Avoid

Steer clear of refined carbohydrates, sugars, and breads. I know this seems like a tough set of restrictions to follow, but you'll quickly learn why making these changes is so important. These are the foods that put you on a blood sugar roller coaster, in which your energy levels zoom up or down, with little control or predictability. They overstimulate your dominant gland (the pancreas), keeping you off balance and eventually overweight.

Cravings for sugar, breads, and refined carbohydrates—all those "goodies" from your morning bagel to cakes, cookies, and those gooey desserts and packaged goods—are a sign that you've overstimulated your pancreas, depleted your short-term energy, and run out of fuel. But these foods burn off instantly for your meta-type, so the pancreas gets on a treadmill, producing more and more insulin, which ferries the fat directly to your worst nightmare spots—your lower half, with its fatty estrogen-primed areas. Also, sugar intensifies your already strong emotional side.

You'll be amazed at how much better you look and feel without these foods literally weighing you down.

The following table gives you an overview of the foods and other substances that do *not* suit your meta-type.

Your *Never* Foods

REFINED CARBOHYDRATES	WHITE-FLOUR PRODUCTS	SUGAR	FATS
All packaged foods: Breads Cakes Cookies Doughnuts Crackers, etc. All foods containing: Synthetic additives Sweeteners	Bread Cakes Pasta Doughnuts Cookies Muffins, etc.	White sugar Beet sugar Cane sugar Brown sugar	Butter Margarine Mayonnaise

What to Fill Up On

Meat, poultry, fish, dairy, seeds, nuts, and legumes are your foods of choice. You see, there are lots of absolutely delectable foods on your eating plan, and they are all just perfect for you. The slow-burning proteins help regulate and stabilize your blood sugar and help you think faster and clearer—while keeping your energy high. All of the foods also help your weaker thymus, thyroid, and adrenal glands to boost energy and eliminate fat. So you'll have plenty of opportunities to enjoy great-tasting meals while watching your excess weight disappear.

The accompanying table lists the foods that best suit your meta-type.

The foods that are required by your specific metabolic type (unsaturated fatty acids and proteins) are exactly the ones that feed and support your weaker endocrine gland, the thymus.

Your *Always* Foods

PROTEINS		CARBOHYDRATES		FATS
Food	Times per Week	Food	Times per Week	
Meat: abundant	2	Grains: abundant	1–2	*Moderate* amount of unsaturated fatty acids— cold-pressed vegetable or nut oils
Fowl: abundant	2	Legumes: abundant	1	
Fish: abundant	2	Starchy vegetables: abundant	1	
Dairy: large variety	1–2	Slightly starchy vegetables: variety	1–2	Choose from your food plan.
Seeds/nuts: abundant	2	Nonstarchy vegetables: small variety	Daily	
Legume protein: abundant	1–2	Fruit: small variety	Daily	

How to Speed Up Weight Loss

Here are a few other tips to stimulate faster weight loss:

- Chew your food slowly and well.
- Try to avoid drinking more than one glass of water or liquid during your meals. Drinking large amounts of liquid during meals dilutes the precious enzymes needed for your digestion.
- Have at least six to eight glasses of water during the day, *not* at mealtimes.
- When eating vegetarian meals, mix 60 percent grains to 40 percent legumes (beans) or tofu (soybean curd) for a complete protein complement. Tofu is an excellent accompaniment to grains.

Keeping Your Pancreas in Balance

As a balanced synthesizer, you are the most vulnerable of the metatypes to stress and can easily be pulled into emotional extremes—anger, exhaustion, depression, and sexual problems—when you're not eating right. And you easily pack on those unwanted, unsightly pounds. Remember how kids "overdose" on candy and ricochet off the walls? Remember the infamous "Twinkie defense"—that a murder was committed while the defendant was allegedly experiencing a sugar-induced psychosis? Well, I wouldn't go that far, but your meta-type, like the synthesizer's, *is* vulnerable to intense sugar-induced emotions.

Your dominant endocrine gland, the pancreas, governs several processes that are essential in controlling your weight—and your repair and rest functions. You know it best, perhaps, as an insulin pump to control blood sugar, creating those spikes and slumps in energy. But it also produces the prized enzymes that break down the carbohydrates, fats, and proteins, and it generates the hormone glucagon, which liberates energy from your liver and muscles. Insulin malfunctions are well known to most of us as diabetes (excessive blood sugar) and hypoglycemia (low blood sugar).

Your pancreas is located in the "center," where your chest meets your stomach in the area where your rib cage separates. In Chinese medicine it's known as your "emotional brain." To Western science it's where the major nerve (vagus nerve) controlling your parasympathetic system is focused, governing your regeneration and repair functions. These pancreatic juices kick in as your food, broken down by stomach acid, moves into the small intestine.

If you are under any kind of stress—and with your somewhat weaker adrenal glands, which control the stress response—you can readily be drawn into the more emotional synthesizer profile. You may even be remarkably open to moderate to severe depressions and allergies when under stress.

Or if you're drawn into the metabolic profile of the mixed synthesizer, you'll tend to be more dominated by your sex glands and could easily be engulfed in sexual activity to burn off that excess or relieve depression—or you may flip to the other extreme and sexually shut down. You must learn to stay in your center—that is, learn balanced moderation.

When you're not in metabolic balance, your reactions to emotional stress, too much mental stimulation, or fatigue tend to bring on those cravings—and you grab the quick fixes for energy, only to crash.

Losing the ability to stabilize blood sugar, you'll overproduce insulin, develop "hyperinsulinemia," or carbohydrate intolerance, and immediately store all that blood sugar as fat. And here's even more trouble: insulin takes excess blood glucose to your lower regions—and fat will suddenly appear in those saddlebags and other places where you've never seen it before.

Too much of the sugar-insulin yo-yo and you'll wind up with instant energy drops and fatigue—and at times even feel paralyzed with lethargy.

If your pancreas becomes hyperactive, you may be overproducing pancreatic enzymes, which could cause bloating, gas, and very loose bowel movements.

Your body's immune system is also on the line when you're out of balance, since your weakest endocrine gland tends to be your energy-producing thymus gland, which is responsible for your body's immune response—fighting off the hostile invaders, from allergy to disease. This, in turn, depends on your heart's action to keep your immune system's lymphatic pathways open and free-flowing.

States of physical and emotional stress increase a person's sensitivity to allergic attacks. The heavy-duty emotions that are the probable cause of an allergic response are anger, fear, resentment, worry, and lack of self-confidence. So if you've fallen into more of the synthesizer profile, you'll be extremely susceptible to allergies. Studies have shown that certain individuals have allergic reactions to a particular allergen when under stressful conditions but experience no reaction to that allergen when the stress is removed. Imagine that.

The good news in all this, of course, is that your strong pancreas responds quickly to restore and regenerate itself. With just a few quick changes, you'll see those pounds fall off and your energy soar.

Your Balanced Synthesizer Secret Weapons

Now I know—from firsthand experience—just how tough it can be to switch to a whole new way of eating. In addition to having to apply a lot of willpower, you have to give your body time to adjust to your new lifestyle. If you find yourself feeling cranky and frustrated, relax; it's par for the course. It's just a sign that you're shedding those extra pounds and getting back into balance.

The teas and elixirs in this chapter were created to help you sail through the transition phase of your meta-type diet while making the pounds melt away even faster.

Hot Tomato Energizer

For each meta-type there is one food or group of foods that helps to speed up the weight-loss process, and the ones in this subsection are just for you. Since the best way to jump-start your fat-burning mechanisms is to make sure you get a certain combination of nutrients each day, I've created a delicious drink that you can use throughout your diet to make sure you get all the proper vitamins and enzymes each morning and afternoon.

Your weaker glands—the thymus, adrenals, and thyroid—respond to your pituitary's morning wake-up call in a less than energetic way, so you have to help them along. They need the stimulus of energy-producing foods to get them going.

The energizing drink I've formulated to help wake up your sleepy energy-producing glands and keep them activated is called the Hot Tomato Energizer. Its dynamic ingredients include kelp or blue-green algae, apple cider vinegar, wheat germ oil, capsicum, and tomato juice.

Kelp or *blue-green algae* contains abundant iodine—the mineral required by your weaker energy-producing thyroid gland. Two-thirds of your body's iodine reserve is used by your thyroid gland to make its potent hormone, thyroxine, which is responsible for activating the way your body burns off or uses energy. It influences your mental, physical, and hormonal growth; metabolizes all of your nutrients; stimulates your energy; and regulates the way you oxidize, or burn off, your fat.

Another ingredient in kelp is mannitol—a natural sugar essential to the composition of thyroxine. Mannitol is also an energizer that helps your weaker endocrine glands produce their hormones, in turn activating all the organs and glands of your body—so you burn fat. Kelp is also rich in calcium, a mineral that is absolutely necessary to provide a stable equilibrium between your thyroid and parathyroid glands; it helps to build your bones, stabilizes your nerves, and enlivens your skin and hair.

Apple cider vinegar has long been known as a cure for weight problems, but not just any vinegar will do. It must be the cider vinegar made from apples that still contain their valuable minerals: phosphorus, chlorine, potassium, sodium, magnesium, calcium, sulfur, iron, fluorine, silicon, and many trace minerals.

Apple cider vinegar's secret is that it raises your metabolic rate—speeds up the way you burn fat—by oxygenating your blood. In other words, it allows your bloodstream to be filled with much more oxygen than is normal, which in turn raises the rate at which your cells burn off fat.

Wheat germ oil is the food for your weakest endocrine gland—your thymus—your immune response, and your heart. It's a fatty acid and is part of all your body's cell membranes. Fatty acids also act as major factors in the production of phospholipids, the "good guys" that break down cholesterol and eliminate it from your bloodstream. But one of their main claims to fame is that they are a major source of the nutrients required by your immune system. Wheat germ oil is also rich in vitamin E, which has been found to strengthen your heart muscle.

Capsicum, known as *Capsicum frutescens*, or cayenne pepper, is one of the best-known stimulants for your weaker glands, especially your thymus and adrenals. This fantastic herb will help stimulate the energy of your adrenals and thyroid, quickly raising your metabolic rate, and you'll soon begin to burn off those excess pounds while stimulating your thymus's immune function. Capsicum also increases your heart's action, increases the power of the apple cider vinegar, and promotes the health of all your organs. It's also high in vitamin A, vitamin C (needed for your adrenals), iron, and calcium and contains magnesium, phosphorus, sulfur, potassium, and some of the all-important energy-producing B-complex family.

Tomato juice is the carrier for your stimulating cocktail. Tomatoes are rich in vitamins A, K (good for your immune system), B (releases energy), and C (needed by your adrenals), as well as calcium, iron, phosphorus, and potassium. Of course, fresh tomato juice is the best, but you may use bottled—*not* canned—juice that contains no added salt.

Mixing all of these ingredients together and taking this drink *before breakfast* will wake you right up, energize you, and literally set your body in motion to melt away those excess pounds. (For the recipe, see Hot Tomato Energizer, on page 406.)

Slimming Tea

Another important part of your plan is the herbal tea formula I've created to meet the needs of each meta-type. Each tea will stimulate, harmonize, or help balance your system. In the weekly menus table later in this chapter, you will find suggestions for when to take your tea. To make the tea, you'll need to add a few special ingredients to my Master Weight Loss Tea (see pages 103–05 for instructions).

These supplementary herbs should be added in equal proportions to the herbs already in the basic formula. I suggest you take one to three cups per day of your special tea. The herbs may be purchased at your local health-food store or ordered from the companies listed in appendix 2.

Balanced Synthesizer Slimming Tea

Basic Formula: One Teaspoon Each

Alisma, poria, rhubarb root, red clover tops, alfalfa leaf, hawthorn berry, radish seed, sargassum, Indian chickweed, evergreen artemesia, astragalus root, fleeceflower root, citrus peel

Balanced Synthesizer Slimming Formula: Add One Teaspoon Each

NAME			FUNCTION
Common	Latin	Eastern	
Licorice root	*Radix glycyrrhizae*	Gan cao	Great for supporting and stimulating the adrenals and thyroid—an energizer for your body.
Codonopsis root (Asiabell root)	*Codonopsis pilosula*	Dang shen	Great stimulator of your immune system and thymus gland.
Laminaria	*Lamineria Japonica aresh*	Kun Bu	Stimulates the thyroid gland, speeding up your metabolism; reduces fat.
White atractylodes	*Atractylodes macrocephala*	Bai zhu	Powerful immune stimulant; also helps to reduce water retention.
Safflower	*Carthamus tinctorius*	Hong hua	Opens the pancreas and liver, energizes, balances insulin levels, helps digestion, burns cholesterol, and stimulates the adrenals.
Fennel fruit	*Foeniculum officinale vulgare*	Hui xiang	Excellent for weight loss, opens digestion and liver function, burns fat, and removes waste and mucus.
Gingerroot	*Zingiber officinalis*	Gan jiang	Raises blood pressure; warms; stimulates digestion.

Notes: The thymus gland is supported additionally by astragalus root, and the heart is supported by hawthorn berry—both in the Master Weight-Loss Tea. If you are pregnant, have high blood pressure, or are allergic to grasses or flowers, it's suggested that these teas not be used. Licorice root and gingerroot should not be used if you have high blood pressure.

Rules of the Road

Your Eating Schedule

Since you have the most *natural rhythm* of all the meta-types, you do best eating carbohydrates in the morning, then a combination of carbohydrates and proteins at lunch to maintain your energy level for the remainder of the day and get you across the cortisol dip in the late afternoon. Proteins for dinner would be appropriate to motivate your dominant metabolic characteristic—the repair and regeneration of your body.

Lunch should be an integration of both energy-producing carbohydrates and slow-burning proteins to bridge the energetic gap during the afternoon cortisol crash, when your weaker sympathetic nervous system retires for the day and before your parasympathetic nervous system takes over.

Dinner should consist mainly of proteins that supply you with ample amino acids, vitamins, and minerals to facilitate the repair and regeneration of your body, which take place during the nighttime hours and under the auspices of your own dominant parasympathetic nervous system. Therefore, the key to your eating schedule would be:

- Light to moderate breakfast
- Moderate to substantial lunch
- Medium dinner

Late Afternoon—Making the Most of Your Energy

As you've learned, your least energetic time is in the morning to mid-morning, and your less energetic time is in the late afternoon. Eating balanced meals in proportionate amounts should stave off any late-afternoon energy crashes. However, if you haven't eaten a good lunch of proteins, you'll really feel your blood sugar drop, and if you've also been under pressure, your weaker adrenals won't be able to sustain your energy. This could result in a devastating cortisol drop in the afternoon. You'll experience fatigue, lethargy, moodiness, drowsiness, headaches, and irritability. Don't take the easy out and reach for the carbohydrates. A late-afternoon protein snack will help stabilize your blood sugar and support your energy. For your meta-type a little caffeine, in the form of green tea, would certainly be acceptable.

YOUR LATE-AFTERNOON SNACK
Protein snack: seeds, nuts, fowl, or fish
Hot herbal tea or green tea

Bedtime—Indulging a Little

If you're following your proper diet, you shouldn't need to eat before bed. But if you'd like a snack, stick to protein. If you want to save your afternoon snack and have it before you go to bed, okay. But no more than that. You can handle proteins, since they digest slowly and are the foods that facilitate cellular regeneration. They won't wake you up by their conversion to energy. But *stay away* from carbohydrates. No cookies, candy, bread, fruit, ice cream, and so forth. They quickly convert to blood sugar, and you don't want that extra energy surging through your bloodstream. It will either wake you right up or turn to fat.

Balanced Synthesizer Meals and Menus

Now you've completed the first part of the plan, and here's your reward: the tailor-made diet for your balanced synthesizer meta-type. If you've reached this point in the book, you know that losing weight and keeping it off take more than just watching what you eat. And I'll bet you know a lot more about yourself than you did when you picked up *Your Body, Your Diet*.

The meals presented in this section are designed to meet all the needs of your metabolism while giving you the chance to eat a delicious, wide variety of fresh, nutritious foods. The first week may seem like a big adjustment, but by week two, I assure you, you'll be making your juices and tossing together your special meals like a pro.

Eating the Right Foods at the Right Times

Eating the *right kinds of food* at the *right times* is another key to the success of your weight-loss and rejuvenation program. With the alkaline nature of your balanced synthesizer metabolism, if you eat a majority of alkaline foods, it will throw you way out of balance and increase your alkalinity. Then you'll want to balance yourself, so you'll reach for the wrong acid-type foods—sugars and starches—that just cause you to retain that extra fat, and you'll feel terrible.

What you require are the right slower-burning acid foods to balance out your body chemistry, just as your counterpart, the balanced accelerator

meta-type, is more acid in nature and requires more of the alkaline forming foods.

You've learned that your metabolism tends to be the most balanced of
all the synthesizer meta-types. Along with the acid foods, such as grains
and animal proteins, needed to stabilize your metabolism, you also need
some of the more alkaline foods, such as vegetables and fruits, to balance
out your equilibrium. You are known as the *alkaline* meta-type, with your
natural body pH tending to be 7.4, the pH of blood. (Chapter 3 has a detailed explanation of the acid-alkaline aspect of your meta-type.)

Therefore, your diet should consist of foods that are strong acid, acid
forming, and weak acid. Foods that are strong alkaline and weak alkaline
forming can be eaten one to three times per week. Foods that are the same
as your own pH tendency—alkaline forming—should be avoided. Appendix 5 lists the full spectrum of foods and their pH factors.

Here We Go!

To make this adventure of slimming down to a new and healthy you
fun, I've taken all the guesswork out of how to shop and prepare your
meals. Before you begin, glance through your weekly menus and balanced
synthesizer elixirs in the accompanying tables and look over the vast array
of food selections in your Balanced Synthesizer Food Choices list. At the
end of this chapter, you will find your own balanced synthesizer shopping
list for a week. Then turn to appendix 1 and take a look at the equipment
list (which includes all the supplies you'll need to make this as simple as
possible), your advance food-preparation suggestions for the week, and
your recipes and food-preparation instructions for both men and women.

For any of the foods specified in the weekly menus and recipes, you
may substitute comparable foods from the Balanced Synthesizer Food
Choices list.

Eat only the foods that are indicated for you on your individual food
choices list. If your favorite isn't on there, don't eat it. You can check the
"General Food Choices and Their Calorie Content for Each Meta-Type" in
appendix 5.

You see, it's all done for you, down to the last detail—and my personal
promise to you is that this eating plan will keep your balanced synthesizer
metabolism in perfect balance while helping you achieve a slender, gorgeous physique.

You're on your way to a bright, new, skinny, energetic you. Treat this as
a ritual in celebrating your beauty and regeneration.

Balanced Synthesizer Omnivore Weekly Menus

Acid to Alkaline-Based Foods

Larger quantities for men are shown in **boldface**.

WHEN	SATURDAY	SUNDAY	MONDAY	TUESDAY
On rising	Hot Tomato Energizer			
Breakfast	Poached Salmon and Egg Delight Poached Eggs on Salmon with Toasted Sesame Seeds 1 cup herbal tea or Balanced Synthesizer Slimming Tea	Chipper Chicken Omelet Chicken and Egg Frittata 1 cup herbal tea or Balanced Synthesizer Slimming Tea	Whole-Grain Cereal Breakfast with Soy Milk, Toast, and Fruit Spread 1 cup herbal tea or Balanced Synthesizer Slimming Tea	Slim and Thin Protein Drink 1 cup herbal tea or Balanced Synthesizer Slimming Tea
Midmorning	½ grapefruit **(½ cup strawberries)** 1 cup herbal tea or Balanced Synthesizer Slimming Tea	½ grapefruit **(½ cup strawberries)** 1 cup herbal tea or Balanced Synthesizer Slimming Tea	2 apricots 1 cup herbal tea or Balanced Synthesizer Slimming Tea	½ cantaloupe 1 cup herbal tea or Balanced Synthesizer Slimming Tea
Lunch	Exotic Vegetables with Couscous Tomatoes, Mushrooms, Zucchini, Yellow Squash, Eggplant, and Red Beans Salad Greens 1 cup herbal tea or Balanced Synthesizer Slimming Tea	Health Salad with Ricotta Cheese with Scallions, Radishes, and Grated Carrots 1 cup herbal tea or Balanced Synthesizer Slimming Tea	Health Salad with Filet of Beef with Tomatoes and Mushrooms Fennel, Dill, and Cucumber Salad 1 cup herbal tea or Balanced Synthesizer Slimming Tea	Exotic Vegetables with Couscous Tomatoes, Mushrooms, Zucchini, Yellow Squash, Eggplant, and Red Beans Salad Greens 1 cup herbal tea or Balanced Synthesizer Slimming Tea
Midafternoon	1 cup cucumber sticks **(4 oz. soy milk)** or 1 oz. seeds or nuts **(4 oz. soy milk)** 1 cup herbal tea or Balanced Synthesizer Slimming Tea	1 cup raw sugar snap peas **(4 oz. soy milk)** or 2 oz. fish or chicken **(4 oz. soy milk)** 1 cup herbal tea or Balanced Synthesizer Slimming Tea	1 cup jicama sticks **(4 oz. soy milk)** or 1 oz. seeds or nuts **(4 oz. soy milk)** 1 cup herbal tea or Balanced Synthesizer Slimming Tea	1 cup carrot sticks **(4 oz. soy milk)** or 2 oz. fish or chicken **(4 oz. soy milk)** 1 cup herbal tea or Balanced Synthesizer Slimming Tea

WHEN	SATURDAY	SUNDAY	MONDAY	TUESDAY

Dinner	Mineral Makeover Dinner
	Ginger Shrimp or Scallops
	  with Sugar Snap Peas
	Tomato, Pepper, and
	  Mushroom Salad
	1 glass Balanced
	  Synthesizer Elixir
	1 cup herbal tea or
	  Balanced Synthesizer
	  Slimming Tea
		Think Thin Dinner
		Seared Filet of Beef
		Sautéed Mushrooms
		  and Onions
		Steamed Asparagus
		Radicchio, Fennel, and
		  Spinach Salad
		1 cup herbal tea or
		  Balanced Synthesizer
		  Slimming Tea
			Tasty Tangier Dinner
			Couscous and Moroccan-
			  Style Vegetables
			Steamed Seaweed
			Celery and
			  Cucumber Salad
			1 glass Balanced
			  Synthesizer Elixir
			1 cup herbal tea or
			  Balanced Synthesizer
			  Slimming Tea
				Saucy Salmon Dinner
				Broiled Salmon
				Roast Garlic Mashed
				  Potatoes with Basil
				Sautéed Cherry Tomatoes
				Green Vegetable
				Spinach and
				  Mushroom Salad
				1 cup herbal tea or
				  Balanced Synthesizer
				  Slimming Tea

WHEN	WEDNESDAY	THURSDAY	FRIDAY
On rising	Hot Tomato Energizer		

Breakfast	Whole-Grain
	  Breakfast Cereal
	  with Soy Milk, Toast, and
	  Fruit Spread
	1 cup herbal tea or
	  Balanced Synthesizer
	  Slimming Tea
		Slim and Thin Protein Drink
		1 cup herbal tea or
		  Balanced Synthesizer
		  Slimming Tea
			Whole-Grain
			  Breakfast Cereal
			  with Soy Milk, Toast, and
			  Fruit Spread
			1 cup herbal tea or
			  Balanced Synthesizer
			  Slimming Tea

Midmorning	½ cantaloupe
	1 cup herbal tea
	  or Balanced
	  Synthesizer
	  Slimming Tea
		1 peach
		(½ pear)
		1 cup herbal tea
		  or Balanced
		  Synthesizer
		  Slimming Tea
			1 peach
			(½ pear)
			1 cup herbal tea
			  or Balanced
			  Synthesizer
			  Slimming Tea

Lunch	Health Salad with Cold
	  Salmon
	  with Tomatoes and
	  Mushrooms
	Fennel, Dill, and Cucumber
	  Salad
	1 cup herbal tea or
	  Balanced Synthesizer
	  Slimming Tea
		Poached Chicken Lunch
		Poached Chicken Breast
		  with Roasted Red Pepper
		  Puree
		Steamed Green Beans
		Salad Greens with Sprouts
		1 cup herbal tea or
		  Balanced Synthesizer
		  Slimming Tea
			Health Salad with Cold
			  Salmon,
			  Tomatoes and
			  Mushrooms
			Fennel, Dill, and Cucumber
			  Salad
			1 cup herbal tea or
			  Balanced Synthesizer
			  Slimming Tea

WHEN	WEDNESDAY	THURSDAY	FRIDAY
Midafternoon	1 cup jicama sticks **(4 oz. soy milk)** or 1 oz. seeds or nuts **(4 oz. soy milk)** 1 cup herbal tea or Balanced Synthesizer Slimming Tea	1 cup raw sugar snap peas **(4 oz. soy milk)** or 2 oz. fish or chicken **(4 oz. soy milk)** 1 cup herbal tea or Balanced Synthesizer Slimming Tea	1 cup celery sticks **(4 oz. soy milk)** or 1 oz. seeds or nuts **(4 oz. soy milk)** 1 cup herbal tea or Balanced Synthesizer Slimming Tea
Dinner	*Cheerful Chicken Dinner* Poached Chicken Breast with Roasted Red Pepper Puree Steamed Green Beans Endive and Watercress Salad 1 cup herbal tea or Balanced Synthesizer Slimming Tea	*Pasta Parade with Artichoke,* and Tofu, Tomatoes, and Basil Arugula, Onion, and Watercress Salad 1 cup herbal tea or Balanced Synthesizer Slimming Tea	*Dijon-Garlic Chicken Dinner* Dijon Mustard Chicken Breast Steamed Asparagus Boston Lettuce with Red Onion Salad 1 cup herbal tea or Balanced Synthesizer Slimming Tea

Balanced Synthesizer Food Choices

Proteins									
MEAT	**FOWL**	**FISH**		**DAIRY**		**NUTS**	**SEEDS**	**LEGUMES**	**FRUIT PROTEIN**
Strong Acid	**Strong Acid**	**Strong Acid**	**Acid Forming**	*Note:* If you have	**Acid Forming**	**Strong Acid**	**Strong Acid**	**Strong Acid**	**Strong Acid**
Venison	Turkey	Mackerel	Crab	allergies,	Soy milk	Pine nuts	Pumpkin	Peanuts	Avocados
Veal	Goose	Roe	Lobster	eliminate	(also under	Water	seeds		
Beef,	Squab	Halibut	Scallops	dairy of	"Legumes")	chestnuts	Sunflower	**Acid Forming**	**Strong Alkaline**
lean	Chicken	Red snapper	Clams and	any kind.		Cashews	seeds		
Lamb,	Duck	Sole	mussels		**Weak Acid Cheeses**	Coconut	Squash	Lentils	Olives
lean	Frog legs	Tuna	Shrimp and	**Weak Alkaline (Use Low-Fat)**	**(Use Low-Fat)**		seeds	Soybeans	
Rabbit	Quail	Bluefish	crayfish			**Weak Alkaline**	Safflower	Soy milk	**AVOID**
Organ	Pheasant	Eel			Camembert		seeds	Adzuki	None
meats		Swordfish	**Weak Acid**	Whey	Brie	Coconut	Sesame	beans	
	Acid Forming	Squid	Oysters	Goat's milk	Edam	milk	seeds	Black beans	
AVOID		(calamari)		Yogurt	Gruyère		Flaxseeds	Kidney	
Pork	Eggs	Cod	**AVOID**	Cow's milk	Cottage	**Acid Forming**	Chia seeds	beans	
(ham,		Mullet	None	Cream	Farmer	**(Nonsalted)**		Navy beans	
bacon,	**AVOID**	Haddock		Buttermilk	Feta		**AVOID**	Pinto beans	
roast)	None	Ocean perch			Ricotta	Pecans	None	Red beans	
		Sturgeon		**Cheeses (Use Low-Fat)**	Muenster	Pistachios			
		Octopus			Monterey	Walnuts		**Weak Alkaline**	
		(scungilli)			Jack	Brazil nuts			
				Parmesan	Provolone	Macadamias		Soybean	
		Acid Forming		Limburger	Mozzarella	Chestnuts		curd	
		Carp		Cheddar	Goat	Almonds		(tofu)	
		Yellowtail		Brick	Blue				
		tuna		Swiss	Gorgonzola	**Weak Acid**		**AVOID**	
		Salmon				Filberts		None	
		Hake			**AVOID**	(hazelnuts)			
		Lake perch			None	Hickory nuts			
		Bass							
		Trout				**AVOID**			
						None			
		Weak Acid							
		Anchovies							
		Caviar							
		Herring							
		Sardines							
		Shellfish Strong Acid							
		Abalone							

Carbohydrates						
GRAINS	HIGH-STARCH LEGUMES	HIGH-STARCH VEGETABLES	SLIGHTLY STARCHY VEGETABLES	NONSTARCHY VEGETABLES		
Strong Acid	**Strong Acid**	**Strong Acid**	**Weak Acid**	**Strong Acid**	**Weak Acid**	**Eliminate If You Have Allergies of Any Kind**
Popcorn	Black-eyed peas (cowpeas)	Field corn	Beets, cooked	Mushrooms	Cauliflower, cooked	Eggplant
Corn grits		Sweet corn	Parsnips	Garlic		Tomatoes
Rice bran	**Acid Forming**	Potatoes	Jicama		Eggplant	Peppers
Millet				**Acid Forming**	Artichokes	
Barley	Lima beans	**Weak Alkaline**	**Weak Alkaline**		Shallots	**AVOID**
Corn meal	Garbanzo beans (chickpeas)	Acorn squash	Carrots	Bamboo shoots	Gingerroot	**Alkaline**
Wheat			Rutabagas	Green peas	Salsify	**Forming**
Couscous	Great northern beans	**Acid Forming**		Sugar peas	Soybean sprouts	
Bulgur (cracked wheat)	Split peas	Yams	**Acid Forming**	Mungbeans and sprouts	Kohlrabi	Yellow dock, cooked
Rye	White (fava) beans	Pumpkin, raw	Beets, raw	Chili peppers	Chicory	Chicory greens
Oats				Asparagus	Onions	Horseradish
Pastinas (egg)		**Weak Acid**	**AVOID**	Celeriac root	Cucumbers	Cabbage, cooked
Sprouted grain bread	**AVOID**	Butternut squash	None	Sweet peppers	Radishes	Okra, cooked
		Hubbard squash		Brussels sprouts	Summer squash, raw	Swiss chard, raw
Acid Forming	None	Sweet potatoes		Cauliflower, raw		Spinach, cooked
		Pumpkin, canned		Tomatoes	**Weak Alkaline**	Kale, raw
Farina					Summer squash, cooked	Lettuce: cos, romaine, dark green, white
Brown rice		**Eliminate If You Have Any Allergies**		**Strong Alkaline**	Leeks	Watercress
Basmati brown rice				Kale, cooked	Garden cress	Alfalfa sprouts
Wild rice		Corn		Collards	Chinese cabbage	Dandelion greens
Buckwheat (kasha)		Corn meal		Swiss chard, cooked	Snap beans	Arugula
Quinoa		Corn grits		Parsley	Yellow beans	Beet greens, raw
		Potatoes		Mustard greens, cooked	Turnips	
Strong Alkaline				Beet greens, cooked	Scallions	
Amaranth grain and flakes		**AVOID**		Turnip greens, cooked	Broccoli	
		None		Lamb's-quarter	Lettuce: butter, Boston, iceberg	
Eliminate If You Have Any Allergies				Mustard spinach	Celery	
					Endive	
Wheat				**Seaweeds**	Radicchio	
Wheat germ					Yellow dock, raw	
Rye				Agar-agar	Cabbage, raw	
Barley				Kelp	Okra, raw	
				Irish moss	Spinach, raw	
AVOID				Dulse	Fennel	
None				Arame		

FRUIT		OILS	CONDIMENTS	TEAS
Acid Forming	**Weak Alkaline**	**Strong Acid**	**Weak Acid**	**Licorice root:** strengthens the adrenals (Don't use if you have high blood pressure.)
Litchis	Lemons	Avocado	Vinegar	
Passion fruit	Cherries	Corn	Honey	
Groundberries	Blackberries	Soybean	Mustard	
Pomegranates	Limes	Peanut		**Juniper berry:** strengthens the adrenals and kidneys
Crab apples		Cottonseed	**Weak Alkaline**	
Peaches	**Melons (Eat Alone)**	Olive	Pickles	
	Watermelon	Safflower		**Fennel:** curbs your appetite and aids digestion
Weak Acid	Muskmelon	Sunflower	**Strong Alkaline**	
Guavas	Cantaloupe	Flaxseed	Molasses: blackstrap or	**Dandelion root:** metabolizes cholesterol
Loquats	Casaba	Walnut	light	
Cherimoya	Crenshaw	Apricot	Sorghum	
Grapes: muscat, Tokay	Honeydew	Almond	Maple syrup	**Burdock root:** regulates insulin levels
Quince				
Tamarinds	**Sweet Fruit**	*AVOID*	**Weak Acid**	**Red clover:** blood cleanser and immune builder
Apples	**Acid Forming**	**(Saturated Fats)**	Soy sauce	
Apricots	Persimmons			
Prickly pears	Plantains	Mayonnaise	*AVOID*	**Alfalfa leaf:** blood cleanser and immune builder
Pears	Bananas	Butter	Yeast—in all forms	
Mangoes		Margarine	Brown sugar	
	Weak Acid		Cane sugar	**Blue flag:** raises your metabolism and clears the liver and skin
Strong Alkaline	Apricots, dried			
Rhubarb	Raisins		**Alkaline Forming**	
	Prunes		Cane syrup	
Weak Alkaline	Dates			**White oak bark:** strengthens the thyroid gland
Boysenberries				
Grapefruit	**Weak Alkaline**			**Wild cherry:** supports your thymus and stimulates production of white blood cells
Raspberries	Figs			
Strawberries				
Plums	*AVOID*			
Acerola cherries	**Alkaline Forming**			
Blueberries	Loganberries			
Nectarines	Oranges			
Gooseberries	Clementines			
Pokeberries	Tangerines			
Papaya	Kumquats			
Grapes: Concord,	Kiwifruits			
Thompson	Pineapple			
Elderberries				
Sapotes				
Cranberries				
Currants				

Balanced Synthesizer Elixirs for Both Women and Men

Adrenal Stabilizer: With carrot juice, parsley is the great adrenal stabilizer and also balances the thyroid gland, cleanses the kidneys, brightens the eyes, and brings oxygen into the body.	Carrots: 6 oz. juice (about 6 carrots) Parsley: 3 oz. juice (about 3 bunches) Water: 2 oz.
Green Superpower: Cucumber juice leads this rich formula, providing you with an abundant silicon and sulfur content along with potassium, calcium, phosphorus, and choline, and it is the best natural diuretic known; celery balances your nerves and clears your skin; parsley balances your adrenals; spinach, full of iron, burns fat; all the minerals rebalance your hormone levels.	Cucumbers: 4 oz. juice (about 1½ cucumbers) Spinach: 3 oz. juice (about 1 bunch) Celery: 3 oz. juice (about 1 bunch) Parsley: 2 oz. juice (about 2 bunches) Water: 2 oz.
Immune Energizer: Full of vitamins and iron, this juice energizes, nourishes, and regenerates your whole immune system. Spinach builds iron-rich blood that nourishes your immune warriors, cleans out toxins, and burns up excess fat. It also supplies the iron needed by your thyroid gland. Dandelion greens clear out a toxic liver and support your thymus gland.	Carrots: 6 oz. juice (about 6 carrots) Spinach: 3 oz. juice (about 1 bunch) Dandelion greens: 2 oz. juice (optional) Water: 2 oz.
Thyroid Energizer: Stimulating both your thyroid and adrenal glands, the carrot juice along with the beet juice builds your blood; provides the nutrients needed by your thyroid gland to produce its hormone, thyroxine; increases your circulation; balances your hormonal levels; and literally rebuilds your skin.	Carrots: 6 oz. juice (about 6 carrots Beets: 3 oz. juice (about 2 beets) Cucumber: 3 oz. juice (about 1 cucumber) Water: 2 oz.
Insulin Balancer: Yes, Brussels sprouts. It's been found that the combination of minerals in this elixir helps to strengthen and regenerate your overworked pancreas cells, especially those that produce insulin. (You may substitute broccoli, collard greens, or cabbage.)	Carrots: 6 oz. juice (about 6 carrots) Lettuce: 4 oz. juice (about 1 head) String beans: 3 oz. juice (about 1 lb.) Brussels sprouts: 3 oz. juice (about 1 lb.) Water: 2 oz.

Your On-Program Cheat Sheet

Naturally there will be days when you just have to cheat. No problem. There's no need to become obsessed with eating perfectly. If you do, you'll only end up out of balance.

For your balanced synthesizer profile, pretzels are your main cheat food. Not the thin, salty, white-flour pretzels that make you retain water and leave you craving more. No, your pretzels of choice are sourdough, without salt. They're easy to find in any supermarket. Snyder's of Hanover is a good brand because its pretzels are baked, not fried, and have absolutely no fat. There are also a few other great-tasting snacks you can indulge in when you just must have something to munch on.

Here's a complete list of your official cheat foods:

- *Hard pretzel:* 1 unsalted
- *Raisins:* ¼ cup, or 2 oz.
- *Dates:* ¼ cup pitted, or 2 oz.
- *Prunes:* ½ cup pitted, or 4 oz.
- *Apricots, dried:* ½ cup pitted, or 4 oz.

You'll need to follow some guidelines in order to make these foods work for you. Otherwise, using these cheat foods in the wrong way could sabotage your goal of losing weight.

CHEAT-FOOD GUIDELINES

- *Eat your cheat foods only at the recommended times.* Cheat foods should be eaten no oftener than once per week, on the weekends (when you're not under stress), and at one meal or one time—only.
- *Eat only the amount suggested.* Your body can handle a small amount of these foods without triggering excessive insulin production. If you eat a large amount, your insulin level will spike and turn your "treat" into a "bad trick" of blubber.
- *Eat only one cheat food at a time.* Don't have several together or you'll wreak havoc with your metabolism and digestion. For instance, raisins *and* pretzels or prunes will send you over the top.
- *Never eat your cheat foods when you're under stress.* I guarantee you that's a surefire way to add pounds, not lose them. Only eat cheat foods when you're relaxed—usually on a weekend. Otherwise, your digestion shuts down and your insulin rises, and you become a veritable fat factory.
- *Never eat your cheat foods late at night.* You'll end up having a restless night's sleep, and it's mandatory for you to sleep deeply so your body can regenerate itself.

Balanced Synthesizer Healers and Helpers: Vitamins, Minerals, and Amino Acids

This section of your program is dedicated to the additions to the food plan that will help you lose weight even faster and improve your overall health and well-being. As I discussed in chapter 13, you can enhance the benefits of your meta-type diet with vitamins, minerals, and supplements tailored for you.

For your balanced synthesizer meta-type, I suggest that you add a gentle, full-spectrum multiple amino acid, vitamin, and mineral complex containing only those essential nutrients that support your weaker sympathetic nervous system. This will speed up your weight-loss program, help tone your muscles, and give you abundant good health. The multiple amino acid, vitamin, and mineral complex can be purchased at your local vitamin store or ordered from the companies listed in appendix 2.

If the controlling endocrine gland governed by your dominant nervous system is out of balance, either hyperactive or hypoactive, you may need some additional nutrients in the form of amino acids, vitamins, or minerals besides the full-spectrum amino acid, vitamin, and mineral formula supporting your opposite nervous system. In your case your dominant endocrine gland is the pancreas.

As you learned earlier, your pancreas plays the vital role in providing hormones and enzymes for digestion as your food moves into the intestine—and for regulating your blood sugar levels and fat absorption. Overworked, it can crash at either extreme—resulting in diabetes or hypoglycemia and creating carbohydrate intolerance.

Remember, among the beneficial workhorses from your pancreas are enzymes that digest carbohydrates, proteins, and fats as well as your two powerhouse hormones that regulate your blood sugar: glucagon and insulin.

Along with your pancreas gland, some additional attention must be focused on your weaker opposite sympathetic endocrine gland, your thymus. Since it controls your immune system, you can be vulnerable to allergies, viral or bacterial invasions, and debilitating diseases. Your thymus is responsible for your body's immune response, which also involves the action of your lymphatic system and the energetic action of your heart and cardiovascular system.

The following nutrients are needed for the health of your pancreas gland: the amino acids glycine, alanine, and methionine; the B-complex complements choline and inositol (prime components in the phospholipids); and the minerals chromium and zinc.

Glycine is known as food for the brain. It helps to regulate your pancreas's function by controlling the release of your pancreatic hormone glucagon, liberating it into your bloodstream in set amounts that help to balance out your insulin levels and stabilize any low blood sugar. It's also involved with the amino acid taurine in the production of bile acid for fat metabolism—so it helps to burn off fat.

Alanine is great at stabilizing blood sugar levels by helping convert the energy-producing pyruvic acid to energy. So your excess blood sugar is turned into energy, not fat. A great bonus for your meta-type is that alanine stimulates the immune system.

Both alanine and glycine can be found in your local health-food store, usually in combination with isoleucine (which also helps to stabilize blood sugar) in specific formulas for blood sugar stability.

Methionine is vital for several reasons. It's essential for the integration of choline in the manufacturing of your parasympathetic nervous system's neurotransmitter, acetylcholine. Working with choline, inositol, and folic acid (all part of the B-complex family), methionine assists in breaking down fats and cholesterol and prevents a buildup of fat in your liver, arteries, and other organs—especially around your heart. This amino acid is also a strong antioxidant and helps to neutralize toxins, heavy metals, and allergic reactions. An added bonus is that methionine helps produce endorphins, which give you euphoric feelings to offset pain, stress, or depression.

Choline and *inositol* are part of the B complex and work as fat busters, breaking down fats and reducing cholesterol. They also soothe nerves. Choline forms acetylcholine—the neurotransmitter needed by your parasympathetic nervous system that keeps your body calm, soothes your nerves, and helps your body run smoothly and in balanced order. Choline and inositol should be taken in equal amounts and occur naturally in the form of lecithin. You can also take plain choline and inositol blended with methionine, called "lipo factors."

Chromium is the magic bullet that regulates your pancreas's insulin production (it's a component of the "glucose tolerance factor" produced by your pancreas) and activates certain pancreatic enzymes. It's a major fat burner, too. Chromium also helps both to synthesize cholesterol in your liver and to lower blood pressure.

Zinc is the other magic key that supports your pancreas and helps your fat melt away by stimulating adequate pancreatic enzyme production. It's an essential component of all the enzyme systems and a required component in the pancreatic enzyme complex. It's also essential for the synthesis and metabolism of proteins. With chromium, zinc supports and stimulates the formation of insulin and helps reduce excess cholesterol.

The following nutrients help strengthen your weaker thymus gland:

• *Essential fatty acids:* These nutrients are the key ingredient for your thymus, needed for cell repair, nerve transmission, energy, and to feed your immune system. They are *the* food for your thymus and immune response. They also manufacture the adrenal and sex glands' steroid hormones and act as a major factor in the production of phospholipids, the good guys that break down cholesterol.

• *Vitamin C:* Not only is vitamin C essential for the health of your immune system, it's also crucial for utilizing the amino acids tryptophan (which produces the calming serotonin) and tyrosine (which helps form the adrenal hormones needed to fight allergies, fend off diseases, and speed healing). Another major function of vitamin C is its ability to control cholesterol because it burns off fat. Since it is not stored in the body, it must be taken daily or several times a day if you're in a continued stress response.

• *B complex:* For your meta-type the B-complex vitamins stabilize your immune system while burning fat. B_2, B_5, B_6, and biotin help form antibodies, and B_3 and B_{15} stimulate the immune response. All the Bs play a role in fat metabolism, especially B_3, B_5, and B_{15}, which reduce cholesterol and fatty deposits.

Special note: When taking any of the B vitamins, it's important to know that you shouldn't take an isolated B—such as pantothenic acid or riboflavin—without taking the whole B-vitamin complement. Otherwise, the lone B constituent will rob your body of the other Bs to activate its energy.

• *Zinc:* This mineral promotes the growth of T cells, those "warriors" that provide the antibodies in your natural immunity. Zinc also accelerates healing and cuts cholesterol and fat.

• *Protein:* The amino acids in protein make hemoglobin, the oxygen carrier in your red blood cells and stem cells, the foundation of your white cells. The amino acid arginine stimulates your thymus gland's output of thymosin. I've formulated your diet to include amino-rich protein to provide the appropriate building blocks for your thymus gland and immune function. (The daily intake level of protein should be about 1 gram to 1.5 grams per pound of body weight, depending on the individual's age and circumstances. To convert grams to ounces, multiply the gram figure by .0353.)

The Bottom Line

By taking a complete amino acid, vitamin, and mineral combination based on the formulation for your general metabolic type, you'll be supplied with the nutrients needed to support your complementary side, the sympathetic nervous system. You may want to add a few of the vitamins and minerals we've just discussed, which are also listed in the accompanying table of recommended nutrients. If you're interested, turn to appendixes 3 and 4 for a more in-depth study of the vitamins, minerals, and amino acids for your meta-type. If you prefer to get all your nutrients from foods, I've listed the foods highest in vitamin, mineral, and amino acid content in the accompanying table.

Balanced Synthesizer Vitamin, Mineral, and Amino Acid Food Sources

Pancreas Gland	
Amino acids: alanine, glycine, and methionine	All animal proteins (meat, fish, and fowl) and soy products
Chromium	Blackstrap molasses, cheese, apple peels, bananas, corn meal, vegetable oils, and wheat bran
Zinc	Spices, wheat bran, crab, and popcorn
Lecithin *or* choline and inositol (called lipotropic factors)	• *Choline:* soybeans, cabbage, wheat bran, navy beans, alfalfa leaf meal, rice polishings, rice bran, whole grains, hominy, turnips, and blackstrap molasses
	• *Inositol:* wheat germ, citrus fruits, blackstrap molasses, fruits, whole grains, bran, nuts, legumes, milk, and vegetables

Thymus Gland	
Essential fatty acids (EFA)—vitamin F	• *Oils:* safflower, sunflower, corn, olive, wheat germ, soy, cottonseed, and cod-liver
	• *Nuts:* walnuts, Brazil nuts, and almonds
Vitamin C	Acerola cherries, rose hips, citrus fruits, guavas, hot green peppers, black currants, parsley, turnip greens, poke greens, and mustard greens
B complex	• B_1: torula yeast, sunflower seeds, rice bran, wheat germ, pine nuts, dried coriander leaf, safflower seeds, soybeans, alfalfa seeds, sesame seeds, and rye flour (dark)
	• B_2: almonds, cheese, turnip greens, wheat bran, and soybeans
	• B_3 *(niacin):* fish, nuts, milk, cheese, bran flakes, sesame seeds, and sunflower seeds
	• B_6: rice bran, wheat bran, sunflower seeds, avocados, bananas, corn, fish, brown rice, soybeans, and whole grains
	• B_{15}: grains, cereals, rice, apricot kernels, and torula yeast
Zinc	As listed under "Pancreas Gland"

There are a few easy things to remember about taking the supplements:

• Try to take amino acids on an empty stomach. (They need adequate amounts of stomach enzymes to be broken down properly.)

• If possible, take enzymes with your meals to aid in your food digestion.

• Take vitamins and minerals after you've eaten, which helps their assimilation.

• The water-soluble vitamins—B complex, vitamin C, and vitamin P (bioflavonoids)—can be taken at any time.

• Your body isn't used to concentrated food substances, so I recommend that you introduce one type of amino acid, vitamin, or mineral into your regimen every few days. Gently and easily is the name of the game.

Balanced Synthesizer Recommended Nutrients

ENDOCRINE GLAND	NUTRIENT	WOMEN			MEN		
		Number	Strength	Times per Day	Number	Strength	Times per Day
Pancreas	Alanine	1	500 mg	1	1	500 mg	2
	Glycine	1	500 mg	1	1	500 mg	2
	Methionine	1	500 mg	1	1	500 mg	2
	Chromium	1	100 mcg	1	1	200 mcg	2
	Zinc	1	30 mg	1	2	30 mg	1
	Choline and inositol	1	500 mg	1	1	500 mg	1–2
Thymus	Essential fatty acids	1	300 mg	2	2	300 mg	2
	or lecithin	1	1,200 mg	1–2	1	1,200 mg	2–3
	Vitamin C (buffered)	1	1,000 mg	2–3	1–2	1,000 mg	3
	B complex	1–2	50–75 mg	2	1–2	100–150 mg	2
	Zinc	See under "Pancreas"	—	—	See under "Pancreas"	—	—

Taking these extra vitamins, minerals, and supplements will require work—there's no mistaking that. Just as you have to plan meals with the right ingredients, you'll need to organize these. But as your metabolic system moves back into balance, you'll reduce the number of pills you'll need. And along the way, you'll discover that the dividend of glowing good health pays off quickly enough to make Wall Street envious.

Stocking Up

You've now finished reading about the program and are well on your way to a brand-new you. Just wait and see—you'll be slim, sexy, and full of bounce to every ounce. To get started, you'll need to stock up and organize. The accompanying list shows all the foods you'll need for the coming week. Double-check this list against your weekly menu and make any adjustments you feel are necessary. Happy regeneration!

Weekly Shopping List for Balanced Synthesizers

Larger quantities for men are shown in **boldface**.

PRODUCE

Fruit
2 Apricots
1 Cantaloupe
(1 Pear)
1 Grapefruit
2 Peaches
4 **(6)** Lemons
1 Lime
(1 pt. Strawberries)

Vegetables
1 Artichoke
1 sm. piece Ginger
2 lb. Sugar snap peas
5 lb. Carrots
2 bunches Celery
7 Cucumbers
3 lb. Spinach
1½ lb., or 3½ cups Green beans
1 lg. Yellow squash
1 lg. Zucchini
4 10-oz. Mushrooms
4 bulbs Garlic
14 **(16)** Plum tomatoes
1 pt. Cherry tomatoes
4 Red peppers
1 Green pepper
1 bulb Fennel
1 sm. Radicchio
1 bunch Scallions
1 bunch Radishes

1 Red onion
1 sm. Japanese eggplant
1 lg. Jicama
1½ **(2)** lb. Asparagus
3 Yukon gold potatoes
2 lg. Beets
1 lb. Brussels sprouts
1 med. Yellow (Spanish) onion

Salad Greens
1 head Red leaf lettuce
1 sm. **(lg.)** Kale
1 Chicory
1 bunch Arugula
1 sm. head Boston lettuce
1 Belgian endive
2 bunches Watercress
6 **(8)** bunches Parsley
1 head Romaine lettuce
1 bunch Dandelion greens
2 boxes Radish sprouts
1 bunch Basil, fresh
1 bunch Dill, fresh

GROCERIES
1 lb. Red kidney beans
1 lb. Couscous
½ lb. Egg pastina
2 qt. Tomato juice, unsalted—in a
   glass bottle
1 jar Dijon mustard
1 bottle Apple cider vinegar
1 bottle Wheat germ oil

1 **(3)** qt. Soy milk
1 container Protein powder
   (whey- or soy-based)
1 container Kelp powder or
   blue-green algae
1 loaf Sprouted grain bread
1 8-oz. jar Fruit spread (your
   choice)
1 package Seaweed of choice
(3 oz. Pecans)
(1 oz. Pumpkin seeds)
(1 oz. Sesame seeds)
1 tube Harissa (hot Moroccan
   spice)
1 package Frozen peas
1 bottle Vanilla or almond extract
Whole-grain cereal of choice
   (enough for 3 cups)
Saffron, dried thyme, nutmeg,
   cardamom seed, turmeric,
   cayenne pepper, black pepper

Soy sauce
Herbal teas
Safflower oil

DAIRY
6 Eggs
1 8-oz. Ricotta cheese, low-fat
1 lb. Tofu, extra firm

MEAT AND FISH
2 pieces: 1 8-oz., 1 4-oz. **(2 pieces:
   1 12-oz., 1 6-oz.)** Salmon
4 oz. Shrimp (or sea scallops)
   **(3 oz. *each* shrimp and sea
   scallops)**
2 pieces: 1 8-oz., 1 7-oz. **(3 pieces:
   2 5-oz., 1 8-oz.)** Chicken breast
   (skin off)
1 8-oz **(12-oz.)** piece Beef
   tenderloin

19 The Mixed Synthesizer Diet

If you are a true mixed synthesizer, keeping your weight under control has probably been an ongoing battle for most of your life. Well, get ready to smile a lot: this diet is the solution to your problem. Once you master your personal diet plan, your constant worries about your weight will be a thing of the past. I am going to introduce you to a whole new way of eating, living, and feeling great. Just a few quick words on how your personal mixed synthesizer diet works, then on to the menus. As you read, remember:

- Your dominant glands are the sex glands (testes for men, ovaries for women).
- Your weakest gland is the adrenals.
- You're most likely to gain weight in your hips, especially the buttocks.

The Science behind Your System

You've already discovered that your metabolism is dominated by the parasympathetic nervous system but receives almost equal influence from the sympathetic nervous system. Similar to the mixed accelerator, your meta-type acts as a "bridge" that integrates *both* nervous systems as well as their aspects.

267

Your energy, and the fuel that keeps your metabolism running smoothly, is primarily generated by nerve stimulation to those glands and organs responsible for the regeneration, repair, and growth of your body: the pituitary gland, sex glands, salivary glands, stomach, pancreas, liver, small and large intestines, kidneys, and bladder. A little less stimulation goes to your organs of energy production: the adrenal gland, thyroid gland, thymus gland, spleen, lungs, and heart.

Your metabolism works hard to keep your sex-hormone levels balanced so that your energy stores and emotions stay on an even keel while those hormones regulate your libido, fertility, and the sex characteristics that make us so appealingly different.

Since, as a mixed synthesizer, you derive your primary strength more from the parasympathetic digestive and regenerative glands and less from the sympathetic energy glands, you tend to be a *slow metabolizer*, like all synthesizer meta-types. In other words, you break down your foods slowly because you generate less energy.

This type of slower absorption allows for the influx of ample oxygen into your digestive tract during your breathing and digestive processes. Therefore, you digest your foods in an aerobic environment (that is, with oxygen present). By the time your oxygen-filled nutrients reach the cells for transformation into energy, they'll burn off (oxidize) at a fairly rapid rate. Remember, "air fans fire."

In the synthesizer category, your unique characteristic is the different way in which you break down your foods and utilize your energy. You break down your foods a bit faster than your synthesizer meta-mates do, but you don't burn them off as rapidly as they do. Your metabolic profile is: you break down your foods semislowly and burn them fairly fast. Happily for you, this means that you can handle more carbohydrates than other synthesizers. However, since your body oxidizes your blood sugar semi-quickly, if you eat a lot of refined carbohydrates you'll experience a brief high, then drop into fatigue.

Synthesizers also produce ample stomach acid (HCl, or hydrochloric acid) and enzymes. Your meta-type tends to produce adequate stomach acid and pancreatic enzymes—less than your fellow synthesizers—so you need the heavier and somewhat slower-burning proteins along with your complex carbohydrates. As you've learned, the lighter carbohydrates digest rapidly and are the fastest-burning foods. Proteins are slower; fats are the slowest.

Since your digestive process takes place in a semioxygenated environment and oxygen burns off the toxic wastes from cells, you tend to retain lower levels of cellular toxins.

Your body chemistry tends to be alkaline in nature. This gives you a *semialkaline-producing* chemistry. So with your somewhat fast digestion and semifast energy burn-off, you'll tend to have:

- Medium to average production of stomach acid—unless it is completely suppressed by the stress response
- A tendency toward a semialkaline body—that is, tissue alkalinity
- Good production of pancreatic enzymes—unless it is suppressed by a continued stress response
- Balanced production of pancreatic insulin

Metabolically speaking, you require foods that are of an acid nature and burn slowly, such as the proteins in fish and fowl. But for your metabolic profile, this doesn't include red meat. You don't need the additional cholesterol in red meat, which would only stimulate higher production of your already bountiful hormones.

Your metabolism can also handle an appropriate amount of the fast-burning grains and foods of a strong alkaline nature, such as green leafy vegetables and some fruits. Your fats should come from only a *moderate* amount of unsaturated oils—*not* saturated fats—in the form of vegetable oils. Therefore, your mixed synthesizer food formula looks like this:

- Protein: 45 percent
- Carbohydrates: 40 percent
- Fat: 15 percent

Mixed Synthesizer Food Choices

After one month on the Your Body, Your Diet plan, you will not only drop excess fat but also be introduced to a level of vitality and good health that you never dreamed possible. Once you have looked at the basic menus, you will see food lists that will show you the wide variety of delicious foods that are best for you. Suggested vitamins, minerals, and supplements for your metabolic makeover are also included, as these can speed up your conversion into perfect balance. The next three subsections give you an overview of the basic principles you'll be following.

What to Avoid

Steer clear of refined carbohydrates, saturated fats, and spicy foods. I know this seems like a tough set of restrictions to follow, but you will adjust. Here's why making these changes is so important. These are the foods that keep your blood sugar and energy levels zooming up or down, with little control or predictability. And they encourage your sleepy synthesizer metabolism to remain sluggish and hold on to weight. Also, spicy and fatty foods overstimulate your sex glands (resulting in increased girth, not desire) and supply much higher levels of cholesterol and sex hormones than your system can handle. You'll be amazed at how much better you look and feel without these foods literally weighing you down.

You are a *sensuous* eater—and fats and creamy foods appeal greatly. But the saturated fats—like butter, mayonnaise, cream, fried foods, chocolate, red meats, and cheese—are exactly what you *don't* need, triggering too much cholesterol for your already-high system. When you reach for stimulating and sweet foods—especially the refined carbohydrates such as cakes, cookies, doughnuts, breads, pasta, and pastry, as well as that wonderful glass of wine—you'll continue to further weaken your energy-producing glands (basically your adrenals and thyroid), too. The refined carbohydrates of alcohol and sugar, together with stress, also raise the levels of the natural cholesterol that your own body produces—and with your meta-type you'll just keep piling on those cholesterol-induced pounds.

Spicy foods only serve to stimulate the production of more estrogen and testosterone. As a mixed synthesizer, you have a natural tendency for your blood vessels to dilate easily, flooding your pelvic region with abundant blood, which adds to the stimulation of your sex glands. Spicy foods will only enhance this stimulation and will automatically expand your blood vessels, letting more of those hormones race through your already stimulated pelvic area, helping burn out your dominant ovaries and testes.

Refined carbohydrates (sugar) heighten emotional responses. If you were to feel an emotional high and consequently grab for the sugars or carbohydrates, you'd have an energy flash and a heightened emotional response, followed by a rapid decline of both your emotions and your energy. Beginning to crave refined carbohydrates, you reach for the sugar, and the cycle begins again. You're at risk on the other side of the emotional coin, too. If you're feeling low and gobble down that excess sugar or starch, you'll get a brief emotional and energetic high, after which you may quickly plunge into fatigue and even depression. When you're in balance, you can tolerate some refined carbohydrates—in small amounts. But until then excess carbohydrates could spell disaster—for your emotions as well as your derriere.

The accompanying table gives you an overview of the foods and other substances that do *not* suit your meta-type.

Your *Never* Foods

SATURATED FATS	REFINED CARBOHYDRATES	SPICY FOODS
Butter	All packaged foods	Chili
Margarine	Synthetic additives	Hot peppers
Mayonnaise	Sweeteners	Hot spices, such as:
Cream	Processed breads and pasta	Curry
Ice cream	Cakes	Ginger
Whole-milk products	Cookies	Tabasco sauce
Fried foods	Doughnuts	Horseradish
Chocolate	White sugar	Mustard
Red meats	Cane sugar	
Cheese	Brown sugar	
	Processed syrup	
	Alcohol	

What to Fill Up On

Poultry, fish, dairy, seeds, nuts, and legumes are your foods of choice. You see, there are lots of absolutely delectable foods on your eating plan, and they are all just perfect for you. The slow-burning proteins help regulate and stabilize your blood sugar while keeping your energy high. All of the foods also help to support your adrenals, which tends to be your weakest gland, as well as your thyroid. So you'll have plenty of opportunities to enjoy great-tasting meals while watching your excess weight disappear.

The accompanying table lists the foods that best suit your meta-type.

As you've learned, the foods that are required by your specific metabolic type (proteins) are *exactly* the ones that feed and support your weaker endocrine gland, the adrenals.

Proteins serve several functions for you. They burn more slowly, so they don't subject you to an energy roller coaster the way fast-burning refined "carbs" do, and they support your meta-type's weaker adrenal gland, helping provide the energy that battles carb-induced fatigue and stress burnout. So beware of the sugar and starches. They burn off too rapidly for you and can intensify your emotionality. Proteins, in contrast, help to stabilize and ground your emotion-prone energy.

Your *Always* Foods

PROTEINS		CARBOHYDRATES		FATS
Food	Times per Week	Food	Times per Week	
Meat: none	0	Grains: abundant	2–3	*Moderate*
Fowl: abundant	2–3	Legumes: abundant	2	amount of
Fish: abundant	2–3	Starchy vegetables: variety	1	unsaturated fatty
Dairy: soy milk (*Avoid*	Daily	Slightly starchy vegetables:		acids—
whole milk and cheese.)		*small* variety	1	cold-pressed
Seeds: variety; nuts:		Nonstarchy vegetables:		vegetable or nut
abundant	1–2	variety (*Avoid* hot and		oils
Legume protein: abundant		spicy vegetables.)	Daily	Choose from your
(*Avoid* tofu.)	2–3	Fruit: *small* variety	Daily	food plan.

How to Speed Up Weight Loss

Here are some other tips to stimulate faster weight loss:

• Chew your food slowly and well.
• Try to avoid drinking more than one glass of water or liquid during your meals. Drinking large amounts of liquid during your meals dilutes the precious enzymes needed for your digestion.
• Have at least six to eight glasses of water during the day, *not* at mealtimes.
• When having a vegetarian meal, mix 60 percent grains to 40 percent legumes (beans) for a complete protein complement.

Keeping Your Sex Glands in Balance

The glands that make you swing and sway, your sex glands, are the dominant endocrine glands for your mixed synthesizer meta-type. These are the great glands of regeneration and reproduction. In fact, their well-known hormones, estrogen from the ovaries and testosterone from the testes, are so important to our functioning that they even have receptors in the brain. To keep your moods stable and uplifted, your attitudes confident, and your thinking clear, you need ample amounts of these precious hormones.

You tend to be the most "volcanic" of the meta-types, since you're under the domination of the more "feeling" parasympathetic nervous system. But you're a bridge type, with the "hormonal essences" that link your parasympathetic and sympathetic nervous systems. If not balanced with the proper foods, you can easily get pulled out of your own meta-type into the more emotional synthesizer profiles, weakening the influence of your sympathetic system's intellectual energy and your powers of rationalization.

Since your meta-type derives its power and energy from the sex glands, it is critical that your cycles—the female menstrual and male rhythmical cycles—be balanced and stable. If they're highly stimulated and overworked, they'll eventually weaken and become sluggish—or shut down entirely.

Of course, these hormones are essential for fertility and for producing our secondary sexual characteristics as well as our sex drive—and they fight aging. The "female hormone," estrogen, gives clear and smooth skin, mental clarity, quick memory recall, deep and wonderful sleep, emotional stability, and steady energy. The "male hormone," testosterone, gives a strong libido, assertiveness, energy, strength, effective mental perception, quickness of mind, healthy muscle tone, and a great gusto for life.

Now both men *and* women produce estrogen and testosterone in varying degrees, and stress can reduce the amounts to critical levels. These hormones are the link between the dominant parasympathetic nervous system and the sympathetic system.

Chinese medicine views the daytime action of your sex hormones as complementing your sympathetic nervous system, keeping your energy focused in the appropriate channels—whether emotional or intellectual. At night, governed by your parasympathetic system, they provide regenerative powers for cellular growth and fertile expression.

Remember puberty—that tender age of thirteen or fourteen when girls suddenly get interested in clothes and makeup, guys find muscles and facial hair, and both are suddenly thinking about each other? As a mixed synthesizer, this was your most powerful time, making sex an important element in your life.

If you were a mixed synthesizer girl, your body unfortunately added pounds where you didn't want them—in your buttocks, hips, and thighs. Your dominant endocrine glands demanded more fat in order to produce their ample cholesterol-based hormones, which stimulate the maturity of your ovum, or egg. Your meta-type *naturally* produces generous amounts of cholesterol, so saturated fats with high cholesterol content just overload your hormone production. And the tendency sticks with you throughout life—if you don't find that dietary balance.

Certain types of estrogen, called catechol estrogens, occur *exclusively* in the brain and are only synthesized there. They influence those dreaded mood swings. If your ovaries are producing the right balance of estrogen, you'll have normal and full menstrual cycles, a healthy sex drive, and hearty emotional stability. If not, you'll have a lowered sex drive, and you will experience erratic mood swings, especially around ovulation. The emotional pathways in your brain have been robbed of their food—estrogen—and the result is tough on you and those around you. Similarly if your estrogen levels are abnormally high, you'll have a heightened sex drive, your mood swings will intensify, and you'll experience high levels of sexual responses, especially around ovulation.

When they reach midlife, women face menopause, with hot flashes and skin and memory changes, and men hit "andropause," with declining sexual interest and performance, fatigue, irritability, and depression.

For normal sexual functioning, secretion of thyroid hormone (thyroxine) *must* be normal and well balanced. Scientists aren't sure of the mechanism that causes these changes, but it's thought that they result from a direct metabolic effect on the sex glands and/or the way in which the excitatory and inhibitory effects in your anterior pituitary's hormones operate. The following connections have been determined:

- In males reduced thyroxine production can cause a complete loss of libido, whereas too much thyroxine can cause impotence.
- In females reduced thyroxine production can disrupt the menstrual cycle, with periods being either too heavy and frequent or absent. As with men, underproduction of thyroid hormone can lower or shut down the sex drive.

It's been found, too, that tumors in the pineal gland can produce excessive quantities of melatonin or end up destroying the gland. These tumors are often associated with serious hypo- or hyperfunctioning (under- or overfunctioning) of the sex glands.

It's also important to look at your weaker gland, the adrenals, and how supporting the adrenals can help you shed pounds fast. The adrenals are your "speed centers," sitting atop your kidneys, generating energy for your action-oriented sympathetic nervous system. While their best-known product is adrenaline (epinephrine), their inner core also produces norepinephrine and dopamine—all used in the stress response and in waking you up in the mornings. The outer core produces cortisol, which regulates carbohydrate, fat, and protein metabolism; androgens, which are varying degrees of male and female hormones; and aldosterone, which regulates the sodium and potassium levels in the body. All these hormones are used in the stress, inflammatory, and allergy responses.

These glands are responsible for coping with everything from a routine wake-up call to fear, anger, rage—and any life-threatening emergency, the "fight-or-flight" syndrome you know so well.

This is why someone with your meta-type tends never to be a "morning person." For you the adrenals produce smaller amounts of those hormones that release stored blood sugar, or glycogen, for conversion into usable blood sugar, or glucose. Waking is hard work, and you'll need to eat to get your energy machine cranking. Once fired up, however, you become a dynamo.

Interestingly enough, the adrenal outer core shares the same cellular structure as your own dominant ovaries and testes. That's why Asian philosophy sees a direct link between the adrenal gland and your sexual functioning.

With the adrenals as your opposing gland, you may be very susceptible to the stress response. With less of their norepinephrine, epinephrine, and dopamine readily available, your body may shut down in continued crisis. Fatigue, allergies, slow healing, and mood swings or depression follow hard on the heels of adrenal burnout. And as your cortisol and its fat-busting duties shut down, the pounds pile on.

But with a diet tailored for your meta-type, you'll see how to shed those hormone-induced pounds—and find a reinvigorated, sexier you.

Your Mixed Synthesizer Secret Weapons

Now I know—from firsthand experience—just how tough it can be to switch to a whole new way of eating. In addition to having to apply a lot of willpower, you have to give your body time to adjust to your new lifestyle. If you find yourself feeling cranky and frustrated, relax; it's par for the course. It's just a sign that you're shedding those extra pounds and getting back into balance.

The teas and elixirs in this chapter were created to help you sail through the transition phase of your meta-type diet while making the pounds melt away even faster.

For each meta-type, there is one food or group of foods that helps to speed up the weight-loss process. The best way to jump-start your fat-burning mechanisms is to make sure you get a certain combination of nutrients each day. I've created two delicious drinks (one cool, smooth milkshake and one warm, energizing tonic) that you can enjoy throughout your diet to make sure you get all of these important vitamins and enzymes each morning and afternoon.

To help wake up your sleepy adrenals and keep them activated, I've formulated an energizing drink of apple cider vinegar, honey, and capsicum. Then, to feed your adrenals the nutrients they need, which keep them pumping out their hormones, I've designed a light protein drink for you to take as breakfast. This will keep your adrenal cortisol levels stable until their normal drop in the late afternoon.

Fat-Buster Tonic

Long favored as a weight-loss drink, the combination of apple cider vinegar, honey, and capsicum is especially good for your meta-type.

Why *honey* for a mixed synthesizer? It's rich in two simple sugars, levulose (fruit sugar) and dextrose (grape sugar), and much lower in sucrose (cane sugar). Levulose is a high-powered energy producer—higher and better than even dextrose and especially sucrose. Honey normally is already predigested, and with these sugars it's able to go right into your bloodstream, giving you the immediate energy needed to raise your blood sugar levels in order to activate your brain, your pituitary, and your adrenals and get you moving into the day.

And no, you won't gain weight from the honey. The honey supplies both your pituitary and adrenals with the needed fuel—glucose—which helps you and your brain to wake up in the morning. Your blood sugar will remain stable because it's followed by a protein breakfast.

The honey will also activate your somewhat sluggish thyroid gland. Honey is rich in the vitamins necessary to feed your weaker adrenals. It's rich in vitamin C from the pollens used by the bees to make it, pantothenic acid—part of the vitamin B complex—and active enzymes. All are essential for the health of your adrenal gland. Honey is also rich in B_1, B_2, B_6, and B_5. The minerals in honey are even more impressive: potassium (which prevents growths), sodium, calcium, magnesium, iron, copper (for liver health), chlorine, manganese, sulfur (a blood purifier), and silica.

Normally the best types of honey are the darker varieties, such as buckwheat and heather, because they have the highest mineral content. Tupelo honey has the highest content of levulose and is a powerful energizer. Honey is truly a perfect food.

Apple cider vinegar, long known as a cure for weight problems, is the second ingredient in your weight-loss drink. Not just any vinegar will do. It must be the cider vinegar made from apples that still contain their valuable minerals: phosphorus, choline, potassium, sodium, magnesium, calcium, sulfur, iron, fluorine, silicon, and many trace minerals.

The beauty of apple cider vinegar is that it's able to raise your metabolic rate—to speed up the way you burn off fat—by oxygenating your blood. In other words, it allows your bloodstream to be filled with much more oxygen, which, as you've learned, will in turn raise the rate at which your cells burn off fat. It also has the unique ability to stimulate your stomach's production of hydrochloric acid, which will help intensify and speed up the way you break down your foods and lessens the oxygenation of your stomach environment.

Capsicum, known as *Capsicum frutescens*, or cayenne pepper, is one of the best-known stimulants in the herbal kingdom. Now I know that I said no stimulants or spicy foods for your meta-type, but in this instance we're making an exception. Used only before breakfast—and not before dinner, when your dominant sex glands are beginning to work at their energetic peak—this fantastic herb will stimulate your energy, your adrenals, and your thyroid gland and also raise your metabolic rate, so you'll begin to burn off those excess pounds quickly during your day's activities. Capsicum also increases your heart's action and your digestive abilities, increases the power of both the honey and the apple cider vinegar, and promotes the health of all your organs. Capsicum is high in vitamins A and C (needed for your adrenals) and the minerals iron and calcium. It also contains magnesium, phosphorus, sulfur, potassium, and some of the B-complex vitamins.

Mixing all of these ingredients in spring water and taking this drink before breakfast will feed your lazy adrenals, wake you right up, energize you, and literally set your body in motion to melt away those excess pounds. (For the recipe, see Fat-Buster Tonic, on page 413.)

Slim and Thin Protein Drink

To feed and nurture your adrenals, we'll give them their favorite food—protein. Now it's important not to overload your system in the morning, since you'll have fairly strong action from your sympathetic nervous system. Once your adrenals get into action, you won't need or probably want a heavy breakfast. So I'll introduce your morning protein in the form of a light and easy protein drink. It won't overload your system and will gently feed your adrenals, keeping them manufacturing their energy-producing hormones. Blended and easily assimilated, it will go right to work keeping your blood sugar stable and supplying you with long-lasting energy.

Low-fat soy milk will be the base of your protein drink. For your meta-type, soy milk is a treasure. It's a protein and is easily digestible and full of glycosides and protease inhibitors, which help to build up your immune system. It also has an abundant supply of folic acid and plant hormones, which balance and stabilize your sometimes overworked hormones, whether you tend to over- or underproduce them.

Soy milk also stabilizes your hormone production. Rich in phytoes-terols—plant estrogens that are weaker versions of human estrogens—these nutrients powerfully balance estrogen levels, whether they are too high or too low. First, phytoesterols have the ability to bind to estrogen receptor sites on your cells' surface, blocking any excess estrogen from entering the cells. Second, these phytoesterols also appear to stimulate the liver's production of a particular protein that binds to blood-circulating es-trogen. Consequently it will decrease the amount of the blood-circulating estrogen and balance your own hormonal levels. Now the estrogenic activity of soy is about 0.1 percent of the estrogen produced by women, which gives your body the ability to absorb what it wants and discard the rest. If your body is too low in estrogen, then the phytoesterols act as a natural and gentle replacement for waning estrogen levels. If it's too high in estrogen, the phytoesterols act as a balancing agent, helping to equalize the out-of-balance hormonal levels. Soy milk is a perfect coordinator.

Supporting the amino acids in your soy milk, I've added a full-spectrum *protein powder*—soy-based or whey-based—which will supply you with all the essential amino acids needed to activate and feed your adrenals and energize and repair your body. There are many protein powders available at health-food stores. I've listed my recommendation in appendix 2.

Next, we'll give your metabolism an added boost by strengthening your other energy-producing gland—your thyroid. Iodine and zinc are the minerals needed to feed and support your thyroid so it can produce enough thyroxine to keep your metabolism active and burn off those ex-cess pounds. *Blue-green algae* and *kelp* are rich sources of the phyto-chemicals needed by your thyroid and are especially bountiful in sea-rich iodine, zinc, and protein. Added to your protein drink, they'll give you extra energy and supply your thyroid with the minerals it requires. Your metabolism will be raised to burn off that fat. As extra benefits, they also contain abundant B_{12}, will help clean out toxic cellular residue, and are powerful antioxidants.

Women over forty or younger women with low or declining estrogen levels may tend to have a deficiency of calcium and phosphorus and therefore have lower activity of the bone-building cells, or osteoblasts. This osteoblastic activity is under the direct control of estrogen, so the more estrogen, the stronger the osteoblastic activity and bones. To protect and strengthen your bones, to balance and calm your nerves if your estrogen levels are low or are coming back into balance, and to support your whole body, a mineral-rich food can be added to your morning drink. *Bone meal,* in powder form, contains abundant calcium, phosphorus, magnesium, and other important minerals. It will be absorbed into the bones, helping to ward off the perils of soft and brittle bones.

Mixing all of these ingredients together and taking this drink *as breakfast* will provide sustaining energy to get your day off to a strong start. (For the recipe, see Slim and Thin Protein Drink, on page 413.)

Slimming Teas

Another important component of your plan is the herbal tea formula I've created to meet the needs of each meta-type. Each tea will harmonize and balance your specific metabolism, facilitating your weight loss. To make yours, you'll need to add a few special ingredients to the basic Master Weight Loss Tea (see the formula and directions on pages 103–105).

These supplementary herbs (see table on page 280) should be added in equal proportions to the herbs already in the basic formula. I suggest you take one to three cups per day of your special tea. The herbs may be purchased at your local health-food store or ordered from the companies listed in appendix 2.

Rules of the Road

Your Eating Schedule

Since your body's natural clock is guided by the parasympathetic nervous system, your body works hardest on regeneration between 4:00 P.M. to 7:00 A.M. This process activates your digestive glands, especially your pancreas and thyroid glands, as well as your liver, gallbladder, large and small intestines, and specifically your sex organs. Your energy is at its peak from early to late afternoon, then in the early evening and sometimes the late evening. The ideal meals for you during these hours are composed of light proteins. Proteins help to stabilize your blood sugar levels as well as strengthen your adrenals.

Mixed Synthesizer Slimming Tea

Basic Formula: One Teaspoon Each
Alisma, poria, rhubarb root, red clover tops, alfalfa leaf, hawthorn berry, radish seed, sargassum, Indian chickweed, evergreen artemesia, astragalus root, fleeceflower root, citrus peel

Mixed Synthesizer Slimming Formula: Add One Teaspoon Each

NAME			FUNCTION
Common	Latin	Eastern	
Licorice root	*Radix glycyrrhizae*	Gan cao	Great for supporting and stimulating the adrenals and energizing your body.
Laminaria	*Lamineria japonica aresh*	Kun bu	Stimulates the thyroid, speeding up your metabolism; reduces water.
Safflower	*Carthamus tinctorius*	Hong hua	Opens the pancreas and liver, energizes, balances insulin levels, helps digestion, burns cholesterol, and stimulates the adrenals.
Fennel fruit	*Foeniculum officinale vulgare*	Hui xiang	Excellent for weight loss, opens digestion and liver function, burns fat, and removes waste and mucus.
Angelica root	*Radix angelica sinensis*	Dang gui	Builds up the blood and energy; balances hormonal levels.

Note: If you are pregnant, have high blood pressure, or are allergic to grasses or flowers, it's suggested that these teas not be used. Licorice root should not be used if you have high blood pressure.

Your less energetic time will be in the morning, since the adrenals are your weaker gland and may respond to your pituitary gland's wake-up call in a less than energetic way. They may be able to supply you with only minimal amounts of hormones and neurotransmitters, so you need to help them along with some outside natural stimulus. This will kick them into high hormone production, stimulating your energy and keeping it at a stable level throughout the day. A little food in the morning goes a long way for you, and once your adrenals are activated, your energy should be strong. Your breakfast should be light and contain protein.

Your best energetic time is from early to mid-afternoon and in the early evening and evening. Although this is your natural energetic time, your specific type of energy can actually stimulate you to indulge in seductive and sensual bingeing. You're a sensual person and need to be satisfied—but with the right kinds of foods for your meta-type. So you'll need a moderate dinner of generally proteins to keep those seductive tastes satisfied. Proteins help to stabilize your blood sugar levels, supply the amino acids needed for your cellular repair and regeneration, and strengthen your adrenals.

Lunch for you needs to be moderate to substantial. Since your adrenals' cortisol production falls swiftly in the late afternoon, you'll feel the effect more severely than others because your adrenal gland may be weak. You'll need the energy liberated from foods to help bridge the "energetic gap" left in the late afternoon when your sympathetic nervous system shuts down for the night just before the parasympathetic system has a chance to take over for the regeneration of your body. The key to your eating schedule is therefore:

- Light breakfast
- Moderate to substantial lunch
- Moderate dinner

Late Afternoon—Stabilizing the Energy Drop

Your less energetic time is in the morning, as you've just learned, and your least energetic time would be the late afternoon. If you haven't eaten a good lunch of proteins, you'll really feel your blood sugar drop. If you've also been under a lot of stress, then this time of day can be really frustrating. You'll experience fatigue, sleepiness, headaches, and irritability. In order to avoid this, you should have a moderate to substantial lunch, and the food of choice for you is protein. To help stave off that cortisol drop, a late-afternoon protein snack will help stabilize your blood sugar and support your energy.

YOUR LATE-AFTERNOON SNACK
Protein snack, 2 oz. fish or chicken; 1 oz. seeds or nuts
Hot herbal tea or green tea

Bedtime Eating—Not a Problem

If you're following your proper diet, you shouldn't need to eat before bed. But if you'd like a snack, stick to protein. If you want to save your afternoon snack and have it before you go to bed, okay. But no more than that. You can handle proteins, since they digest slowly and are the foods that facilitate cellular regeneration. They won't wake you up by their conversion to energy. *Stay away* from carbohydrates. Don't reach for the cookies, candy, bread, fruit, ice cream, and so forth. They break right down into glucose, or blood sugar, and you don't want that extra energy liberated into your bloodstream. It will either wake you right up or turn to fat.

Mixed Synthesizer Meals and Menus

Now you've completed the first part of the plan, and here's your reward: the tailor-made diet for your mixed synthesizer meta-type. If you've reached this point in the book, you know that losing weight and keeping it off take more than just watching what you eat.

The meals presented in this section are designed to meet all the needs of your metabolism while giving you the chance to eat a delicious, wide variety of fresh, nutritious foods. The first week may seem like a big adjustment, but by week two, I assure you, you'll be making your juices and tossing together your special meals like a pro.

Eating the Right Foods at the Right Times

Eating the *right kinds of food* at the *right times* is another key to the success of your weight-loss and rejuvenation program. With the semialkaline nature of your mixed synthesizer metabolism, if you eat a majority of alkaline foods, it will throw you way out of balance and increase your alkalinity. Then you'll want to balance yourself, so you'll reach for the wrong acid-type foods—sugars and starches—that just cause you to retain that extra fat, and you'll end up feeling terrible.

What you require are the correct acid foods to help balance out your body chemistry, just as your counterpart, the mixed accelerator meta-type, is semiacid in nature and requires the alkaline forming foods.

Your metabolism tends to be the least alkaline of all the synthesizer meta-types, which bridges to the more acid sympathetic system. You need some of the alkaline foods, such as vegetables and fruits, to stabilize your metabolism, but you also require the acid forming foods, such as grains and animal protein. You need protein to strengthen your adrenals. You are known as the *weak alkaline* meta-type, with your natural body pH tending to be 6.8. (Chapter 3 has a detailed explanation of the acid-alkaline aspect of your meta-type.)

Therefore, your diet should consist of foods that are strong acid, acid forming, and strong alkaline forming ash. Foods that are weak acid and alkaline forming can be eaten two to three times per week. Foods that are your own pH tendency—weak alkaline forming—should be avoided. Appendix 5 lists the full spectrum of foods and their pH factors.

Here We Go!

To make this adventure of slimming down to a new and healthy you fun, I've taken all the guesswork out of how to shop and prepare your meals. Before you begin, glance through your weekly menus and mixed synthesizer elixirs in the accompanying tables and look over the vast array of food selections in your Mixed Synthesizer Food Choices list. At the end of this chapter, you will find your own mixed synthesizer shopping list for a week. Then turn to appendix 1 and take a look at the equipment list (which includes all the supplies you'll need to make this as simple as possible), your advance food-preparation suggestions for the week, and your recipes and food-preparation instructions for both men and women.

For any of the foods specified in the weekly menus and recipes, you may substitute comparable foods from the Mixed Synthesizer Food Choices list.

Eat only the foods that are indicated for you on your individual food choices list. If your favorite isn't on there, don't eat it. You can check the "General Food Choices and Their Calorie Content for Each Meta-Type" in Appendix 5.

You see, it's all done for you, down to the last detail—and my personal promise to you is that this eating plan will keep your mixed synthesizer metabolism in perfect balance while helping you achieve a slender, gorgeous physique.

You're on your way to a bright, new, skinny, energetic you. Treat this as a ritual in celebrating your beauty and regeneration.

Mixed Synthesizer Semiomnivore Weekly Menus

Acid to Alkaline-Based Foods

WHEN	SATURDAY	SUNDAY	MONDAY	TUESDAY
On rising	Fat-Buster Tonic			
Breakfast	Slim and Thin Protein Drink 1 cup herbal tea or Mixed Synthesizer Slimming Tea			
Midmorning	1 orange 1 cup herbal tea or Mixed Synthesizer Slimming Tea	1 peach 1 cup herbal tea or Mixed Synthesizer Slimming Tea	2 apricots 1 cup herbal tea or Mixed Synthesizer Slimming Tea	1 orange 1 cup herbal tea or Mixed Synthesizer Slimming Tea
Lunch	Sensational Vegetables and Couscous Couscous with Moroccan- Style Vegetables Tomato, Mushrooms, Eggplant, and Red Beans Seaweed Salad 1 glass Mixed Synthesizer Elixir 1 cup herbal tea or Mixed Synthesizer Slimming Tea	Mushroom and Tomato Omelet 3-Egg Fritatta with Mushrooms, Tomatoes, and Basil Salad Greens ½ hour after lunch: ½ small cantaloupe 1 cup herbal tea or Mixed Synthesizer Slimming Tea	Turkey Delight Roast Turkey Baked Sweet Potato Steamed Kale Watercress and Sprout Salad ½ hour after lunch: ½ cup each: pineapple, orange, and mango 1 cup herbal tea or Mixed Synthesizer Slimming Tea	Moroccan Salad Couscous Moroccan-Style Vegetables with Salad Greens 1 glass Mixed Synthesizer Elixir 1 cup herbal tea or Mixed Synthesizer Slimming Tea
Midafternoon	8 oz. fat-free soy milk or 4 oz. regular soy milk 1 cup herbal tea or Mixed Synthesizer Slimming Tea	8 oz. fat-free soy milk or 4 oz. regular soy milk 1 cup herbal tea or Mixed Synthesizer Slimming Tea	8 oz. fat-free soy milk or 4 oz. regular soy milk 1 cup herbal tea or Mixed Synthesizer Slimming Tea	8 oz. fat-free soy milk or 4 oz. regular soy milk 1 cup herbal tea or Mixed Synthesizer Slimming Tea
Dinner	Delicious Brown Rice Health Salad Brown Rice Salad with Tomatoes, Peas, Red Kidney	Turkey Jamboree Dinner Roast Turkey Steamed Spinach Cauliflower and Tomato Salad	Simple Chicken Dinner Poached Chicken with Roasted Red Pepper Puree String Beans and Zucchini	Simple Simon Salmon Broiled Salmon Asparagus Raw Veggie Salad Zucchini and Yellow

WHEN	SATURDAY	SUNDAY	MONDAY	TUESDAY
Dinner *(cont'd)*	Beans, Garlic, and Basil 1 cup herbal tea or Mixed Synthesizer Slimming Tea	1 cup herbal tea or Mixed Synthesizer Slimming Tea	Tomato and Mushroom Salad 1 cup herbal tea or Mixed Synthesizer Slimming Tea	Squash with Greens 1 cup herbal tea or Mixed Synthesizer Slimming Tea

WHEN	WEDNESDAY	THURSDAY	FRIDAY
On rising	*Fat-Buster Tonic*		
Breakfast	*Slim and Thin Protein Drink* 1 cup herbal tea or Mixed Synthesizer Slimming Tea		
Midmorning	2 kiwifruits 1 cup herbal tea or Mixed Synthesizer Slimming Tea	1 peach 1 cup herbal tea or Mixed Synthesizer Slimming Tea	2 apricots 1 cup herbal tea or Mixed Synthesizer Slimming Tea

Lunch	*Fabulous Fish Fiesta*
	Broiled Salmon
	Sautéed Cherry Tomatoes
	Steamed Spinach
	Arugula, Red Pepper and
	  Onion Salad
	
	½ hour after lunch:
	1 cup sliced fresh peaches
	1 cup herbal tea or Mixed
	  Synthesizer Slimming Tea
		Chicken with Red Pepper
		Puree Dinner
		Poached Chicken Breast
		  with Red Pepper Puree
		Sugar Snap Peas
		Radish Sprout and
		  Watercress Salad
		
		1 cup herbal tea or Mixed
		Synthesizer Slimming Tea
			Seared Tuna Lunch
			Cold Seared Tuna
			Asparagus
			Arugula and Cucumber
			  Salad
			
			½ hour after lunch:
			1 cup sliced fresh peaches
			1 cup herbal tea or
			  Mixed Synthesizer
			  Slimming Tea

Midafternoon	8 oz. fat-free soy
	milk (or 4 oz.
	  regular soy milk)
	1 cup herbal tea or
	  Mixed Synthesizer
	  Slimming Tea
		8 oz. fat-free soy
		milk (or 4 oz.
		  regular soy milk)
		1 cup herbal tea or
		  Mixed Synthesizer
		  Slimming Tea
			8 oz. fat-free soy
			milk (or 4 oz.
			  regular soy milk)
			1 cup herbal tea or
			  Mixed Synthesizer
			  Slimming Tea

Dinner	*Delicious Brown Rice*
	* Health Salad*
	Brown Rice Salad with
	  Tomatoes, Peas,
		Tasty Tuna Delight
		Seared Tuna
		Carrots, Celery, and Parsnips
		Cauliflower and
			Easy Egg Salad with
			* Mushrooms and Tomatoes*
			1 cup herbal tea or
			  Mixed Synthesizer

WHEN	WEDNESDAY	THURSDAY	FRIDAY
Dinner *(cont'd)*	Red Kidney Beans, Garlic, and Basil 1 cup herbal tea or Mixed Synthesizer Slimming Tea	Red Onion Salad 1 cup herbal tea or Mixed Synthesizer Slimming Tea	Slimming Tea

Mixed Synthesizer Food Choices

Proteins								
MEAT	FOWL	FISH		DAIRY	NUTS	SEEDS	LEGUMES	FRUIT PROTEIN
None	**Strong Acid**	**Strong Acid**	**Acid Forming**	**Acid Forming**	**Strong Acid**	**Strong Acid**	**Strong Acid**	**Strong Acid**
	Turkey Squab Chicken Frog legs Quail Pheasant	Mackerel Roe Halibut Red snapper Sole Tuna Bluefish Eel Swordfish Squid (calamari) Cod Mullet Haddock Ocean perch Sturgeon Octopus (scungilli)	Carp Yellowtail tuna Salmon Hake Lake perch Bass Trout	Soy milk (also under "Legumes")	Pine nuts Water chestnuts Cashews Coconut	Pumpkin seeds Sunflower seeds Squash seeds Safflower seeds Sesame seeds Flaxseeds Chia seeds	Peanuts	Avocados
	Acid Forming		**Shellfish Strong Acid**	*AVOID*	**Acid Forming (Nonsalted)**		**Acid Forming**	**Strong Alkaline**
	Eggs		Abalone	All Cheeses	Pecans Pistachios Walnuts Brazil nuts Macadamias Chestnuts Almonds		Lentils Soybeans Soy milk Adzuki beans Black beans Kidney beans Navy beans Pinto beans Red beans	Olives
	AVOID **Fatty Strong Acid**		**Acid Forming**	**Weak Alkaline**		*AVOID*		*AVOID*
	Goose Duck		Crab Lobster Scallops Clams and mussels Shrimp and crayfish	Goat's milk Yogurt Cow's milk Cream Buttermilk Whey		None		None
		Weak Acid			**Weak Acid**		*AVOID* **Weak Alkaline**	
		Anchovies Caviar Herring Sardines	**Weak Acid**		Filberts (hazelnuts) Hickory nuts		Soybean curd (tofu)	
			Oysters		*AVOID* **Weak Alkaline**			
			AVOID		Coconut milk			
			None					

Carbohydrates

GRAINS	HIGH-STARCH LEGUMES	HIGH-STARCH VEGETABLES	SLIGHTLY STARCHY VEGETABLES	NONSTARCHY VEGETABLES	
Strong Acid	**Strong Acid**	**Strong Acid**	**Weak Acid**	**Strong Acid**	**Weak Acid**
Popcorn	Black-eyed peas	Field corn	Beets, cooked	Mushrooms	Cauliflower, cooked
Corn grits	(cowpeas)	Sweet corn	Parsnips	Garlic	Eggplant
Rice bran		Potatoes	Jicama		Artichokes
Millet	**Acid Forming**			**Acid Forming**	Shallots
Barley		**Acid Forming**	**Acid Forming**		Salsify
Corn meal	Lima beans			Bamboo shoots	Soybean sprouts
Wheat	Garbanzo beans	Yams	Beets, raw	Green peas	Kohlrabi
Couscous	(chickpeas)	Pumpkin, raw		Sugar peas	Chicory
Bulgur (cracked	Great northern beans		**AVOID**	Mungbeans and	Onions
wheat)	Split peas	**Weak Acid**	**Weak Alkaline**	sprouts	Cucumbers
Rye	White (fava) beans			Asparagus	Radishes
Oats		Butternut squash	Carrots	Celeriac root	Summer squash, raw
Pastinas (egg)	**AVOID**	Hubbard squash	Rutabagas	Sweet peppers	
Sprouted grain		Sweet potatoes		Brussels sprouts	**Alkaline Forming**
bread	None	Pumpkin, canned		Cauliflower, raw	
				Tomatoes	Yellow dock, cooked
Acid Forming		**Eliminate If You**			Chicory greens
		Have Any Allergies		**Strong Alkaline**	Cabbage, cooked
Farina					Okra, cooked
Brown rice		Corn		Kale, cooked	Swiss chard, raw
Basmati brown rice		Corn meal		Collards	Spinach, cooked
Wild rice		Corn grits		Swiss chard, cooked	Kale, raw
Buckwheat (kasha)		Potatoes		Parsley	Lettuce: cos,
Quinoa				Mustard greens,	romaine, dark
		AVOID		cooked	green, white
Strong Alkaline		**Weak Alkaline**		Beet greens, cooked	Watercress
				Turnip greens,	Alfalfa sprouts
Amaranth grain and		Acorn squash		cooked	Dandelion greens
flakes				Lamb's-quarter	Arugula
				Mustard spinach	Beet greens, raw
Eliminate If You					
Have Any Allergies				**Seaweeds**	**Eliminate If You**
					Have Allergies of
Wheat				Agar-agar	**Any Kind**
Wheat germ				Kelp	
Rye				Irish moss	Eggplant
Barley				Dulse	Tomatoes
				Arame	Peppers
AVOID					
None					

NONSTARCHY VEGETABLES	FRUIT		OILS	CONDIMENTS	TEAS
AVOID **Weak Alkaline**	**Acid Forming**	**Sweet Fruit Acid Forming**	**Strong Acid**	**Weak Acid**	Licorice root: strengthens the adrenals (Don't use if you have high blood pressure.)
Summer squash, cooked	Litchis	Persimmons	Avocado	Vinegar	
Leeks	Passion fruit	Plantains	Corn	Honey	
Garden cress	Groundberries	Bananas	Soybean		
Chinese cabbage	Pomegranates		Peanut	**Strong Alkaline**	**Dong quai (Angelica sinensis):** tonic to balance the regenerative and reproductive organs
Snap beans	Crab apples	**Weak Acid**	Cottonseed	Molasses: blackstrap or light	
Yellow beans	Peaches	Apricots, dried	Olive	Sorghum	
Turnips		Raisins	Safflower	Maple syrup	
Scallions	**Weak Acid**	Prunes	Sunflower		
Broccoli	Guavas	Dates	Flaxseed	**Weak Acid (Salty)**	**Yellow dock:** great blood builder
Lettuce: butter, Boston, iceberg	Loquats		Walnut		
Celery	Cherimoya	**Alkaline Forming**	Apricot	Soy sauce	**Red clover:** tonic for the reproductive system
Endive	Grapes: muscat, Tokay	Pineapple	Almond		
Radicchio	Quince			*AVOID*	
Yellow dock, raw	Tamarinds	*AVOID* **Weak Alkaline**	*AVOID* **(Saturated Fats)**	Yeast—in all forms	**Hibiscus and rose hips:** tonic for the reproductive glands; also reduces water retention
Cabbage, raw	Apples			Brown sugar	
Okra, raw	Apricots	Boysenberries	Mayonnaise		
Spinach, raw	Prickly pears	Grapefruit	Butter	**Spicy**	
Fennel	Pears	Raspberries	Margarine	Mustard	
	Mangoes	Strawberries		Cane syrup	**Lemon grass:** reduces cellulite
Hot and Spicy		Plums			
Chili peppers	**Melons (Eat Alone)**	Acerola cherries		**Weak Alkaline**	**Nettle:** stabilizes blood sugar levels
Gingerroot	Watermelon	Blueberries		Cane sugar	
Horseradish	Muskmelon	Nectarines		Pickles	**Fennel:** curbs your appetite and aids digestion
	Cantaloupe	Gooseberries			
	Casaba	Pokeberries			
	Crenshaw	Papaya			
	Honeydew	Grapes: Concord, Thompson			
		Elderberries			
	Strong Alkaline	Sapotes			
	Rhubarb	Cranberries			
		Currants			
	Alkaline Forming	Lemons			
	Loganberries	Cherries			
	Oranges	Blackberries			
	Clementines	Limes			
	Tangerines	Figs			
	Kumquats				
	Kiwifruits				

Mixed Synthesizer Elixirs for Both Women and Men

Potassium Powerhouse: Carrot juice leads this potassium-rich formula full of vitamins A, D, B, C, E, and K; celery balances your nerves and clears your skin; parsley balances your adrenals; spinach, full of iron, burns fat; all the minerals rebalance your hormone levels.	Carrots: 6 oz. juice (about 6 carrots) Spinach: 3 oz. juice (about 1 bunch) Celery: 3 oz. juice (about 1 bunch) Parsley: 2 oz. juice (about 2 bunches) Water: 2 oz.
Energizer: Full of vitamins and iron, this juice energizes, nourishes, cleans out, and regenerates your whole endocrine system. Spinach builds iron-rich blood, which nourishes your ovaries, cleans out toxins, and burns up excess fat. It also supplies the iron needed by your thyroid gland.	Carrots: 6 oz. juice (about 6 carrots) Spinach: 3 oz. juice (about 1 bunch) Water: 2 oz.
Adrenal Stabilizer: With carrot juice, parsley is the great adrenal stabilizer and also balances the thyroid gland, cleanses the kidneys, brightens the eyes, and brings oxygen into the body.	Carrots: 6 oz. juice (about 6 carrots) Parsley: 3 oz. juice (about 3 bunches) Water: 2 oz.
Skin Beautifier: Feeding the ovaries and adrenal glands, the carrot juice along with the beet juice builds the blood, increases your circulation, and balances your hormonal levels; the cucumber improves and literally rebuilds your skin.	Carrots: 6 oz. juice (about 6 carrots) Beets: 3 oz. juice (about 2 beets) Cucumber: 3 oz. juice (about 1 cucumber) Water: 2 oz.

Your On-Program Cheat Sheet

Naturally there will be days when you just have to cheat. No problem. There's no need to become obsessed with perfection. You can be yourself and still succeed at weight loss on your meta-type diet. Besides, if you try to be flawless, you'll only end up frustrated and out of balance.

You've got to forget about bread, sugar, and refined carbohydrates, but there are other great-tasting treats that are just ideal for you.

Interestingly enough, for your mixed synthesizer profile, the best snack food is what your meta-mate the balanced synthesizer needs—pretzels, which are your main cheat food. These pretzels can be whole-grain, sourdough, or otherwise, but always baked and salt-free.

Here's a complete list of goodies that you can use to put a stop to the munchies—fast:

- *Hard pretzel:* 1 unsalted
- *Raisins:* ¼ cup, or 2 oz.
- *Dates:* ¼ cup pitted, or 2 oz.

- *Prunes:* ½ cup pitted, or 4 oz.
- *Apricots, dried:* ½ cup pitted, or 4 oz.

The list looks pretty good, right? But you have to make a deal with me. You need to follow some guidelines so that you can have these great goodies and really enjoy them. Otherwise, eating these cheat foods at random would undermine your goal for creating a beautiful body.

CHEAT-FOOD GUIDELINES
- *Eat your cheat foods only at the recommended times.* Cheat foods should be eaten no oftener than once per week, on the weekends (when you're not under stress), and at one meal or one time—only.
- *Eat only the amount suggested.* Your body can handle a small amount of these foods without triggering excessive insulin production. If you eat a large amount, your insulin level will spike and turn your "treat" into a "bad trick" of blubber.
- *Eat only one cheat food at a time.* Don't have several together or you'll wreak havoc with your metabolism and digestion. For instance, raisins *and* pretzels will send you over the top.
- *Never eat your cheat foods when you're under stress.* I guarantee you that's a surefire way to add pounds, not lose them. Only eat cheat foods when you're relaxed—usually on a weekend. Otherwise, your digestion shuts down and your insulin rises, and you become a veritable fat factory.
- *Never eat your cheat foods late at night.* You'll end up having a restless night's sleep, and it's mandatory for you to sleep deeply so your body can regenerate itself.

Mixed Synthesizer Healers and Helpers: Vitamins, Minerals, and Amino Acids

This section of your program is dedicated to the additions to the food plan that will help you lose weight even faster and improve your overall health and well-being. As I discussed in chapter 13, you can enhance the benefits of your meta-type diet with vitamins, minerals, and supplements tailored for you.

For your mixed synthesizer meta-type, I suggest that you add a gentle, full-spectrum multiple amino acid, vitamin, and mineral complex containing only those essential nutrients that support the sympathetic nervous system. This will speed up your weight-loss program, help tone your muscles, and give you abundant good health. The multiple amino acid, vitamin, and mineral complex for your meta-type can be purchased at your local vitamin store or ordered from the companies listed in appendix 2.

If the controlling endocrine gland governed by your dominant nervous system is out of balance, either hyperactive or hypoactive, more supplements may be needed. The following information should help you understand just what role each amino acid, vitamin, and mineral in your program plays in helping regulate your dominant sex glands—for a woman, your ovaries, and for a man, your testes. Then you can be your own best judge when choosing which nutrients to take to support their health.

As you have learned, your strength comes from these glands of reproduction—and regeneration. They control not just your fertility but your sex drive, your emotional stability, and your ability to fend off those unwanted excess pounds as well. Estrogen and testosterone, your glands' main hormones, also play a role in mental ability long after the fertility issues are history. Estrogen also is made from the breakdown of fat, so as you're stripping off weight, it's important to stay in balance.

A further incentive—your brain is stimulated to release its antiaging "growth" hormones when you're in metabolic balance, so you keep a youthful, not haggard, look as you shed pound after unwanted pound.

Remember, stress is the enemy here especially, lowering testosterone levels for men and boosting them in women.

With the news filled with questions about Viagra and prostate cancer for men, and estrogen replacement and breast and uterine cancer for women, it's important to know all you can about ways to support your own natural system.

For men there are several nutrients that are basic for your sexual health: the mineral selenium and the amino acids arginine and ornithine. Selenium is often called "the man's mineral" because one-half of the body's selenium is found in the testicles and a great deal is lost in the semen during ejaculation. It helps to alleviate prostate problems and is very synergistic with vitamin E. Ladies, you can get some benefit from selenium as well. It's been known to help with hot flashes and other menopausal problems as your body begins to shift its hormones during menopause.

Now menopause may be one time when women find that extra fat pays a dividend. That's because fatty tissue provides about 40 percent of the estrogen when your ovaries are functioning. As the menstrual cycle diminishes and the ovaries no longer produce eggs and estrogen, the customary hot flashes, headaches, fatigue, irritability, and volatile emotions can follow. If your weaker adrenals are already worn out from other stress, the male hormones may dominate. With proper balance restored, serenity and even a renewed libido are terrific payoffs.

For men flab and disinterest in sex can be a consequence of the "male menopause," or andropause, as your sex hormones diminish. If the already weak adrenals can't compensate, you'll face emotional slumps or depression, too.

A formula of amino acids, vitamins, and minerals will support your weaker opposite sympathetic endocrine gland, your adrenals. For male and female mixed synthesizers alike, you'll need to combat your normally sluggish wake-up, fight stress, and strip away those excess pounds.

In the mornings you need a bigger jolt of energy, to release stored blood sugar, or glycogen, and to cope with daily stresses. The action hormones—norepinephrine, epinephrine (adrenaline), and dopamine—provide the ultimate fight-or-flight surge.

And as you're battling to free yourself of those too-generous "curves," you'll need extra adrenal help from cortisol, the powerful fat-busting, energy-generating hormone. But it doesn't stop there, because if your weaker adrenals burn out, you'll find your once-strong sex hormones abruptly declining.

The nutrients needed to gently support your mixed synthesizer dominant sex glands are vitamin E; the B-complex components niacin (B_3), pantothenic acid (B_5), folic acid, and choline; and the minerals zinc, calcium, and selenium—especially for men. You don't need the essential fatty acids since you produce plenty of cholesterol on your own.

Vitamin E is essential for the health of both the ovaries and testes as well as for fertility and reproduction, and it provides many other benefits as you shed excess weight. It balances the hormonal output of estrogen for women and testosterone for men, helping you maintain that youthful glow, while providing more oxygen to improve your skin. If that's not enough, it helps regulate menstrual cycles, eases the effects of menopause, dissolves blood clots, and boosts your immune system. Vitamin E inhibits fatigue, improving the endurance that your meta-type usually lacks. Also this megavitamin is essential in preventing the oxidation of fats.

The *B-complex vitamins*—niacin (B_3), pantothenic acid (B_5), and folic acid—similarly are vital for healthy ovaries or testes, especially on a weight-loss regimen in which estrogen-rich fat is broken down and eliminated. Without them women may face irregular menstrual cycles, and men may have low libido. Niacin is necessary for estrogen, progesterone, and testosterone production; pantothenic acid and folic acid are essential for hormone synthesis and reproduction; and pantothenic acid is needed to transform your mixed synthesizer's abundant cholesterol into your sex hormones.

Choline is manufactured from the amino acid methionine and the B-complex components B_{12} and folic acid. It works with inositol (another part of the B-complex components) as a fat buster, breaking down fats and regulating the liver and gallbladder to reduce your meta-type's abundant cholesterol. Choline and inositol should be taken in equal amounts and occur naturally in the form of lecithin. You can also take them in capsule form with the amino acid methionine, called "lipo factors."

If you've been under a great deal of stress or are recovering from an illness, you may want to take more of the above nutrients.

Zinc, the magic mineral of the sex glands, is *vital* for supporting all reproductive organs, boosting fertility and male potency and easing menopausal or prostate problems. It works with calcium to cause proper bone calcification—essential to combat osteoporosis or other bone problems.

Calcium (as just mentioned) is important for building and protecting bones. But for your meta-type, it's needed for your sex glands, for toning and tightening muscles as you lose all that extra weight. It helps muscle growth and contractions and soothes nerves, ends excess water retention, relieves premenstrual and menstrual symptoms, and alleviates anxieties usually accompanying significant weight loss. Too much stress inhibits the flow of blood calcium—and may trigger cravings and binge eating. Calcium should be balanced with magnesium in a two-to-one ratio for cardiovascular and gonad health.

The benefits of *selenium* were discussed earlier in this section (see page 291).

Special note: When taking any of the B vitamins, it's important to know that you shouldn't take an isolated B—such as pantothenic acid or riboflavin—without taking the whole B-vitamin complement. Otherwise, the lone B constituent will rob your body of the other Bs to activate its energy. If you've been under a great deal of stress, are in a continued stress response, or are recovering from an illness, you may want to take more of these nutrients.

I also recommend the following nutrients for your weaker adrenal gland:

• *Vitamin C:* This key vitamin enhances your adrenals' ability to reduce allergic reactions and fight inflammation. It's essential for the synthesis of two amino acids—tryptophan, to help form the calming serotonin, and the energizing tyrosine (the precursor to the adrenal hormones dopamine, epinephrine, and norepinephrine). During adrenal activity or in a continued stress response, vitamin C is quickly depleted, and since it's not stored in the body, it must be taken daily or several times a day.

• *Pantothenic acid:* Vital to your adrenal health, pantothenic acid functions as two enzymes—CoA (coenzyme A) and ACP (acyl carrier protein)—to produce and burn fat and synthesize carbohydrates and proteins, especially in converting cholesterol into the steroid hormones formed by your adrenals and sex glands. It also aids in maintaining your insulin levels. It's needed to calm nerves, boost antibodies, and spark regeneration for great skin. As noted earlier, don't take just one component of the Bs. Be sure to get the full complement for them to work properly.

• *Tyrosine:* This amino acid is especially effective for exhausted adrenals. It's metabolized from the amino acid phenylalanine and is the basic ingredient in the production of your energizing adrenal hormones: dopamine, epinephrine, and norepinephrine. A deficiency almost guarantees your meta-type a slide into fatigue and depression—after triggering those binge cravings of sugar and bread.

The Bottom Line

By taking a complete amino acid, vitamin, and mineral combination based on the formulation for your general metabolic type, you'll be supplied with the nutrients needed to support your complementary side, the sympathetic nervous system. Then you may want to add a few of the vitamins and minerals we've just discussed, which are summarized in the accompanying table of recommended nutrients. If you prefer to get all your nutrients from foods, I've listed the foods highest in vitamin, mineral, and amino acid content in the accompanying table.

There are a few easy things to remember about taking the supplements:

• Try to take amino acids on an empty stomach. (They need adequate amounts of stomach enzymes to be broken down properly.)
• If possible, take enzymes with your meals to aid in your food digestion.
• Take vitamins and minerals after you've eaten, which helps their assimilation.
• The water-soluble vitamins—B complex, vitamin C, and vitamin P (bioflavonoids)—can be taken at any time.
• Your body isn't used to concentrated food substances, so I recommend that you introduce one type of amino acid, vitamin, or mineral into your regimen every few days. Gently and easily is the name of the game.

Mixed Synthesizer Vitamin, Mineral, and Amino Acid Food Sources

Sex Glands (Ovaries/Testes)	
Vitamin E	Oils (except coconut), alfalfa seeds, nuts, sunflower seed kernels, asparagus, avocados, blackberries, green leafy vegetables, oatmeal, rye, seafood (lobster, shrimp, tuna), and tomatoes
Zinc	Wheat bran, crab, and popcorn.
Calcium	Wheat flour, blackstrap molasses, almonds, Brazil nuts, caviar, cottonseed flour, dried figs, fish, green leafy vegetables, hazelnuts, oysters, soybean flour, and yogurt
B complex	• B_1: torula yeast, sunflower seeds, rice bran, wheat germ, pine nuts, dried coriander leaf, safflower seeds, soybeans, alfalfa seeds, sesame seeds, and rye flour (dark)
	• B_2: almonds, turnip greens, wheat bran, and soybeans
	• B_3 (niacin): fish, nuts, bran flakes, sesame seeds, and sunflower seeds
	• B_6: rice bran, wheat bran, sunflower seeds, avocados, bananas, corn, fish, brown rice, soybeans, and whole grains
	• B_{15}: grains, cereals, rice, apricot kernels, and torula yeast
Choline and inositol or lecithin	• Choline: soybeans, cabbage, wheat bran, navy beans, alfalfa leaf meal, rice polishings, rice bran, whole grains, hominy, turnips, and blackstrap molasses
	• Inositol: wheat germ, citrus fruits, blackstrap molasses, fruits, whole grains, bran, nuts, legumes, and vegetables
Selenium	Brazil nuts, butter, lobster, smelt, blackstrap molasses, cider vinegar, clams, crab, eggs, lamb, mushrooms, oysters, garlic, cinnamon, nutmeg, Swiss chard, turnips, wheat bran, and whole grains
Adrenals	
B complex	Listed under "Sex Glands"
Pantothenic acid (B_5)	Cottonseed flour, wheat bran, rice bran, rice polishings, nuts, soybean flour, buckwheat flour, lobster, sunflower seeds, and brown rice
Vitamin C	Acerola cherries, rose hips, citrus fruit, guavas, black currants, parsley, turnip greens, poke greens, and mustard greens
Tyrosine	All animal proteins (meat, fowl, and fish) and soy products

Mixed Synthesizer Recommended Nutrients

ENDOCRINE GLAND	NUTRIENT	WOMEN			MEN		
		Number	Strength	Times per Day	Number	Strength	Times per Day
Sex glands	Vitamin E	1	200–400 IU	1	1	400–800 IU	1
(ovaries/	Zinc	1	30 mg	1	2	30 mg	1
testes)	Calcium-						
	magnesium	1	500 mg	3	1–2	500 mg	3
	B complex	1	50–75 mg	2	1	100–125 mg	2
	Lipo factors	1	500 mg	1	1	1,000 mg	1
	or lecithin	1	1,200 mg	1–2	1	1,200 mg	3
	Selenium	optional	—	—	1	200 mcg	1
Adrenals	B complex	See under "Sex glands"	—	—	See under "Sex glands"	—	—
	Pantothenic acid	1	250 mg	1–2	1	500 mg	2
	Vitamin C						
	(buffered)	1	1,000 mg	3	2	1,000 mg	3
	Tyrosine	1–2	250 mg	2–3	1–2	500 mg	2–3

Although, as indicated in the accompanying table, women don't normally require selenium, you may wish to take 50 micrograms per day if you're experiencing menopausal problems.

Taking these extra vitamins, minerals, and supplements will require work—there's no mistaking that. Just as you have to plan meals with the right ingredients, you'll need to organize these. But as your metabolic system moves back into balance, you'll reduce the number of pills you'll need. And along the way, you'll discover that the dividend of glowing good health pays off quickly enough to make Wall Street envious.

Stocking Up

You've now finished reading about the program and are well on your way to a brand-new you. Just wait and see—you'll be slim, sexy, and full of bounce to every ounce. Now to get started, you'll need to stock up and organize. The accompanying list shows all the foods you'll need for the coming week. Double-check this list against your weekly menu and make any adjustments you feel are necessary. Happy regeneration!

Weekly Shopping List for Mixed Synthesizers

Larger quantities for men are shown in **boldface**.

PRODUCE

Fruit

2 Kiwifruits
2 Apricots
1 package (approx. 4 slices)
   Pineapple, precut
½ sm. Cantaloupe
4 Oranges
1 sm. Mango
7 Peaches
4 Lemons

Vegetables

4 lb. Carrots
1 bunch Celery
2 Cucumbers
3 lb. Spinach
2 sm. Yellow squashes
2 sm. Zucchini
2 lg. bunches Kale
3 10-oz. Mushrooms
1 bulb Garlic
14 Plum tomatoes (if on diet)
2 pt. Cherry tomatoes
4 Red peppers
2 sm. Sweet potatoes
1 sm. Cauliflower
1 Red onion
1 sm. Eggplant
2 lb. Asparagus
¼ lb. Peas, fresh or frozen
¼ lb. Sugar snap peas

Salad Greens

1 head Romaine lettuce
1 head Red leaf lettuce
1 Swiss chard
2 bunches Arugula
2 bunches Watercress
6 bunches Parsley
2 boxes Alfalfa sprouts
1 box Radish sprouts
1 bunch Cilantro, fresh

GROCERIES

1 lb. Red kidney beans
½ lb. Couscous
½ lb. Brown rice
1 loaf Sprouted grain bread
1 bottle Apple cider vinegar
1 16-oz. jar Tupelo honey
4 qt. Soy milk, fat-free
1 container Protein powder
   (whey- or soy-based)
1 container Kelp powder or
   blue-green algae
1 container Bone meal
   (optional)
1 package Seaweed of choice
Cayenne pepper, cumin, dried
   thyme, cinnamon, nutmeg,
   cardamom seed, paprika
Soy sauce
Herbal teas
Safflower oil

DAIRY
6 Eggs

MEAT AND FISH
2 4-oz. **(2 6-oz.)**
   cutlets Turkey breast

2 pieces: 1 5-oz., 1 4-oz. **(2 pieces: 1 6-oz., 1 5-oz.)** Salmon
2 pieces: 1 4-oz., 1 5-oz. **(2 pieces: 1 5-oz., 1 6-oz.)** Tuna
2 cutlets: 1 6-oz., 1 4-oz. **(2 6-oz.)** Chicken breast

Part five

Strategies for Success

To keep those pounds steadily melting away, diet alone isn't enough for most people on weight-loss plans. My specialized programs include three strategically important techniques, based on both Western and Eastern concepts, that will help those pounds evaporate.

These powerful techniques, when added to your meta-type's food program, will dramatically enhance the effects of your rapid weight loss and increase your feelings of glowing health while keeping you emotionally centered, energized, and motivated to follow through to the end of your goal.

From the West comes the first technique: Aromatherapy and Bach flower remedies help balance, energize, or calm your mind and emotions, whatever your meta-type, as you go through the day's trials and tribulations. We all know that everyday life—exacerbated by our reaction to pressures and the stress response—can be emotionally and physically damaging, causing us to hit those walls of total resistance. We end up falling off the wagon and plunging into bingeing on exactly what we don't need: comfort foods that pile on those excess pounds we worked so hard to shed. Using the essential oils of aromatherapy and Bach flower remedies in these situations will keep you centered, calm, energized, and stabilized while preventing you from plummeting into an eating abyss.

From the East comes the second technique: acupressure. By using gentle finger pressure on specific areas of the body—called acupuncture points (reserves, or "wells," of energy throughout your body)—you can affect the way you gain or lose weight and can electrify or calm your energies. As you've learned, the results of the stress response cause energetic chaos in your body, even blocking your ability to digest food, eliminate properly, and consequently burn off fat. Daily stimulation of the appropriate points for your meta-type will restore and release your body's correct energetic flow, allowing you to run as a highly effective machine and in turn rapidly burn off those pounds.

From both East and West comes the third technique, one of the basic foundations of a successful weight-loss program: exercise. The body *must* move and burn off calories or your program will come to a screeching halt. But one type of exercise is not good for all. Accelerator meta-types need to calm and balance their intense energies; heavy aerobic exercise would overstimulate their highly overactive body, causing a burnout effect. They need the calming and relaxing types of exercises that are brought to us by Eastern traditions; these exercises will bring their overactive systems into balance and harmony. Synthesizer meta-types need to stimulate and speed up their slower energies. The movements they love, Yoga or T'ai Ch'i, aren't stimulating enough to speed up their slower metabolisms. They need what the West brings: methods of stimulating exercise, such as aerobics, weight training, or Dancercize.

Incorporating my three Strategies for Success into your individual program—on a *daily basis*—will guarantee that your *individualized* program will be a total success, and you will have been given a great gift: *the ability to move the energies in your own body*.

20 Easing Weight Loss with Aromatherapy and Bach Flower Remedies

Believe it or not, *essential oils* are some of the most powerful weapons against unwanted weight gain. They are natural stress busters that can help you balance your mind and emotions. And as you've learned, that's extremely important in your weight-loss program. In this chapter you will find essential-oil formulas developed especially for each metatype. Let's start with a quick primer on how they work.

For years scientists have used many of these liquid essences as active ingredients in drugs. For instance, peppermint oil is an anti-inflammatory used to treat arthritis and rheumatism. It is also marketed as a remedy for digestive discomfort under the trade name Colperin. These amazing oils can also be antiseptics, antineuralgics, antispasmodics, antitoxics, antidepressants, analgesics, and even great sources of energy.

But what do these oils have to do with our emotions and weight loss? Do we drink them or take them in pill form? Good questions! We *smell* the aromas of the essential oils and *drink* minute amounts of the Bach flower remedies in small amounts of water.

Aromatherapy

Here's how aromatherapy works. When we inhale any kind of odor, some 20 million nerve endings in our nose become excited and are stimulated to telegraph their message to the olfactory bulb and its tract, which enters the brain's limbic system (that center part of the brain that tightly surrounds your hypothalamus and pituitary gland). Housed within the limbic system are areas known as the amygdala and hippocampus, which act as your memory and emotional centers and are responsible for eliciting emotional responses.

The odor's aromatic message and the emotional response it automatically triggers from your limbic system are then telegraphed to your major control center—the hypothalamus, which regulates your circadian rhythms. The hypothalamus also controls your metabolism, since one of its main functions is to integrate your sympathetic and parasympathetic nerve fibers and systems, as well as your emotions and thoughts. It's also responsible for activating the release or inhibition of your hormones based on your internal time clock or emotions. This is how the mind-body connection works.

When it receives the aromatic message and emotional response, your hypothalamus decides which part of your brain should receive the communication. For example if a euphoric oil, such as jasmine, has been inhaled, the hypothalamus might direct the message to the thalamus (right in back of the hypothalamus), instructing it to secrete enkephalins, which act as painkillers and make you feel terrific by inducing feelings of elation.

Your pituitary gland might be alerted to produce endorphins, which are painkillers as well as aphrodisiacs, when a scent such as ylang-ylang has been absorbed. Through these odorous messages the pituitary can also alert your other endocrine glands—such as your thyroid gland, adrenal gland, pancreas, thymus, and sex glands—to produce their precious secretions. Pretty powerful stuff!

The more sedative odors, such as sandalwood, will trigger the hypothalamus to stimulate the brain's raphe nucleus, which releases serotonin, the neurochemical sedative. Excitatory oils, such as juniper, urge the hypothalamus to contact the brain's locus coeruleus, which stimulates your adrenals to use their powerful hormones norepinephrine and epinephrine, your natural "wake-up call" stimulators.

Essential oils are divided into four basic categories: stimulants, sedatives, euphorics, and regulators. The regulators are important because they act as natural adaptogens—in other words, they work to achieve a natural state of balance in the body regardless of whether the situation is "hyper" or "hypo." Their actions affect the autonomic nervous system and the endocrine system as well as blood pressure stabilization.

How does this work in your weight-loss program? Let's say you've had a rough day at the office and are really tempted to reach for that bagel, bread, or a drink. Instead, you can take a sniff of a calming essential oil. The results are almost instantaneous. You immediately begin to calm down and relax. Take another sniff and you're ready to go home to a relaxing bath and healthy dinner. You've won. You didn't let your stress and anxiety get you down. The same is true if you need added energy. Wave a bottle of one of the stimulant oils under your nose and you'll soon feel ready to get up and go.

The best way to use essential oils is through inhalation or external application on the body. You can inhale them by using a diffuser, putting them in a humidifier, or just taking a sniff from a small bottle. You can put them in massage oils or in your bath. I even had one client who just set a basin of water on her radiator and put the drops of oil right in the water.

Since these oils are so potent, they have to be used in a *base oil* if they are going to be applied to the body in any way. Base oils are vegetable, nut, or seed oils that have therapeutic properties, such as *sweet almond oil*, which is rich in proteins, vitamins, and minerals. It helps to relieve itching, soreness, dryness, and inflammation. Then there is *apricot kernel oil*—one of my favorites. It's full of minerals and vitamins and is great for all skin types, especially to prevent premature aging of the skin as well as to soothe sensitive, inflamed, or dry skin.

Next comes *avocado oil*, which is rich in vitamins, proteins, lecithin, and fatty acids. It is especially beneficial for dry and dehydrated skin and for eczema. This oil needs to be used as an addition to a base oil in a 10 percent dilution; otherwise, it's too rich and heavy. *Carrot oil* is also rich in vitamins, minerals, and the much-touted beta-carotene, so wonderful for prematurely aging skin, itchiness, dryness, psoriasis, and eczema. It's also rejuvenating and reduces scarring but, like avocado oil, must be used as a 10 percent dilution in another base oil.

Grapeseed oil is rich in vitamins, minerals, and protein and is excellent on all skin types, while *jojoba oil*—another favorite of mine—not only is protein- and mineral-rich but also contains a waxy substance similar to collagen that is excellent on inflamed skin, psoriasis, eczema, and acne. Additionally it is great for hair care and is highly penetrative. Again, like carrot and avocado oils, jojoba oil needs to be used as a 10 percent dilution in a base oil. Other oils that need to be used at a 10 percent dilution are borage seed oil, evening primrose oil, olive oil, sesame oil, and wheat germ oil.

The most commonly used base oils are corn oil, hazelnut oil, peanut oil, safflower oil, soya bean oil, and sunflower oil. You can also use oils found around your home, although they may not be as effective. Be sure to look at your own individual meta-type food choices list to see which oils are recommended for you.

Here are some quick guidelines to help you blend a small amount of your base oil with essential oils:

Amount of Essential Oil	IN	Amount of Base Oil
2 to 5 drops		1 teaspoon
6 to 15 drops		1 tablespoon
1 teaspoon		2 ounces
1 tablespoon		6 ounces

When buying essential oils, it's also useful to know that 20 drops is equivalent to ⅓ teaspoon of the essential oils and 60 drops is equivalent to 1 teaspoon of the oils. As a rule of thumb, use 5 drops of essential oil to each teaspoon of base vegetable oil.

These measurements are for your general use if you're buying any essential oils that are not included in your specific meta-type formula. I've listed the exact amount of essential oils needed for your base oils in the specific formulas, which are presented in the next subsection.

Whether you want to create magical moments by using the euphorics, relieve your stress by calming with the sedatives, energize your nervous system or alleviate your depressive moods by using the stimulants, or balance your energies by applying the regulators, you can't go wrong. They'll serve you well as important tools in keeping your program in high gear and keeping you right on track toward your goal-oriented weight loss. The following list shows some of the more important essential oils, categorized according to their functions:

Stimulants	Sedatives	Euphorics	Regulators
Peppermint	Chamomile	Clary sage	Bergamot
Eucalyptus	Lavender	Grapefruit	Frankincense
Juniper	Marjoram	Jasmine	Geranium
Rosemary	Orange blossom	Rose otto	Rose absolute
Tea tree	Sandalwood	Ylang-ylang	Rosewood
Black pepper	Hyacinth	Patchouli	Lemon
Lemon	Jonquil		Peppermint
Lemongrass	Narcissus		Hyssop
Cardamom			
Grapefruit			
Melissa			
Mandarin orange			
Coriander			
Ginger			

Stress-Buster Aromatherapy Formulas

The formula for each meta-type contains several essential oils, and I have a few suggestions about how you might use them. First, put the appropriate number of drops—which I'll give you in the following subsections—in a small, airtight container filled with about 4 ounces of the base oil of your choice. Pour about 2 ounces of that solution into a smaller container and keep it in your briefcase, pocket, or purse throughout the day. Pull it out anytime you feel harried, anxious, or tempted to reach for the wrong food or drink. Rub a small amount over your hands, around your neck, and under your chin. The essence will penetrate deeply into your pores and be absorbed into your skin by osmosis, ready to go into those deeper cellular layers to do your fat-busting work. The smell of the essential oils sends those messages into your brain to release the appropriate neurotransmitters to rebalance your body, keep that fat burning away, and temper the way in which you react to stress.

My second suggestion is that you keep a larger container of the base oil and formula in your home and apply it sparingly all over your body both morning and evening. During the day its continued aroma will help keep you calm and relaxed while stimulating those extra pounds to be turned into energy. In the evening it will help you to unwind from your hectic day, relax, and get a good night's sleep. You might want to massage it deeply into those areas that are holding on to fat—the stomach, waist, hips, thighs, or upper torso. It will help to break apart those fatty tissues and flush them out of your body.

Or put five to six drops of your concentrated essential oil formula directly into a nice, warm bath. Soak and relax in it before going to bed and let those oils just permeate your body.

If you don't want to do any of the preceding, then just keep a small vial or container of the essential oil formula itself in your pocket. Pull it out when needed and take a sniff. It will go to work right away directing your brain to produce the right secretions, helping your body and nerves rebalance and realign themselves, all the while stimulating your continued weight loss.

When making up your individual formula, put the essential oil drops in the bottom of an airtight container, fill it with the base oil, close tightly, shake, and use. Or make up the formula by itself and keep it in a small, airtight bottle. Then you can add the appropriate amount of formula drops to anything you wish—base oil, bathwater, or even a diffuser or bowl of hot water.

The following list shows the proportions of essential oil combination to base oil that you can use to mix various amounts of your special aromatherapy formula. The boldfaced proportion (120 drops of essential oil combination to 4 ounces of base oil) is the one on which the meta-type formulas in the following subsections are based.

Amount of Essential Oil Combination	IN	Amount of Base Oil
30 drops		1 oz. (2 tbs.)
60 drops (1 tsp.)		2 oz.
120 drops (2 tsp.)		**4 oz.**
180 drops (1 tbs.)		6 oz.

You can purchase the essential oils at your health-food store as well as at some pharmacies and drugstores, or order them from the suppliers listed in appendix 2.

Once you've read the subsection below on the aromatherapy formula that's tailor-made for your meta-type, turn to page 316 and learn about the benefits of Bach flower remedies.

Accelerator

Now since we know that your meta-type is prone to anxiety, our objective is to keep you calm enough so that those excitatory neurotransmitters you're always pumping out won't suppress the growth hormones your pituitary releases at night to help you burn off fat. You see, when you're sleeping, you actually regenerate and rebuild your cells and burn off those extra pounds.

For you highly active accelerators, I've put together a special formula that not only calms, relaxes, and soothes that harried mind of yours but also helps to burn off those extra pounds. It will help you to be less irritable and resentful, relieve your anxiety, bring your blood pressure down, reverse the aging process, relieve premenstrual tension, induce sleep, and give you a feeling of general well-being. I've used this formula for years, and my accelerator clients leave my office feeling great.

I call your formula (shown in the accompanying table) the Accelerator Balancer, and it's composed of those essential oils that relax your highly active sympathetic nervous system while stimulating your parasympathetic nervous system—your alter ego. Remember, the parasympathetic nervous system is responsible for your regeneration, your new body, and how it redistributes your weight.

Accelerator Balancer Formula

ESSENTIAL OIL	DROPS	FUNCTION
Base Formula ("The Big Guns")		
Chamomile*	24	Powerful tonic and relaxer; also stimulates digestion.
Lavender	24	"The healer": a tonic; also attacks fat and calms anxiety.
Marjoram	16	Stimulates parasympathetic activity and calms anxiety.
Neroli	16	"Fat burner" and strong tonic; also calms anxiety.
The Regulators		
Bergamot	12	Tonic that stimulates digestion and burns fat.
Frankincense	10	Tonic that calms, is a digestive, and is slightly euphoric.
The Euphorics		
Clary sage	10	Soothes your nerves and raises your spirits and sexuality.
Ylang-ylang	9–10	Relaxes but stimulates sexuality and fertility—a *must!*

*If you have any tendency to ragweed allergy, I recommend that you substitute sandalwood, hyacinth, or narcissus for the chamomile.

Other essential oils to help your accelerator meta-type are for:

- *Stimulating sexuality:* jasmine
- *Antiaging:* grapefruit
- *Calming impatience:* rose absolute
- *Opening emotionally:* jasmine
- *Insomnia:* rosewood
- *Muscle aches (from exercise):* eucalyptus, peppermint, and rosemary
- *Added stress:* sandalwood
- *Added anxiety:* rose absolute, geranium, jasmine, Melissa (lemon balm), and sandalwood

Balanced Accelerator

As a balanced accelerator, you know you're prone to tensions and anxieties. You tend to live in the world of the stress response. Our objective is to keep you calm enough to moderate those excitatory neurotransmitters you're always pumping out.

For you balanced accelerators, I've put together a special formula that excites, stimulates, and regenerates that tired body of yours. You'll be less irritable and stressed and will feel your worries and depression just melt away.

Your formula, which I call the Balanced Accelerator Stabilizer (shown in the accompanying table), contains those essential oils that activate your less active parasympathetic system and rebalance your overworked sympathetic system. Use it anytime you feel harried, worried, or tempted to reach for fatty food.

Balanced Accelerator Stabilizer Formula

ESSENTIAL OIL	DROPS	FUNCTION
Base Formula ("The Big Guns")		
Lavender	24	"The healer": a tonic; also attacks fat and calms anxiety.
Chamomile*	16	Powerful tonic and relaxer; also stimulates digestion.
Neroli	16	"Fat burner" and strong tonic; also calms anxiety.
Marjoram	12	Stimulates parasympathetic activity and calms anxiety.
Lemongrass	12	Gastric stimulator; also balances parasympathetic activity.
The Regulators		
Bergamot	8	Tonic that stimulates digestion and burns fat.
Frankincense	8	Tonic that calms, is a digestive, and is slightly euphoric.
Rose absolute	6	Tonic, sedative, and aphrodisiac; also stimulates the liver.
The Euphorics		
Clary sage	4	Soothes your nerves and raises your spirits and sexuality.
Ylang-ylang	4	Relaxes but stimulates sexuality and fertility—a *must!*
Jasmine	6	Tonic, sedative, and aphrodisiac; also stimulates creativity.
Sandalwood	6	Tonic, sedative, and aphrodisiac; also balances hyperactivity.

*If you have any tendency to ragweed allergy, I recommend that you substitute sandalwood, hyacinth, or narcissus for the chamomile.

Other essential oils to help your balanced accelerator meta-type are for:

- *Antiaging:* grapefruit
- *Muscle aches (from exercise):* eucalyptus, peppermint, and rosemary
- *Fertility:* rose otto
- *Insomnia:* rosewood
- *Added anxiety:* rosewood, geranium, and Melissa (lemon balm)

Mixed Accelerator

As a mixed accelerator, you know you're vulnerable to stress and anxiety. You easily get pulled into the world of the stress response. Our objective is to keep you calm enough to balance those excitatory neurotransmitters you're always pumping out with the calming neurotransmitters from your parasympathetic system. Then they won't suppress the growth hormones your sluggish pituitary releases at night, which redistribute and burn off your fat. It's only when you sleep that your body regenerates, your cells rebuild, and you burn off those extra pounds.

For you more active mixed accelerators, I've put together a special formula that will help keep you tranquil and peaceful as you're hurrying through your hectic day. It will also help to burn off those extra pounds. You'll be less irritable and less tense about your day and diet, and you'll feel your anxieties melt away. This formula will help you sleep, will give you a feeling of general well-being, and can even reverse the aging process. I've used this formula for years, and my mixed accelerator clients love it.

Mixed Accelerator Balancer Formula

ESSENTIAL OIL	DROPS	FUNCTION
Base Formula ("The Big Guns")		
Chamomile*	20	Powerful tonic and relaxer; also stimulates digestion.
Lavender	20	"The healer": a tonic; also attacks fat and calms anxiety.
Marjoram	12	Stimulates parasympathetic activity and calms anxiety.
Neroli	12	"Fat burner" and strong tonic; also calms anxiety.
Juniper	8	Tonic and diuretic; also invigorates, energizes, and regulates insulin.
Fennel	8	General tonic and diuretic; also energizes.
The Regulators		
Bergamot	12	Tonic that stimulates digestion and burns fat.
Frankincense	10	Tonic that calms, is a digestive, and is slightly euphoric.
The Euphorics		
Clary sage	6	Soothes your nerves and raises your spirits and sexuality.
Ylang-ylang	6	Relaxes but stimulates sexuality and fertility—a *must!*
Grapefruit	6	Stimulates enkephalins, combats aging, and burns fat; also a diuretic.

*If you have any tendency to ragweed allergy, I recommend that you substitute sandalwood, hyacinth, or narcissus for the chamomile.

I call your formula (shown in the accompanying table) the Mixed Accelerator Balancer, and it's composed of those essential oils that relax your highly active sympathetic nervous system while energizing your parasympathetic nervous system. Remember, the parasympathetic nervous system is responsible for your regeneration, your new body, and how it redistributes your weight.

Other essential oils to help your mixed accelerator meta-type are for:

- *Stimulating sexuality:* jasmine
- *Opening emotionally:* jasmine
- *Calming impatience:* rose absolute
- *Muscle aches (from exercise):* eucalyptus, peppermint, and rosemary
- *Insomnia:* rosewood
- *Added anxiety:* rose absolute, rosewood, geranium, jasmine, Melissa (lemon balm), and sandalwood
- *Added stress:* sandalwood

Synthesizer

As a synthesizer, you know you're vulnerable to stress and depression. You have extremely poor defenses against the stress response because of your weaker energy-producing glands, your adrenals, your thymus, and especially your thyroid. Our objective is to keep you energized by helping you to produce excitatory neurotransmitters from your sympathetic system. They will balance the calming neurotransmitters you're always pumping out.

For you less active synthesizers, I've put together a special formula that not only excites, stimulates, and regenerates that tired body of yours but helps to energize it as well. You'll be less irritable and depressed and less moody, and it will help to give you an upbeat attitude toward life. You'll feel your worries and depression just melt away. This formula will stimulate your possible low blood pressure (don't use it if you have high blood pressure) and give you a feeling of general well-being, and can even reverse the aging process. I've used this formula for years, and my synthesizer clients love it.

I call your formula (shown in the accompanying table) the Synthesizer Stimulator. It contains those essential oils that activate your less active sympathetic system as well as energize your own dominant parasympathetic system. Remember, the sympathetic nervous system is responsible for your energy production and the way your body burns off those excess pounds. We still want your own dominant parasympathetic system active, since it's responsible for your body's regeneration and for the redistribution of your fatty tissues.

Synthesizer Stimulator Formula

ESSENTIAL OIL	DROPS	FUNCTION
Base Formula ("The Big Guns")		
Cardamom	12	Powerful energizer and diuretic; also stimulates digestion.
Juniper	12	Tonic, energizer, and digestive; also regulates blood sugar.
Lemongrass	16	Gastric stimulator; also balances parasympathetic activity.
Rosemary	12	Stimulates the adrenals; energizer and cardiotonic.
Peppermint	12	Stimulates the sympathetic nervous system; also a strong tonic.
Basil	10	Stimulates the adrenal cortex and digestion; also a nerve tonic.
Special Additions		
Clove	8	Tonic and mental stimulant; also stimulates the adrenals.
Neroli	8	"Fat burner" and strong tonic; also calms anxiety.
The Regulators		
Geranium	4	Tonic; also stimulates the adrenal cortex and regulates insulin.
Rose absolute	4	Antidepressant, tonic, aphrodisiac, and hepatic.
Clary sage	4	Tonic; also stimulates the adrenals and regulates the parasympathetic nervous system.
Bergamot	4	Tonic that stimulates digestion and burns fat.
The Euphorics		
Ylang-ylang	6	Antidepressant, tonic, and aphrodisiac; also calms.
Jasmine	4	Antidepressant, tonic, and aphrodisiac.
Rose otto	4	Tonic, euphoric, aphrodisiac, and antidepressant.

Other essential oils to help your synthesizer meta-type are for:

- *Insecurity:* sandalwood
- *Nightmares:* frankincense
- *Mood swings:* rosewood
- *Muscle aches (from exercise):* eucalyptus, peppermint, and rosemary
- *Added anxiety:* rosewood, Melissa (lemon balm), and sandalwood
- *Added stress:* sandalwood
- *Fears:* frankincense and sandalwood

Balanced Synthesizer

As a balanced synthesizer, you know you're vulnerable to stress, anxiety, and depression. You have extremely poor defenses against the stress response because of your weaker energy-producing glands, your adrenals, your thyroid, and especially your thymus. Our objective is to keep you energized enough by helping you produce those excitatory neurotransmitters from your sympathetic system to balance out the calming neurotransmitters you're always pumping out. Then, when your pituitary releases its growth hormones at night to redistribute and burn off your fat, your body will be able to regenerate and rebuild as you adjust those extra pounds.

Balanced Synthesizer Stabilizer Formula

ESSENTIAL OIL	DROPS	FUNCTION
Base Formula ("The Big Guns")		
Cardamom	12	Powerful energizer and diuretic; also stimulates digestion.
Juniper	12	Tonic, energizer, and digestive; also regulates blood sugar.
Lemongrass	16	Gastric stimulator; also balances parasympathetic activity.
Rosemary	12	Stimulates the adrenals; energizer and cardiotonic.
Peppermint	12	Stimulates the sympathetic nervous system; also a strong tonic.
Basil	10	Stimulates the adrenal cortex and digestion; also a nerve tonic.
Special Additions		
Marjoram	8	Stimulates parasympathetic activity and calms anxiety.
Neroli	8	"Fat burner" and strong tonic; also calms anxiety.
The Regulators		
Geranium	6	Tonic; also stimulates the adrenal cortex and regulates insulin.
Rose absolute	6	Antidepressant, tonic, aphrodisiac, and hepatic.
Bergamot	4	Tonic that stimulates digestion and burns fat.
The Euphorics		
Grapefruit	6	Stimulates enkephalins, combats aging, and burns fat; also a diuretic.
Jasmine	4	Antidepressant, tonic, and aphrodisiac.
Rose otto	4	Tonic, euphoric, aphrodisiac, and antidepressant.

I call your formula (shown in the accompanying table) the Balanced Synthesizer Stabilizer. It contains those essential oils that activate your less active sympathetic system as well as energize your own dominant parasympathetic system. Remember, the sympathetic nervous system is responsible for your energy production and the way your body burns off those excess pounds. We still want your own dominant parasympathetic system active, since it's responsible for your body's regeneration and for the redistribution of your fatty tissues.

Other essential oils to help your balanced synthesizer meta-type are for:

- *Depression:* clary sage, ylang-ylang
- *Insecurity:* sandalwood
- *Mood swings:* rosewood
- *Muscle aches (from exercise):* eucalyptus, peppermint, and rosemary
- *Added anxiety:* rosewood, Melissa (lemon balm), and sandalwood
- *Nightmares:* frankincense
- *Added stress:* sandalwood
- *Fears:* frankincense and sandalwood

Mixed Synthesizer

As a mixed synthesizer, you know you're vulnerable to stress, anxiety, and depression. You can easily get pulled into the world of the stress response because of your weaker adrenal gland. Our objective is to keep you energized by helping you to produce excitatory neurotransmitters from your sympathetic system. They will balance the calming neurotransmitters you're always pumping out. Then your pituitary will be able to release its growth hormones at night, which redistribute and burn off your fat. It's only when you sleep that your body regenerates, your cells rebuild, and you burn off those extra pounds.

For you less active mixed synthesizers, I've put together a special formula that not only excites, stimulates, and regenerates that tired body of yours but helps to energize it as well. You'll be less irritable and depressed and less moody, and it will help to give you an upbeat attitude toward life. You'll feel your worries and depression just melt away.

I call your formula (shown in the accompanying table) the Mixed Synthesizer Balancer. It contains those essential oils that activate your less active sympathetic system as well as energize your own dominant parasympathetic system. Remember, the sympathetic nervous system is responsible for your energy production and the way your body burns off those excess pounds.

Mixed Synthesizer Balancer Formula

ESSENTIAL OIL	DROPS	FUNCTION
Base Formula ("The Big Guns")		
Cardamom	14	Powerful energizer and diuretic; also stimulates digestion.
Juniper	16	Tonic, energizer, and digestive; also regulates blood sugar.
Lemongrass	18	Gastric stimulator; also balances parasympathetic activity.
Rosemary	14	Stimulates the adrenals; energizer and cardiotonic.
Peppermint	16	Stimulates the sympathetic nervous system; also a strong tonic.
Basil	12	Stimulates the adrenal cortex and digestion; also a nerve tonic.
The Regulators		
Geranium	8	Tonic; also stimulates the adrenal cortex and regulates insulin.
Rose absolute	8	Antidepressant, tonic, aphrodisiac, and hepatic.
The Euphorics		
Grapefruit	8	Stimulates enkephalins, combats aging, and burns fat; also a diuretic.
Jasmine	6	Antidepressant, tonic, and aphrodisiac.

Other essential oils to help your mixed synthesizer meta-type are for:

- *Depression:* clary sage, rose otto, ylang-ylang
- *Insecurity:* sandalwood
- *Immunity:* neroli
- *Mood swings:* rosewood
- *Muscle aches (from exercise):* eucalyptus, peppermint, and rosemary
- *Nightmares:* frankincense
- *Confusion:* rose otto
- *Added anxiety:* rosewood, Melissa (lemon balm), and sandalwood
- *Grief:* rose otto
- *Added stress:* sandalwood
- *Fears:* frankincense and sandalwood

Bach Flower Remedies

The Bach flower remedies are the *diluted essences* of the essential oils put in solutions at very small dosages. They work on the same principle as *homeopathy*—which is basically that a very little bit goes a long way. In this form the essential oils *can* be taken into the body. Bach flower remedies also help to balance your nervous system, which has the effect of stimulating your weight loss.

The Bach flower remedies help keep you emotionally stable when the going gets tough. You're exhausted from the day's frenetic pace, and you don't think you can take one more minute of the craziness! You reach for a destructive tension reliever—starches or sweets—and you've really blown your diet. Stop! You don't have to do that. Three or four drops of one of the flower remedies in a small glass of water will help you through that moment of intensity and bring you back into your center of calmness.

There are some thirty-eight remedies in all, and I've chosen the five that are best suited to the energy of each meta-type. Keep them in your pocket or purse and use them when the need arises—even three to four times per day. I have some of my clients use one or two remedies at the same time, but I find it best to alternate them every few days or every week. By then most of the situations have come under control or have passed, and you've learned how to cope with stress in a more balanced way.

Take a look at the ones I've chosen for your meta-type and see which best seem to fit your needs. You can use one or all of them for your specific requirements. Made out of nonpoisonous flowers and prepared under the principle of homeopathy (in which less is better, so two or three drops is much better than the whole bottle), they are absolutely safe to use. You could drink a whole bottle with no bad effects. If it's not the right formula for you, you won't feel any effects, but when it's the correct remedy for your metabolic type, the results are miraculous. Here we go.

Accelerator

- *Cherry plum:* When you're ready to burst from those intense feelings after a hectic day or stressful experience and are just about to blow your diet, reach for cherry plum.
- *Clematis:* If you've had too much anxiety and are in one of your escapist fantasies in which anything is possible and even a hot fudge sundae is okay, clematis brings you back to reality. It helps to ground you and keep you focused on your weight-loss goal.
- *Gorse:* When you're tired, have had a hard day, and are starting to get pessimistic about your ability to reach your goal, gorse will wipe that defeatism away. Keep it handy and don't let yourself dip into those negative feelings.
- *Pine:* You, the overachiever, set high standards for yourself, and if you don't feel you're perfect, you may dump the whole program. So you

fell off the program. Get back on and erase those guilty feelings. Pine helps you take responsibility for your life, set realistic goals, take the needed time for yourself, and keep more focused on your program.

- *Sweet chestnut:* You've reached your mental limits and have become brain-dead. You've lost your ability to endure, and now it's time for a reward—a no-no food. Stop! Sweet chestnut will pick you and your spirits up and keep you away from those foods that constantly pad you with fat.

Balanced Accelerator

- *Oak:* You've struggled tirelessly through the day despite opposition, throwing yourself into your work and neglecting to eat the right foods or take care of yourself. Out of desperation you reach for the sugars. No! Reach for oak instead to keep you stable under any conditions.
- *Impatiens:* Impatiens for impatience. You're tired and have worked all day, and now you're losing patience, becoming tense and irritable—especially with those around you who can't go as fast as you can. You've reached your point of exasperation and are ready to get that coffee and roll and calm down. Reach for impatiens instead to help calm you down in action and thought and keep you focused on your weight-loss program.
- *Elm:* You've overextended yourself on your commitments and obligations. You've taken on a full plate and may feel overwhelmed by all you have to do even though you know you're extremely capable. You've reached your limit and are about ready to get off your program and give yourself some sugary rewards. Use elm instead to calm yourself down and bring back that capable, intuitive, and efficient you.
- *Cherry plum:* When you're ready to burst from intense feelings after a hectic day or stressful experience and are just about to blow your diet, reach for cherry plum.
- *Sweet chestnut:* You've reached your mental limits and have become brain-dead. You've lost your ability to endure, and now it's time for a reward—a no-no food. Stop! Sweet chestnut will pick you and your spirits up and keep you away from those foods that constantly pad you with fat.

Mixed Accelerator

- *Agrimony:* When those feelings of frustration and anxiety start erupting and your old habit is to reach for the sweets—don't! Reach for agrimony. It helps to fuse your thinking mind and your feeling body.
- *Mustard:* When anxiety has got the best of you and is beginning to turn in on itself and become depression, reach for mustard to lift your spirits, energize your soul, and help you trust your instincts again. It gives you that extra energy boost when temptation is at hand.
- *Wild oat:* It's been going well, then something hits you out of the blue and you lose your focus on your weight-loss program. Reach for wild oat to put you right back on your path again, full of determination to reach your goal. Keep it handy and don't let yourself go down the primrose path.
- *Cherry plum:* When you're ready to burst from intense feelings after a hectic day or stressful experience and are just about to blow your diet, reach for cherry plum.
- *Willow:* Willow helps you to relax and open up to your creativity. It will spark your interest in yourself again and help you let go of those negative feelings of bitterness and resentment, which have been a motivating force in your carbohydrate binges. It will also help you to see the sunny side of your life and keep you motivated toward your weight-loss goal.

Synthesizer

- *Scleranthus:* When you've become uncertain about your ability to stick with your weight-loss program or are beginning to vacillate or weaken, reach for scleranthus. It will help you maintain your inner balance and keep focused on your goal.
- *Sweet chestnut:* You've tried and tried, but things look bleak after those first two days on the diet. Reach for sweet chestnut to clear away your despair. Then you will hold on until the end.
- *Elm:* When you want to see yourself thin but have a hard time visualizing the possibility, reach for elm to turn your ideas into reality. It supports your self-confidence and reinforces your decision to stay on your diet and reach your goals.

- *Mustard:* That dark cloud of doom is beginning to descend on you, and you think that if you can never eat sugar again, you'll just die. Reach for mustard to bring you out of that gloom and get you right back on your path to your body's awareness.
- *Star of Bethlehem:* It helps to keep your adrenals pumped up after a stressful situation and keeps you centered under any adverse circumstances.
- *Mimulus:* When those old fears start creeping into your consciousness, reach for mimulus. It helps to eliminate negative emotions and stimulates you to enjoy life without depression or fears.
- *Olive:* You've had a pretty tough day, and for you the stress was intense. You can't bear it, and you begin to cave in, fatigued, exhausted, and feeling hopeless. Reach for olive to put the zest back into your life and restore your fervent desire to reach your goal.

Balanced Synthesizer

- *Aspen:* When those feelings of fear and negativity begin to take over, persuading you to believe that you won't be able to accomplish your weight-loss goal, reach for aspen. It helps to allay those unfounded fears and anxieties that hit you out of the blue.
- *Hornbeam:* It helps to keep you focused on achieving your personal weight-loss goals. It won't allow you to procrastinate and put off your diet another day, and instead stimulates you into activity.
- *Impatiens:* You're getting closer to your goal, but you're beginning to lose patience with yourself and your program. Reach for impatiens to dispel your irritability, cultivate more patience, and calm your fears.
- *Star of Bethlehem:* It helps to keep your adrenals pumped up after a stressful situation and keeps you centered under any adverse circumstances.
- *Scleranthus:* When you've become uncertain about your ability to stick with your weight-loss program or are beginning to vacillate or weaken, reach for scleranthus. It will help you maintain your inner balance and keep focused on your goal.
- *Larch:* When your fears are starting to creep up and you're feeling a definite lack of self-confidence, reach for larch. It helps to wipe away that fear of failure and increases your self-awareness!

Mixed Synthesizer

- *Crab apple:* When you really want to cleanse your mind and body of those unwanted thoughts about your self-image, reach for crab apple. It will help you see things in the right perspective and get rid of those feelings you find hard to digest.
- *Elm:* When you want to see yourself thin and have a hard time visualizing the possibility, reach for elm to turn your ideas into reality. It supports your self-confidence and reinforces your decision to stay on your diet and reach your goals.
- *Mimulus:* When those old fears start creeping into your consciousness, reach for mimulus. It helps to eliminate those negative emotions and stimulates you to enjoy life without depression or fears.
- *Oak:* When you've had a tough day, you're tired, and your inner strength and determination to stay on your diet begin to wane, reach for oak. It will bolster your strength and your determination to reach your weight-loss goal.
- *Vervain:* If you've become prone to anxiety, irritability, or tension and you're tempted to reach for those awful fat-building comfort foods, reach for vervain instead. It will calm and relax you while stimulating your inner courage to stay focused on your weight-loss goal.
- *Wild rose:* You're starting to dip into depression, beginning to become apathetic about your program. Immediately reach for wild rose to pull you out of the doldrums and keep you focused on your goal.

We all know that hidden emotions begin to spring up, especially when you start losing weight. That's for another discussion. But for now use the Bach flower remedies to help keep you grounded and focused on your weight-loss program when those unexpected feelings tempt you to sway from your goal.

21 Strengthening Your Body with Meta-Type Body Points

We've talked about the differences between synthesizers and accelerators—the differences between their personalities, preferences, and ways in which they metabolize their food. They each have a different type of energy—more of either the slower yin regenerative energy or the yang active energy.

This energy runs throughout the body in regular patterns that are called *meridians*. How effectively these meridians function is critical because they activate your body's organs and systems. If there is an obstruction in any part of these energy flows, it can constrict the energy in one part of your body and inhibit it in another. For instance, if there's a block in your Stomach meridian, it will restrict the way in which you digest your food and ultimately affect how you lose or gain weight.

There are twelve main meridians in your body, each of which corresponds to a particular organ system and endocrine gland. Meridians and organs run in pairs, based on their yin or yang function. For example, the yin Lung meridian is paired with the yang Large Intestine meridian. Along each of these meridians are certain areas where the energy gathers and runs closer to your body's surface. These areas, called the *points* of the meridians, act as wells, or pools, that hold or store your energy.

It's within these points that the energetic flows of the meridian can be influenced. For instance, stimulating these points can unblock any obstructions in the meridians and help reestablish their proper energetic flow. That, in turn, enhances how your body will function energetically. That means you'll be able to burn off those excess pounds at a faster rate.

These points can easily be stimulated with gentle finger pressure in the form of massage. Each meta-type has a unique set of points. I find it best to have my clients manipulate these points when they first get out of bed in the morning. This helps to correct any imbalance in their energies and prepares them for the day. This way their bodies can be activated to burn off those pounds speedily during their action-oriented day.

I also suggest that my clients take five or ten minutes before going to bed to massage their specific points again. Their bodies are then prepared to relax and regenerate during the nighttime hours of peaceful sleep.

Try massaging your body points. It works wonders. Not only will it help you lose weight, but it will stimulate your general health and well-being, your energy, your healing abilities, and your emotional and mental health.

GUIDELINES FOR META-POINT MASSAGE

- Gently press against the point on the surface of your skin and rotate it clockwise in small, circular movements about two to three cycles per second.
- Start with one point at a time. Then, when you've mastered the technique, you can simultaneously work two points at the same time, one with each hand.
- You can spend from one to five minutes on each point, depending on your preference.
- Don't dig in deeply and hurt yourself. Generally light to medium pressure will suffice.
- You may find that one or two of your points are sore or tender. That could be an indication of an energy block or weakness in your meridian. Just work gently and slowly. Soon the tenderness will disappear, and your energy will once again flow unobstructed.
- If you find it difficult to massage any of the points on your back, use a small piece of doweling or an eraser top on a pencil or even roll on a small ball lying flat on your back to stimulate that particular area.

Wonder Points

Wonder Points for All Meta-Types

The three wonder points for general balance (shown in the accompanying table) can miraculously equalize and correct any energetic imbalance in your body. They stimulate the general energetic flow of yang or yin energy, stabilizing both the parasympathetic and sympathetic nervous systems. The great thing about them is that they can be used by any of the meta-types to rebalance themselves, creating a foundation of energetic balance in the body.

Wonder Points for General Balance

NAMES AND NUMBER	IMPORTANCE	LOCATION	
Ge Shu Diaphragm Point *Urinary Bladder 17 (UB17)*	Creates general balance for all the yin and yang meridians and is the reunion point of all yin and yang energies in the body.	1¼ inches lateral to the seventh thoracic vertebra, directly adjacent to the lower border of your scapula, or shoulder blade	**GE SHU** Bladder 17
Neiguan Inner Gate Broken Heart Gate Gate to Success *Pericardium 6 (P6)*	Balances yin to yang equilibrium on a larger scale. Pulls all yin energy into the yang meridians and restores balance between the body and mind.	About 2 inches above the inner crease on your wrist on the inside of your arm in the middle of the tendons	**NEIGUAN** P. 6
Weiguan Outer Gate Conserver of Yang *Triple Warmer 5 (TW5)*	Balances yang to yin equilibrium on a large scale. Balances the whole endocrine system. Brings all yang energy into yin meridians and brings physical, mental, and emotional warmth to the body.	About 2 inches above the outer wrist crease on the outside of your arm between your two arm bones (radius) and ulna); directly adjacent to Neiguan	**WEIGUAN** TW. 5

Note: Neiguan and Weiguan can be worked simultaneously with your thumb on Neiguan and your index finger on Weiguan.

Accelerator Parasympathetic Wonder Points for Balancing Yin Energies

The actions of these next five points (shown in the accompanying table) are similar to those of the three wonder points for general balance, except they are used to stimulate the parasympathetic nervous system and yin energies. I use these points on clients of any meta-type if they have hot and highly active yang energies. All the accelerator types can use these points freely to help stabilize their erratic systems.

Wonder Points for Balancing Yin Energies

NAMES AND NUMBER	IMPORTANCE	LOCATION	
Jiu Wei Dove's or Pigeon's Tail *Conception Vessel* *15 (CV15)*	The reunion point of all the body's vital energetic centers and the main source point for activating all the yin energy in the upper part of the body. Stimulates the pituitary gland.	About 7 inches above the umbilicus, just below the xiphoid process of your chest, directly in the middle between the ribs	JIU WEI CV. 15
Chi Hai Sea of Chi Hara Point *Conception Vessel 6 (CV6)*	The point that activates the *hara*, or the body's energy source. Center of energy for both the body and mind. Main source point for activating all the yin energy in the lower part of the body. Balances the thyroid gland.	About 1½ inches below your umbilicus	umbilicus CHI HAI CV. 6
Wuli Hands 5 Miles *Large Intestine 13* *(LI13)*	Influential point for all the yin organs and helps to balance the lungs, heart, liver, spleen, and kidney.	About 3 inches up from your elbow crease on the inner border of your arm bone when your arm is slightly bent at the elbow.	WULI LI. 13
Jianshi The Intermediary The Passenger *Pericardium 5 (P5)*	Balances all the yin meridians and organs in the upper part of the body and stimulates the metabolism. Controls all digestive functions.	About 3 inches above the inner crease on your wrist on the inside of your arm in the middle of the tendons—or just about 1 inch above Neiguan (Pericardium 6; see page 324)	JIANSHI P. 5
San Yin Chao The Three Yin Crossings Reunion of Yin Strengthening and Calming Point Master of the Blood *Spleen 6 (SP6)*	Balances all the yin meridians and organs in the lower part of the body and balances and heals male or female disorders, both physical and emotional. Balances the adrenals, pituitary, ovaries, and testes.	About 3 inches above the inside anklebone on your inner lower leg just at the back edge of your leg bone (tibia)	SAN YIN CHAO SP. 6

Synthesizer Sympathetic Wonder Points for Balancing Yang Energies

The six points shown in the accompanying table stimulate the sympathetic nervous system and yang energies. These points are great for the slow, sluggish synthesizers and can be generally used by all of the synthesizer meta-types.

Wonder Points for Balancing Yang Energies

NAMES AND NUMBER	IMPORTANCE	LOCATION	
Kuan Yuan Gate of Origin First Gate Gate of Life Elixir of Long Life *Conception Vessel 4 (CV4)*	Works on a very deep level to balance and tone all the yang energy. Great to combat aging!	About 3 inches below the umbilicus on the midline of your abdomen	umbilicus KUAN YUAN CV. 4
Tai Chu or *Da Zhui* Big Hammer Big Vertebra *Governor Vessel 14 (GV14)*	Meeting point of all the yang meridians. The potent and revitalizing point for energetic activation.	On the back of your neck, right where your neck sits on your shoulders just above the large "knob" of the vertebrae (between the seventh cervical vertebra and the first thoracic vertebra)	TAI CHU GV. 14
San Yang Luo Three Yang Junction *Triple Warmer 8 (TW8)*	Meeting point for all the yang in the upper part of your body. Moves and opens all the upper yang meridians; energizes.	About 4 inches above the outer wrist crease on the outside of your arm directly between your two arm bones (radius and ulna), or about 2 inches above Weiguan (Triple Warmer 5; see page 324)	SAN YANG LUO TW. 8
Xuanzhong or *Jeugu* Suspended Bell Hanging Clock *Gallbladder 39 (GB39)*	Meeting point for all the yang in the lower part of your body. Connects and activates all the lower yang meridians.	About 3 inches above your outside anklebone (external malleolus) just on the outside or back border of your leg bone (fibula)	XUANZHONG GB. 39

NAMES AND NUMBER	IMPORTANCE	LOCATION	
Chung Kuan Middle Channel Middle Bowl Stomach Center *Conception Vessel* *12 (CV12)*	Influential point and meeting place for all the yang organs: large intestine, small intestine, gallbladder, urinary bladder, and stomach. Helps to activate them; energizes all digestive functions.	About 4 inches above the umbilicus on a direct line connecting the xiphoid process of the chest with the umbilicus, or about 3 inches below Jiu Wei (Conception Vessel 15; see page 325)	
Lieque or *Lieh* *Ch'ueh* Every Deficiency Series of Vacancies Listening Deficiency Displaced Creek Narrow Defile Lung 7 (LU7)	Balances all deficiencies and all meridians, and keeps a balance between all the organs and meridians. Pulls all the energy from the lungs (energized air) into all the yang meridians. Stimulates the sex hormones.	On the edge of your arm that is next to the body when your arm is hanging down by your side, about 1½ inches above your inner wrist crease on the edge of your inner arm just above the wrist protuberance in a small depression	

Specific Points for Each Meta-Type

To activate your energetic meridians for weight loss, you must first balance your body by stimulating your dominant nervous system's counterpart—either the parasympathetic or sympathetic nervous system—manifesting as yin or yang energies. Second, you must equalize your governing meridian—the one controlled by your dominant endocrine gland—and stimulate the meridian governing your weaker gland.

For instance, the accelerator meta-types would first stimulate some of the wonder points that would activate the parasympathetic nervous system, their nervous system counterpart. Then they would activate the points that would balance their dominant gland, the adrenals, which are governed by the Kidney meridian. Finally they would activate their weaker endocrine glands by stimulating the points that strengthen the ovaries or testes, mainly the Conception Vessel and Spleen meridians.

It's not as hard as it sounds. Just follow the easy steps outlined below, then look at your individual meta-type tables in the following subsections and massage those pounds away.

1. Stimulate your nervous system's counterpart by massaging the wonder points shown in the preceding section to activate either the parasympathetic or sympathetic nervous system.
2. Equalize and stabilize your dominant endocrine gland by massaging the points shown in the table for your meta-type.
3. Stimulate your weaker endocrine gland by massaging the points shown in the table for your meta-type.

Accelerator Meta-Points to Balance the Adrenals and Stimulate the Sex Glands

Remember, your dominant glands are the adrenals, and your weaker glands are the sex glands. As shown in the accompanying tables, the adrenals are governed by the Kidney meridian, and the sex glands are regulated by points on the Conception Vessel, Kidney, and Spleen meridians.

Accelerator Points to Stabilize the Adrenals

NAMES AND NUMBER	IMPORTANCE	LOCATION	
Fuliu Returning Current Returning Flow *Kidney 7 (K7)*	Helps to regulate and tone kidney and adrenal energies.	On the inside of the calf about 2 inches above the anklebone (medial malleolus) on the outer border of the leg bone (tibia)	FULIU K. 7
Shenshu Kidney Position Kidney Shu *Urinary Bladder 23* *(UB23)*	Helps to readjust the kidney and adrenal energies.	About 1½ inches to the side of the second lumbar vertebra You can find this point easily by putting your hands on your waist, thumbs to the back, and continuing to reach with your thumbs until you come near the vertebra.	 SHENSHU B. 23

Accelerator Points to Stimulate the Sex Glands

NAMES AND NUMBER	IMPORTANCE	LOCATION	
Kuan Yuan Gate of Origin First Gate Gate of Life Elixir of Long Life Conception Vessel 4 (CV4)	Stimulates and regulates the continued functioning of the ovaries and testes.	About 3 inches below the umbilicus on the midline of your abdomen	
Chi Hai Sea of Chi Hara Point Conception Vessel 6 (CV6)	Regulates all the energy in the body and promotes the stimulation of the sex hormones.	About 1½ inches below your umbilicus	
Qixue Cave of Qi Hall of Fullness Kidney 13 (K13)	Balances and stimulates the ovaries and testes.	On your lower abdomen, about ½ inch lateral to Kuan Yuan (Conception Vessel 4; see above)	
San Yin Chao The Three Yin Crossings Reunion of Yin Strengthening and Calming Point Master of the Blood Spleen 6 (SP6)	One of the yin wonder points, which you should utilize to stimulate and balance the ovaries and testes.	About 3 inches above the inside anklebone on your inner lower leg just at the back edge of your leg bone (tibia)	

Balanced Accelerator Meta-Points to Balance the Thymus and Stimulate the Pancreas

Remember, your dominant gland is the thymus, and your weaker gland is the pancreas. As shown in the accompanying tables, your thymus is governed by several points on the Large Intestine, Lung, Conception Vessel, and Heart meridians, and your pancreas is regulated by points on the Liver, Spleen, Kidney, and Triple Warmer meridians.

Balanced Accelerator Points to Stabilize the Thymus

NAMES AND NUMBER	IMPORTANCE	LOCATION	
Shanzhong or *Shan Zhong* Center of Chest Center of Smell *Conception Vessel 17 (CV17)*	Balances thymus gland activity. Opens up the energetic pathways between the upper and lower body energy levels. All the *qi*, or energy, is concentrated at this point.	Located at the middle of the chest between the nipples	SHANZHONG CV. 17
Hegu or *Ho Ku* Meeting Point of the Valleys Great Assembly Point Harmonious Valleys Grain Valleys *Large Intestine 4 (LI4)*	Balances the thymus and immune system by acting as the source point for the immune system's Large Intestine meridian.	At the highest spot of the muscle when the thumb and index finger are brought close together	HEGU LI. 4
Lieque or *Lieh Ch'ueh* Every Deficiency Series of Vacancies Listening Deficiency Displaced Creek Narrow Defile *Lung 7 (LU7)*	Harmonizes the thymus and immune system by acting as the connecting point linking the immune system's meridians—the Lung and Large Intestine.	On the edge of your arm that is next to the body when your arm is hanging down by your side, about 1½ inches above your inner wrist crease on the edge of your inner arm just above the wrist protuberance in a small depression	LIEQUE LU. 7
Shenmen Gate of the Gods Gate of Heart Gate of Mind *Heart 7 (H7)*	Soothes and balances the thymus gland.	On the outside edge of the inner wrist in the depression where the hand meets the wrist	SHENMEN H. 7

Balanced Accelerator Points to Stimulate the Pancreas

NAMES AND NUMBER	IMPORTANCE	LOCATION	
T'ai Ch'ung Supreme Rushing Supreme Assault *Liver 3 (LIV3)*	Brings total balance and equilibrium to the body. Balances and harmonizes the pancreas's secretion of insulin and enzymes.	In the web between your first and second toes, about 1½ inches from the margin of the web	T'AI CH'UNG LIV. 3

NAMES AND NUMBER	IMPORTANCE	LOCATION	
T'ai Pai Supreme Whiteness Extreme Whiteness Cerebral Calm Equilibrium and Joy *Spleen 3 (SP3)*	Stimulates the pancreas both to secrete its enzymes and to produce a balanced insulin level.	On the inside border of the foot about 2½ inches from the tip of the big toe, right under the protrusion of the metatarsal bone just where the skin of the top of the foot meets the skin of the bottom of the foot	T'AI PAI SP. 3
T'ai Ch'i or *Taixi* Greater Mountain Stream Supreme Valley Reflecting Sea Bigger Sea *Kidney 3 (K3)*	Can really wake you up and has a strong effect on the pancreas; also balances out the kidney energy.	Right in the hollow on the inside of your ankle between your anklebone and the outside edge of your leg	T'AI CH'I K. 3
Chung Chu or *Zhongzhu* Middle of the Pond Middle Islet Warm Joy Point *Triple Warmer 3 (TW3)*	Helps to lift and balance the energies; stimulates both the pancreas and the thyroid.	On the top of the hand, in the hollow between the little and fourth fingers just under the knucklebone	CHUNG CHU TW. 3

Mixed Accelerator Meta-Points to Balance the Thyroid and Stimulate the Pituitary

Remember, your dominant gland is the thyroid, and your weaker gland is the pituitary, the master gland of the body. As shown in the accompanying tables, your thyroid is governed by several points on the Conception Vessel, Triple Warmer, and Large Intestine meridians, while your pituitary is regulated by points on the Governor Vessel, Conception Vessel, Spleen, and Pericardium meridians, including a secret, or extra, point.

Mixed Accelerator Points to Stabilize the Thyroid

NAMES AND NUMBER	IMPORTANCE	LOCATION	
			TIEN T'U CV. 22
T'ien T'u Heaven Rushing Out *Conception Vessel 22 (CV22)*	Regulates and supports the body's energy; also stimulates the thyroid.	In the hollow right at the junction where your throat meets your collarbone	

NAMES AND NUMBER	IMPORTANCE	LOCATION	
Shang Kuan Upper Channel *Conception Vessel 13 (CV13)*	Has a direct effect on the balance and stimulation of the thyroid.	About 5 inches above your umbilicus on the midline of your stomach	SHANG KUAN CV. 13
Chi Hai Sea of Chi Hara Point *Conception Vessel 6 (CV6)*	The point that stimulates the stored energy of the *hara*, or the body's energy source. Has a direct effect on the balance and stimulation of the thyroid.	About 1½ inches below your umbilicus	umbilicus CHI HAI CV. 6
Chung Chu or **Zhongzhu** Middle of the Pond Middle Islet Warm Joy Point *Triple Warmer 3 (TW3)*	Helps to lift and balance the energies; stimulates both the pancreas and the thyroid.	On the top of the hand, in the hollow between the little and fourth fingers just under the knucklebone.	CHUNG CHU TW. 3
Hegu or **Ho Ku** Meeting Point of the Valleys Great Assembly Point Harmonious Valleys Grain Valleys *Large Intestine 4 (LI4)*	An important revival point and power point for the throat and neck that stimulates and balances the thyroid.	At the highest spot of the muscle when the thumb and index finger are brought close together	HEGU LI. 4

Mixed Accelerator Points to Stimulate the Pituitary

NAMES AND NUMBER	IMPORTANCE	LOCATION	
Bai Hu Hundred Unity Meeting Point for 100 Vessels 100 Meeting Point *Governor Vessel 20 (GV20)*	Stimulates all the yang energies. Stimulates the pituitary and hypothalamus.	In the small depression on top of the skull	BAI HU GV. 20
Yingtang Where Yin and Yang Meet *Extra Point 1 (EX1)*	Stimulates the pituitary and hypothalamus.	Midway between the eyebrows just above the nose	YING TANG EX. 1

NAMES AND NUMBER	IMPORTANCE	LOCATION	
Tz'u Kung Purple Palace Purple Matrix Conception Vessel 19 (CV19)	Stimulates both the thyroid and the pituitary.	About 3 inches above the midpoint between the nipples	TZ'U KUNG CV.19
San Yin Chao The Three Yin Crossings Reunion of Yin Strengthening and Calming Point Master of the Blood Spleen 6 (SP6)	Balances all the yin meridians and organs in the lower part of the body. Balances the adrenals, pituitary, ovaries, and testes.	About 3 inches above the inside anklebone on your inner lower leg just at the back edge of your leg bone (tibia)	SAN YIN CHAO SP 6
Jiu Wei Dove's or Pigeon's Tail Conception Vessel 15 (CV15)	Main source point for activating all the yin energy in the upper part of the body. Stimulates the pituitary gland.	About 7 inches above the umbilicus, just below the xiphoid process of your chest, directly in the middle between the ribs	JIU WEI CV. 15
Jianshi The Intermediary The Passenger Pericardium 5 (P5)	Balances all the yin meridians and organs in the upper part of the body. Controls all digestive functions; helps raise the body's metabolism.	About 3 inches above the inner crease on your wrist on the inside of your arm in the middle of the tendons—or just about 1 inch above Neiguan (Pericardium 6; see page 335)	JIANSHI P. 5

Synthesizer Meta-Points to Balance the Pituitary and Stimulate the Thyroid

Remember, your dominant gland is the pituitary, the body's master gland, and your weaker gland is the thyroid, which is responsible for the body's ability to metabolize foods and the way in which you burn off fat. As shown in the accompanying tables, your pituitary is governed by several points on the Governor Vessel, Conception Vessel, and Spleen meridians plus an extra, or secret, point, while your thyroid is stimulated by several points on the Conception Vessel, Stomach, Kidney, Pericardium, and Governor Vessel meridians.

Synthesizer Points to Stabilize the Pituitary

NAMES AND NUMBER	IMPORTANCE	LOCATION	
Bai Hu Hundred Unity Meeting Point for 100 　Vessels 100 Meeting Point *Governor Vessel 20 (GV20)*	Stabilizes all the yang energies. Balances the pituitary and hypothalamus.	In the small depression on top of the skull	BAI HU GV. 20
Yingtang Where Yin and Yang Meet *Extra Point 1 (EX1)*	Balances the pituitary and hypothalamus.	Midway between the eyebrows just above the nose	YING TANG EX. 1
Shanzhong or **Shan Zhong** Center of Chest Center of Smell *Conception Vessel 17* 　*(CV17)*	Opens up the energetic pathways between the upper and lower body energy levels. Pulls hyperactive upper body energy to the point.	Located at the middle of the chest between the nipples	SHANZHONG CV. 17
San Yin Chao The Three Yin Crossings Reunion of Yin Strengthening and 　Calming Point Master of the Blood *Spleen 6 (SP6)*	Balances all the yin meridians in the lower part of the body. Pulls hyperactive upper body energy down and "grounds it."	About 3 inches above the inside anklebone on your inner lower leg just at the back edge of your leg bone (tibia)	SAN YIN CHAO SP 6

Synthesizer Points to Stimulate the Thyroid

NAMES AND NUMBER	IMPORTANCE	LOCATION	
T'ien T'u Heaven Rushing Out *Conception Vessel 22* 　*(CV22)*	Regulates and supports the body's energy; also stimulates the thyroid.	In the hollow right at the junction where your throat meets your collarbone	T'IEN T'U CV. 22

NAMES AND NUMBER	IMPORTANCE	LOCATION	
Tz'u Kung Purple Palace Purple Matrix *Conception Vessel 19* (CV19)	Stimulates both the thyroid and the pituitary.	About 3 inches above the midway center between the nipples in the middle of your chest	TZ'U KUNG CV.19
Renying or *Jen Ying* Welcomes People Stomach 9 (ST9)	Directly stimulates the thyroid.	On the front of your throat, on each side of the windpipe almost at the midpoint between your collarbone and chin	RENYING ST. 9
Fuliu Returning Current Returning Flow Kidney 7 (K7)	Helps to stimulate and tone kidney, adrenal, and thyroid energies.	On the inside of the calf about 2 inches above the anklebone (medial malleolus) on the outer border of the leg bone (tibia)	FULIU K. 7
Neiguan Inner Gate Broken Heart Gate Gate to Success Pericardium 6 (P6)	Takes all yin energy to the yang meridians; restores balance between the body and mind; stimulates thyroid function.	About 2 inches above the inner crease on your wrist on the inside of your arm in the middle of the tendons	NEIGUAN P. 6
Tai Chu or *Da Zhui* Big Hammer Big Vertebra Governor Vessel 14 (GV14)	One of the yang wonder points, which you should energize again to stimulate the thyroid's action.	On the back of your neck, right where your neck sits on your shoulders just above the large "knob" of the vertebrae (right between the seventh cervical vertebra and the first thoracic vertebra)	TAI CHU GV. 14

Balanced Synthesizer Meta-Points to Balance the Pancreas and Stimulate the Thymus

Remember, your dominant gland is the pancreas, and your weaker gland is the thymus, which governs your immune system. As shown in the accompanying tables, your pancreas is stabilized by several points on the Spleen, Liver, and Bladder meridians, while your thymus is governed by several points on the Conception Vessel, Spleen, Stomach, Large Intestine, and Lung meridians.

Balanced Synthesizer Points to Stabilize the Pancreas

NAMES AND NUMBER	IMPORTANCE	LOCATION	
T'ai Pai Supreme Whiteness Extreme Whiteness Cerebral Calm Equilibrium and Joy *Spleen 3 (SP3)*	Has the unique ability to balance the pancreas, whether it's hypo- or hyperactive.	On the inside border of the foot about 2½ inches from the tip of the big toe, right under the protrusion of the metatarsal bone just where the skin of the top of the foot meets the skin of the bottom of the foot	T'AI PAI SP. 3
T'ai Ch'ung Supreme Rushing Supreme Assault *Liver 3 (LIV3)*	Brings total balance and equilibrium to the body. Balances and harmonizes the pancreas's secretion of insulin and enzymes.	In the web between your first and second toes, about 1½ inches from the margin of the web	T'AI CH'UNG LIV. 3
Pishu Spleen Position *Urinary Bladder 20 (UB20)*	The major point for balancing the pancreas energy.	On your back, about 1½ inches to either side of the eleventh thoracic vertebra. Put your hands on your ribs at the midpoint between your underarm and the bottom edge of your rib cage, thumbs facing backward. Move your hands to the back just to about 1½ inches from the vertebra.	PISHU B. 20

Balanced Synthesizer Points to Stimulate the Thymus

NAMES AND NUMBER	IMPORTANCE	LOCATION	
Shanzhong or **Shan Zhong** Center of Chest Center of Smell *Conception Vessel 17 (CV17)*	Stimulates thymus gland activity. Opens up the energetic pathways between the upper and lower body energy levels. Pulls the energy to the point.	Located at the middle of the chest between the nipples	SHANZHONG CV. 17

NAMES AND NUMBER	IMPORTANCE	LOCATION	
Tai Yuan Large, Deep Abyss *Lung 9 (LU9)*	Stimulates the thymus and immune system by acting as the source point for one of the immune system's main pathways, the Lung meridian.	On the inner wrist just near the outside in the depression where the wrist meets the thumb	
Hegu or **Ho Ku** Meeting Point of the Valleys Great Assembly Point Harmonious Valleys Grain Valleys *Large Intestine 4 (LI4)*	Stimulates the thymus and immune system by acting as the source point for the immune system's second pathway, the Large Intestine meridian.	At the highest spot of the muscle when the thumb and index finger are brought close together	
San Yin Chao The Three Yin Crossings Reunion of Yin Strengthening and Calming Point Master of the Blood *Spleen 6 (SP6)*	One of the yin wonder points, this is also a powerful point for immune and thymus stimulation.	About 3 inches above the inside anklebone on your inner lower leg just at the back edge of your leg bone (tibia)	
Dai Bao or **Ta Pao** Large Envelope Big Wrap *Spleen 21 (SP21)*	Powerful immune stimulant. Connects all the yang and yin energies.	Directly down from your armpit in the sixth rib's intercostal space	
Tsu San Li or **Zu San Li** Three Miles from the Foot *Stomach 36 (ST36)*	Long called the longevity point, this is one of the most important points, especially for immune and thymus stimulus.	About 3 inches below the knee joint in a depression on the semiouter part of the calf	

Mixed Synthesizer Meta-Points to Balance the Sex Glands and Stimulate the Adrenals

Remember, your dominant glands are the sex glands, and your weaker gland is the adrenals, which govern how you create energy in the body. As shown in the accompanying tables, your sex glands are stabilized by several points on the Triple Warmer, Gallbladder, Liver, and Conception Vessel meridians, while your adrenals are stimulated by several points on the Governor Vessel, Bladder, Small Intestine, and Kidney meridians.

Mixed Synthesizer Points to Stabilize the Sex Glands

NAMES AND NUMBER	IMPORTANCE	LOCATION	
Weiguan Outer Gate Conserver of Yang *Triple Warmer 5 (TW5)*	Balances the yang and yin energies within the body. This is a main point on a special meridian, called Yang Wei Mai (The Yang-Regulating Channel), which particularly balances the production of the sex hormones.	About 2 inches above the outer wrist crease on the outside of your arm between your two arm bones (radius and ulna)	WEIGUAN TW. 5
Foot Linqi or *Tsu Lin Ch'l* Foot above Tears Foot Just before Weeping Lying Down to Weep *Gallbladder 41 (GB41)*	The exit, or last point, of the special Yang Wei Mai meridian.	On the top of your foot, in the depression just in front of the junction where the little toe and fourth toe meet	FOOT LINQI GB. 41
Zhangmen The Gate of Law *Liver 13 (LIV13)*	A powerful balancing point for the ovaries and testes; also the meeting point of all the five yin or parasympathetic organs.	On the free end of the eleventh rib	ZHANGMEN LIV. 13
Kuan Yuan Gate of Origin First Gate Gate of Life Elixir of Long Life *Conception Vessel 4 (CV4)*	Stimulates and regulates the continued functioning of the ovaries and testes.	About 3 inches below the umbilicus on the midline of your abdomen	umbilicus KUAN YUAN CV. 4

Mixed Synthesizer Points to Stimulate the Adrenals

NAMES AND NUMBER	IMPORTANCE	LOCATION	
Ming Men Gate of Life Second Youth Point *Governor Vessel 4 (GV4)*	Directly stimulates the adrenals for energy and stamina.	In between the second and third lower lumbar vertebrae. You can find this point easily by putting your hands on your waist, thumbs to the back, and continuing to extend your thumbs until you reach the vertebra.	
Shen Mei Extended Meridian Vessel of the Hour of Chen—3:00 to 5:00 P.M. Calm Sleep *Urinary Bladder 62 (UB62)*	The first point on a special meridian that particularly stimulates the adrenals called Yang Chiao Mai (The Yang Motility Channel).	On the outside of your foot, directly below the tip of your anklebone (malleolus)	
Houxi or **Hou Chi** Black Stream Black Ravine Vitality Point *Small Intestine 3 (SI3)*	The exit, or last point, of the special Yang Chiao Mai meridian, which powerfully stimulates the adrenals.	On the outside and outer edge of your hand, in the depression right under your little finger's knuckle when your fingers are bent	
Fuliu Returning Current Returning Flow *Kidney 7 (K7)*	Helps to stimulate and tone kidney and adrenal energies.	On the inside of the calf about 2 inches above the anklebone (medial malleolus) on the outerborder of the leg bone (tibia)	
Shenshu Kidney Position Kidney Shu *Urinary Bladder 23 (UB23)*	Helps to stimulate and rebalance the kidney and adrenal energies.	About 1½ inches to the side of the second lumbar vertebra. You can find this point easily by putting your hands on your waist, thumbs to the back, and continuing to reach with your thumbs until you come near the vertebra.	

22 Sculpting Your Body with Meta-Type Exercises

The Breath

At the moment of birth, the first food taken in by a baby is *oxygen*—not water or its mother's milk. Oxygen is our first and foremost food. It is the first physical condensation of cosmic energy in an organic form that is vital to the very essence of our life. It is the activator that energizes our meridians—those energetic pathways in our bodies that keep our organs functioning. Without it we don't live.

Breathing—and the way in which you use your breath—directly affects the harmonious operation of your nervous system, your brain's capacity, and your respiratory and circulatory functions. This in turn activates the way in which your body energetically operates. With abundant energy those excess pounds burn right off. Without energy you can bet you'll be stuck with mountains of fat. Proper breathing and different ways of breathing can absolutely alter how your body functions.

Regardless of their meta-type, excess weight gain usually causes people to breathe very shallowly, using only the upper part of their lungs, which has a direct negative impact on both health and weight gain. To properly activate the body's energy, the full capacity of the lungs must be utilized. You can do this with the Yogic Complete Breath (shown in the accompanying box), which can be used by both accelerators and synthesizers.

Yogic Complete Breath

The first step is to work your abdominal muscles in a uniform push-pull technique to gain some definite movement in your stomach. Sitting or standing comfortably erect, push your abdomen out as far as you can, then contract it quickly, pulling it in as far as you can. Do this repeatedly four or five times until you get the idea and feel the rhythmic movement in your stomach walls. To begin the breath, follow the instructions below in *one continuous, uniform movement*:

First, begin to slowly inhale while simultaneously pushing out your abdomen as far as you can—as you've just practiced—which allows air to enter the lower part of your lungs, activating your digestive organs. A *must* for weight loss!

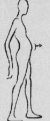

Second, fill the middle part of your lungs by pushing out the lower ribs, breastbone, and chest. This lifts the chest, including the upper pairs of ribs.

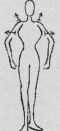

Third, slightly pull in the lower part of your abdomen. This fills the highest part of your lungs, giving them support. Fill your lungs up with as much air as possible.

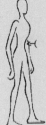

Retain the breath for a few seconds.

Slowly begin to exhale, simultaneously contracting your stomach while allowing all of your muscles to relax, emptying your lungs.

Without a pause start the next deep breath and continue for at least five complete breaths.

The *speed*, *depth*, and *length* of breathing can help to increase or decrease your metabolism, influencing your weight loss or gain. The faster your breath, the faster you raise your metabolism and body temperature. The slower your breath, the slower you lower your metabolism and body temperature. These techniques are essential to help both synthesizers and accelerators regulate their metabolism. The slower synthesizers would use the faster breathing techniques to help raise their metabolism, while the slower breathing will help the accelerators modify their more rapid metabolism.

Accelerator Breathing Techniques

The accelerator breath (shown in the following box) involves slower, deeper, and longer breathing.

Slower breathing helps your physical metabolism slow down while slightly lowering your body temperature. This in turn helps to produce a tranquil and peaceful state, giving you clearer thinking, calmer understanding, and wider perceptions. It even helps you develop deeper insights. *Deeper breathing* harmonizes the balance between your metabolism and organ systems. This enhances your emotional stability, increasing your confidence, producing more inner satisfaction, and even helping you develop greater thoughtfulness toward others. *Longer breathing* helps to stabilize your body temperature and coordinates the various functions of your more rapid metabolism. This helps to relieve anxiety, giving you a more peaceful feeling and increasing your endurance, patience, and quietness. You'll develop more objective and wider perceptions, with deeper understanding of yourself and others.

Accelerator Breath: The Peacemaker

Using the Yogic Complete Breath, inhale very slowly and *deeply*— using a count of ten to complete the inhalation. Retain your breath for a few seconds, then slowly exhale, taking three times as long to exhale as you did to inhale.

Do this very quietly for five to ten minutes in such a way that if you visualized a turquoise silk scarf in front of your face, your breath would not cause it to move at all. This breath will bring you into balance and harmony physically, mentally, and emotionally. Done for a longer period of time, this breathing technique can lead to a deep meditative state, producing a profound state of inner awareness.

Synthesizer Breathing Techniques

The synthesizer breath (shown in the following box) involves faster, deeper, and shorter breathing.

Faster breathing increases your body's metabolism while slightly raising your body temperature. It helps to energize and excite your nervous system. You will also develop more subjective observations about yourself and your surroundings. *Deeper breathing* harmonizes the balance between your metabolism and organ systems, which in turn helps to increase your emotional stability and confidence and produces more faith and inner satisfaction. *Shorter breathing* helps to speed up your metabolism and increase your body temperature. It also helps to energize your mind and will help to produce more frequent changes of images and thoughts.

Synthesizer Breath: The Energizer

Using the Yogic Complete Breath, inhale rapidly and *deeply* through your nose. Retain your breath for a few seconds, then quickly exhale, taking twice as long to exhale as you did to inhale.

Do this gently and *smoothly* for five to ten minutes in such a way that if you visualized a red silk scarf in front of your face, it would flutter quickly as you inhale and exhale. This breath will heighten the balance among your physical, mental, emotional, and spiritual functions and help you release any physical and mental stagnation.

The Exercises

Along with using the proper breathing techniques to help you speedily burn off those excess pounds, doing exercises that are beneficial to your individual meta-type is also vital to your weight-loss program. Not only will exercise speed up or balance your metabolism, but it's a great stress releaser as well.

Not all types of exercises are appropriate for everyone. Different kinds of exercises that require bending and stretching of the body in certain ways have different effects on the energy flows along the meridians of the body. These exercises will either energize or calm the way energy flows along your meridians, thereby enhancing your body's ability to function in optimum balance, which is essential for weight loss.

Fast metabolizers—those who have one of the accelerator meta-types—are already speedy enough working on their excess nervous energy. What they do not need are the types of exercise that would increase their already high energy or anxiety levels, such as aerobics. The slower metabolizers—the synthesizers—need to speed up their metabolism. For them aerobics is the perfect type of exercise.

The Accelerator, Balanced Accelerator, and Mixed Accelerator Meta-Types

The faster metabolizers—the accelerators, balanced accelerators, and mixed accelerators—need to learn to calm and balance their intense energies. They're prone to erratic energy flows and anxiety. Exercises to stimulate them would only cause them to burn out very quickly. For them the best forms of exercise are yoga, tai chi chuan, stretches, bending, or even ballet. These activities involve a system of slow, flowing, and subtle energetic motions or movements. They not only energize the body in a calm way but strengthen and tone it as well.

The more calming system of tai chi may be better suited to the accelerator, while qi gong could be useful to the balanced accelerator, and yoga would be very appropriate for the mixed accelerator. However, yoga can be used by all three meta-types. My suggestion is that you browse through the current selections in your local bookstore or video store to see what might intrigue or excite you.

But you can get started right away. I've chosen a short series of yoga movements preceded by some warm-up exercises especially suited for all the accelerator metabolisms. I've arranged these exercises into two routines, which you can alternate, with each routine taking approximately twenty to thirty minutes to complete. Pick the same time and place to exercise each day. That way your energy builds up in your particular space, which enables you to exercise easily and quickly. Breath is important, so be conscious and focused as you complete your movements and inhale or exhale where indicated. You'll feel invigorated, calm, energized, and balanced.

Days One, Three, and Five

Accelerator Breath: The Peacemaker

Sit calmly and quietly in the special area you've chosen for your exercises and perform the accelerator breathing technique for at least five minutes before you exercise.

Accelerator Warm-Up Exercises

SHOULDER AND CHEST STRETCH

Opens the chest meridians, which stimulates energy, breathing, and proper elimination

Standing comfortably, with your weight evenly distributed between both feet, bring your arms up to shoulder height, holding them straight out. Then begin swinging each arm horizontally in front of your chest, alternating your arms each time you swing to the front. Inhale as each arm crosses in front of your body; then exhale as the arm swings back out to the side. Do this eighteen times.

KIDNEY MASSAGE

Tones the waist; opens the hips, chest, and shoulders; and stimulates knee and ankle circulation

Still standing, spread your feet about 1 foot apart at the heels and slightly bend your knees as if you were skiing. Clasp your hands together and begin swinging your arms in a clockwise direction in front of your body, turning at your waist until you can feel the muscle tension at the back of the hip area. Swing back the same way toward the other side. Inhale as your arms are in front of you and exhale at the back of each turn, adding a "ha" sound. Extend the movement out and around you as far as possible until you're looking behind you. Do this nine times.

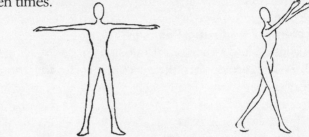

Hip Movement
Good for your waist, hips, and pelvis

Continue standing in a relaxed way and place your hands on your hips, with your heels about 3 inches apart. Inhale and push with your thighs out toward the front and circle them in a clockwise direction, coming back toward your pelvis, then back to your starting position. Exhale with a "ha" sound when you swing in at the end of the movement while pulling your body forward. Then change the swing to a counterclockwise direction. Do this nine times each way.

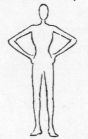 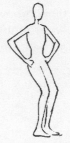

Accelerator Reducing Postures

These five postures are for losing those excess pounds and taking off inches. They are performed in a *continuous slow motion*, with no holding of the forms.

Tall Tower Side Bend
Takes inches off the hips

Standing easily and gracefully, place your heels together. Inhale and raise your arms overhead, palms facing each other. Slowly lean to the left as far as you can go *without strain* and exhale, arms remaining parallel. Without a pause inhale and straighten to an upright position; then lean to the right as far as you can go without strain and exhale. Do this exercise five to eight times in a slow, continuous motion.

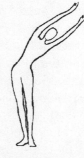

Seated Tall Tower Side Bend
Trims inches from your waist and stomach

From the previous standing position, sit down in a comfortable cross-legged position. *Don't strain.* Raise your arms and clasp your hands behind your head. Inhale and slowly twist to the left as far as possible, then bend forward, bringing your right elbow as close as possible to your left knee. Exhale and straighten to an upright position. Again, inhale and slowly lower your right elbow as close to the floor as possible without strain. Exhale and immediately raise yourself to an upright position. Now inhale and slowly twist to the right as far as possible, then bend forward, bringing your left elbow as close as possible to your right knee. Exhale and straighten to an upright position. Inhale and again slowly lower your left elbow as close to the floor as you can without strain. Exhale and immediately raise yourself to an upright position. Repeat the exercise five to eight times in a slow, continuous movement.

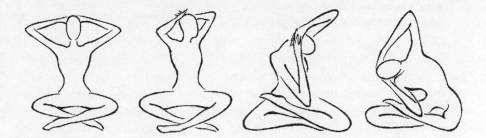

COBRA

Takes inches off the stomach and buttocks

Lie down gracefully. Rest your forehead on the floor, arms at your sides. Relax your body. Inhale and slowly bring your arms up and place them beneath your shoulders—fingers together, pointing at right angles to the shoulders. Exhale. Inhale and *very slowly* begin to raise your head and bend it backward. Simultaneously push against the floor with your hands and begin to raise your body. Bend your head far backward, with your spine continually curving as you bend as far back as possible *without straining yourself*. Exhale. With your elbows now straight, inhale and bend *only* your right elbow and slowly twist your body as far to the left as possible, attempting to see your left heel. Exhale. Without a pause inhale, return to the front, and bend *only* your left elbow, slowly twisting your body as far to the right as possible, attempting to see your right heel. Exhale. Inhale and immediately return to the front. Exhale. Now in very slow motion, inhale and reverse the process as you slowly lower your body back down until your forehead rests on the floor. Exhale. Gently lower your arms to your sides. Repeat the exercise five times in a continuous, rhythmic motion.

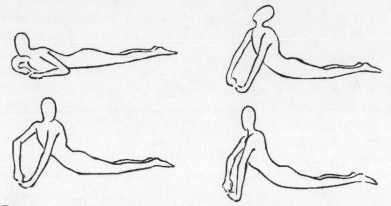

BOW
Reduces your waist, stomach, back, and thighs

Still on your stomach, now rest your chin on the floor. Inhale and gently bend your knees, bringing your feet toward your back. Reach behind you and grab each foot with each hand. Exhale. (If your excess weight precludes this, put a towel or cloth around each foot and hold onto it with each hand.) Inhale and slowly raise your head and body, pulling against your feet. Keeping your knees together, raise your body as far as you can, bringing your knees an inch or so off the ground if possible. *Do not strain* and go *only* as far as is comfortable. Exhale as you attempt to rock forward and backward on your abdomen. Inhale with the backward swing and exhale with the forward swing. When rocking forward, try to bring your chin close to the floor. When rocking backward, try to bring your knees as close to the floor as possible. Try to rock smoothly five times. *Do not strain!* Without a pause inhale and very slowly lower your knees, body, and chin back to the floor. Exhale. Repeat the exercise three to five times in a continuous slow and rhythmic movement. Release your feet and lower them to the floor. Relax.

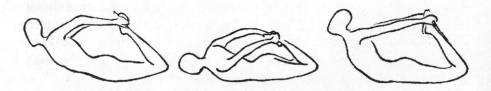

DOUBLE LEG LIFT AND STRETCH FORWARD
Reduces the waist

Coming to a seated position, inhale and grasp your thighs firmly. Exhale as you slowly lower your back onto the floor. With arms down by your sides, inhale, bring your knees up to your chest, and slowly straighten your legs up into the air. Exhale as you lower your legs to the floor as *slowly* as possible. Inhale and tense your abdominal muscles. Exhale and bring yourself into an upright seated position. (Use your hands if necessary to help in the beginning.) Inhale and, in a slow, fluid movement, grasp your calves just below the knee, your ankles, or your feet and pull your body down as far as possible onto your legs, bending your elbows outward as you exhale. Without a pause inhale and straighten to an upright position. Exhale and relax. Repeat five times.

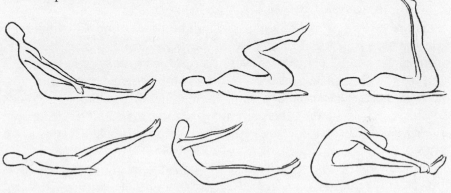

Accelerator Firming and Toning Postures

These postures are for toning and strengthening your muscles. They are performed in slow motion, but you'll also *hold* the extreme positions in a motionless way. This helps to tighten and firm all those flabby muscles as you begin to lose your excess weight.

Leg Clasp
Firms the stomach, waist, and hips

Rise gently to a standing position and place your heels together. Inhale and slowly bend forward, clasping your hands behind your knees or your calves or your ankles—whichever is the easiest for you. *Don't strain yourself!* If all you can grab is your knees, fine. You'll be able to get down to your ankles in time. Now exhale and very slowly draw your body down as far as possible without strain. You must have your neck relaxed, your knees not bent, and your forehead aimed at your knees. When you've reached your extreme position, inhale and hold the position for a count of ten. Now raise your body several inches, exhale, and relax but still retain the clasp on your legs. Then inhale, repeat the pull forward, and hold for a count of ten. Exhale. Repeat the exercise five times. Inhale and unclasp your hands very slowly. Exhale, raising your body to an upright standing position, and relax.

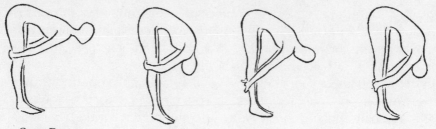

SIDE RAISE

Firms the abdomen, arms, and thighs

From your previous standing position, lie down gently on your right side, keeping your legs together, with your right arm and hand bent and supporting your right cheek with your palm. Move your left arm in front of you, bent, with your left palm on the floor. Inhale while pushing against the floor with your left hand as you raise your left leg as high as possible. Exhale as you are holding this extreme position for a count of ten. Inhale and lower your leg back to the beginning position. Exhale. Do this three times.

Inhale while pushing against the floor with your left hand as hard as you can and raise both legs as high as possible. Exhale as you're holding this extreme position for a count of ten. Inhale and lower both legs back to the beginning position. Exhale. Do this three times.

Relax, then slowly turn over on your left side and repeat the entire exercise.

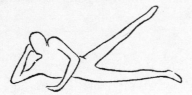 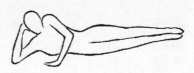

Days Two, Four, and Six
Accelerator Breath: The Peacemaker

Sit calmly and quietly in the special area you've chosen for your exercises and perform the accelerator breathing technique for at least five minutes before you exercise.

Accelerator Warm-Up Exercises

FORWARD LEAN

Opens up both the yang and yin meridians

Standing in an upright position, with your weight evenly distributed between both feet, inhale as you raise both arms over your head. Exhale as you "fall" forward as far as possible, bending at your waist. Inhale as you come back to your original position. Exhale as you lower your arms back to your sides. Do this exercise five times.

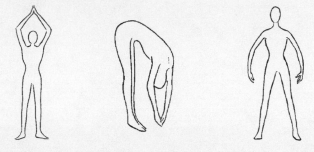

THE BOB
Increases energetic circulation
Still standing with your weight evenly distributed between both feet, heels together, place your hands on your hips. Focus your eyes on an imaginary spot on the wall or ceiling. Inhale, breathing in through the mouth and feeling your breath go down to your navel, and fall forward as far as you can. Exhale with a "ha" sound as you reach the bottom. Bring only your head up and look at your imaginary spot, keeping your spine straight, and begin bobbing gently up and down. Inhale and increase the bobbing as you begin to feel your body loosening. Exhale. Then inhale and bob three times to the right. Exhale and return to the front. Inhale and bob three times to the left. Exhale and return to the front.

Lower your head, looking down until you feel the tension reach your lower back, for three inhalations and exhalations. Inhale as you bring your body back to a standing position and exhale. Repeat the exercise three times.

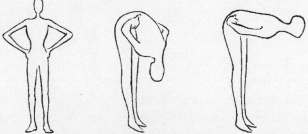

HANDS OF LIGHT
Opens up a horizontal energy flow and strengthens the arms
Not changing from your standing position, bring both arms up gently, stretching them out in front of you. With your hands extended, begin circling your hands and arms to the right up toward the ceiling, starting with small circles and increasing their size until they are about 1½ feet in diameter. Then begin to come back down, gradually making the circles smaller until

you get down to 6 inches. In a continuous motion, change the direction and begin circling to the left, repeating the procedure. Inhale and exhale slowly and rhythmically during the exercise. Repeat the exercise twice. You will begin to sense energy in your hands, coming up your arms to your chest.

Accelerator Reducing Postures

TALL TRIANGLE

Reduces the waist, sides, and hips

Stand with your feet about 2 feet apart or as far apart as they can go. Inhale and raise your arms, stretching them out to your sides at shoulder level. Exhale as you bend to the left, placing your left hand against the left knee, calf, or ankle (whichever is easiest for you to reach) as your right hand and arm come up and over your head parallel to the floor. Inhale and bend your body to the left as far as it can go. (Keep your knees straight, your neck relaxed.) Without a pause exhale and straighten to an upright position. Do the movement again, bending to the right this time. Repeat the exercise six times.

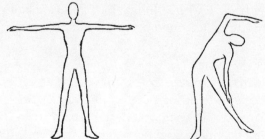

TWIST

Reduces the waist and hips

Still in your standing position, put your heels together and place your hands on your hips. Inhale and bend forward as far as you can. As you begin to exhale, slowly roll your body to the right as far as you can—not bending but twisting it. Inhale and roll your body backward as far as it can go; then exhale. Inhale and twist to the left, going to the farthest point you can maintain; then exhale as you bring your body back to the beginning position. Now reverse the process. The bigger the circle you can make, the more inches disappear off your waist. Repeat the exercise six times.

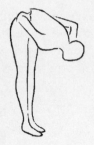
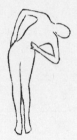

Spinal Twist
Reduces the waist

From your standing position, sit comfortably on the floor and stretch your legs straight out in front of you. Cross your right leg over your left knee with your right foot planted firmly on the floor. Place your right hand firmly on the floor behind you for balance and hold your right knee with your left hand. Inhale while slowly twisting your head and body as far to the right as possible. Exhale while returning to the forward position. Repeat nine times. In a continuous movement, change your legs and repeat the same exercise with your left leg over your right knee. Repeat nine times. Stretch your legs forward and relax.

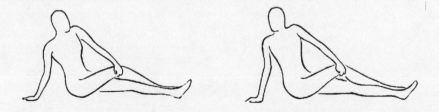

Leg Windmill
Reduces the waist, hips, and buttocks

From your sitting position, gently lie back until your back is resting comfortably on the floor. Stretch your arms out on the floor to each side, keeping them at shoulder height. Inhale, bringing your left knee bent up to your chest, then straighten your leg toward the ceiling. Exhale as you slowly bring your left leg over your right leg, touching the floor as high toward your head as you can possibly reach. *Keep your shoulders on the floor.* Inhale as you bring your left leg back up, then exhale as you lower your left leg to the floor. Repeat with the right leg. Do this exercise nine times.

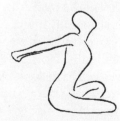

Accelerator Firming and Toning Postures

WAIST AND LEG TONER

Tones the waist, back, and legs

Sit upright, with your legs outstretched in front of you, feet touching. Inhale, raising your arms over your head, and lean backward. Exhale as you fall quickly forward, grabbing your calves, ankles, or feet—whichever are easiest for you to reach. *Don't strain!* Inhale as you pull forward on your legs, bringing your body down as far as it can comfortably go, with your elbows bent outward and your neck relaxed. Exhale and hold for a count of eighteen. Inhale, raising your body to an upright position and keeping your arms overhead. Repeat the exercise six times.

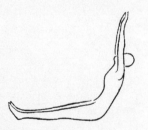

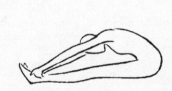

BACK AND SHOULDER RAISE

Tones the chest and bust

Still seated, relax in a cross-legged position. Put your arms behind your back and interlace your fingers. Inhale and raise your arms as far as you possibly can. Exhale while holding for a count of nine. Inhale while lowering your arms; then exhale and relax. Repeat six times.

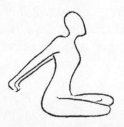

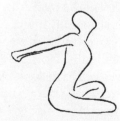

DOUBLE LEG LIFT

Firms the stomach, hips, and buttocks

Turn over and roll slowly onto your stomach, resting your chin on the floor. Make fists with your hands and put each fist under each leg. Inhale, push against the floor with *both* fists, and slowly raise your left leg as high as it can comfortably go, keeping your knee straight. Exhale and hold for a count of nine. Inhale and lower your leg; then exhale. Repeat the same process with your right leg.

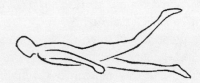

Then inhale, pushing hard against the floor with your fists, and raise both legs as far as you can comfortably go. Exhale and hold for a count of nine. Inhale and slowly lower your legs. Exhale. Repeat the entire exercise six times.

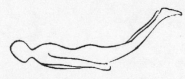

These yogic movements will not only help you achieve the weight loss you desire but can also provide you with a lifetime plan of energetic rejuvenation and keep your weight permanently regulated.

The Synthesizer, Balanced Synthesizer, and Mixed Synthesizer Meta-Types

The slower metabolizers—the synthesizers, balanced synthesizers, and mixed synthesizers—need to stimulate, speed up, and activate their slower energies. They're prone to very low dips in energy as well as diving into depression. Their thyroid and adrenals tend to be weaker, which means a slower-acting body. They need exercises to activate them, stimulating their lazier endocrine glands, the thyroid and adrenals. For them the best forms of exercise are aerobics, Dancercise or Jazzercise classes, step classes, treadmills, NordicTrack, weight training, or any type of exercise that involves active movement.

Dancercise or Jazzercise classes are more suited to the balanced and mixed synthesizers, since these exercises keep their more active minds entertained and stop them from getting bored with repetitious aerobic movements. The synthesizers seem to be completely happy with aerobic step classes, movement, and weight training. My suggestion is to browse through the current selections in your local bookstore or video store to see what might intrigue or excite you.

But you can get started right away. I've chosen a short series of aerobic exercises preceded by some warm-up exercises especially suited for all the synthesizer metabolisms. I've arranged these exercises into two routines, which you can alternate, with each routine taking approximately twenty to thirty minutes to complete. Pick the same time and place to exercise each day. That way your energy builds up in your particular space, which enables you to exercise easily and quickly. Breath is important, so be conscious and focused as you complete your movements and inhale or exhale where indicated. You'll feel invigorated, calm, energized, and balanced.

Days One, Three, and Five
Synthesizer Breath: The Energizer

Sit calmly in the special area you've chosen for your exercises and perform the synthesizer breathing technique for at least five minutes before you exercise.

Synthesizer Warm-Up Exercises
HEAD ROLLS
Stretches and opens the neck muscles

Stand comfortably with your feet about 2 feet apart, shoulders relaxed, stomach and buttocks muscles tightened, arms at your sides. Inhale while rotating your head to the right, stretching the left side of your neck; exhale and hold for a count of five. Inhale while rotating your head to the back; exhale and hold for a count of five. Inhale while rotating your head to the left, stretching the right side of your neck; exhale and hold for a count of five. Inhale and drop your head forward, stretching your chin to your chest; exhale and hold for a count of five. Repeat the same procedure turning in the opposite direction. Repeat three times to the left and three times to the right.

SIDE STRETCHES

Stretches the muscles in your upper body

Still standing comfortably with your feet about 2 feet apart, shoulders relaxed, and arms at your sides, inhale as you open your arms, extending them out to the sides and bringing them up to your shoulder height and over your head; then exhale. Inhale as you reach your right arm up toward the ceiling as far as you can; exhale as you hold for a count of five. Inhale as you then reach your left arm up toward the ceiling, reaching as far as you can; exhale and hold for a count of five. Repeat each reach six times.

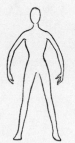 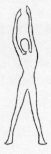

LEG STRETCHES

Opens your lower back, hips, and legs

In the same beginning stance as in your previous warm-up, inhale as you bring your arms up to shoulder height. Exhale and keep your arms at shoulder level as you bend straight forward, stretching your chin outward and pushing your buttocks toward the ceiling. Inhale and "bounce" the small of your back in little bobbing motions for a count of ten as you exhale. Inhale and return to your beginning stance; then exhale. Repeat the exercise five times.

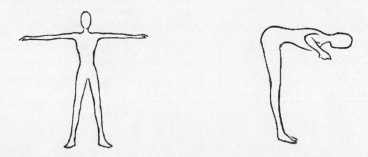

JOGGING IN PLACE

Helps to increase your pulse rate

Standing erect, place your feet together and begin to jog in place for twenty counts. Both the right and left foot should touch down in each count. Breathe at a normal rate throughout this exercise. Repeat three times.

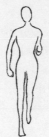

JUMPING JACKS

Begins to burn off those excess pounds

Still standing erect, inhale, jump up, and open your legs, parting them in a triangle as you land, swinging your arms out and up over your head. Exhale as you jump up again, landing with your feet together and bringing your arms back down to your sides. Jump for ten counts. Repeat three times.

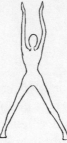

Synthesizer Reducing Exercises

WAIST THINNER

Stand erect, feet about 1 foot apart, stomach and buttocks muscles tight, hands and arms crossed in front of your chest, palms facing your body, and inhale. Exhale while reaching out and down with your right hand and arm pulling you down as far toward the floor as you can go, letting your left elbow bend up as far as it can go. Inhale while coming back up to the beginning position. (Do *not* let your upper body pull you forward.) Repeat for twenty counts. Then change to the left side and repeat for twenty counts.

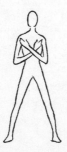

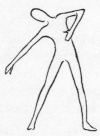

STOMACH SLIMMER

Sit comfortably on the floor. Then lie down on your back, with your knees bent and your feet flat on the floor. Keep your feet and knees parallel and about 1 foot apart. Inhale as you bring your hands up behind your head with your elbows out to the sides. Exhale while lifting your head and upper back off the floor as far as you can reach, keeping your stomach muscles tight. Inhale as you lower yourself *almost* to the floor—but without touching it. Exhale and lift again. Repeat twenty times.

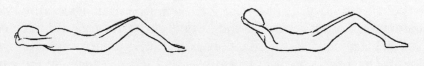

BICYCLE

Strengthens the lower abdomen

Still lying on your back, with your hands under your head, inhale. Exhale as you extend your left leg out as far as it can go, lifting it slightly off the ground, toes pointed. Simultaneously bring your right leg with knee bent up to your chest, reaching out your left elbow to touch your right knee. Inhale and bring your right leg back down to its original position. Exhale. Inhale and switch sides. Exhale as you extend your right leg out as far as it can go, lifting it slightly off the ground, toes pointed. Simultaneously bring your left leg with knee bent up to your chest, reaching out your right elbow to touch your left knee. Inhale and bring your left leg back down to its original position. Exhale. Repeat ten times.

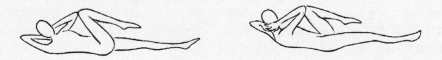

HIPSTER

Reduces the hips and thighs

From your lying position, roll over to your left side, raising yourself on your left elbow, with both hands on the floor, fingers lightly touching, palms down. Extend both your legs out straight—one on top of the other—in a line with your upper body and inhale. Exhale, lifting your right leg up as far as possible, with toes pointed. Inhale, lowering your right leg *almost* to your left leg but without letting it touch. Repeat this movement ten times with your toes pointed and ten times with your toes flexed forward. Turn over to your right side and repeat the exercise.

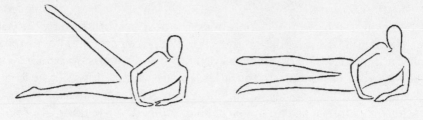

INNER THIGH THINNER

Turn over to your left side and raise yourself by bending your left elbow to support your weight. Grab your right foot with your right hand, bringing it in front of your left leg. Inhale and extend your left leg out as far as it can go, raising it about 1 inch off the floor and pointing your toes. Exhale and raise your left leg; then inhale, lowering it *almost* to the floor. Continue the raising and lowering of your left leg for a count of ten with your toes pointed. Then repeat for a count of ten with your foot flexed forward. (Your inner thigh must face the ceiling.) Turn over on your right side and repeat the exercise.

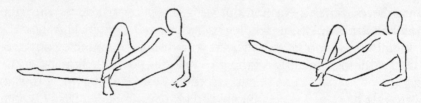

BUTTOCKS BUSTER

Turn with your back on the floor, feet parallel about 1 foot apart, and your arms by your sides. Inhale, shifting your weight onto your shoulders. Exhale, lifting up your buttocks; inhale, lowering them *almost* back to the floor. Continue for ten counts.

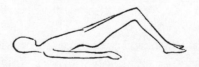

Lift your arms and clasp them behind your head. Turn your knees and feet to the outside and continue the lifting for another ten counts.

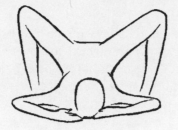

Bring your knees together, feet still apart, and continue the lifting for ten more counts.

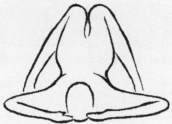

Days Two, Four, and Six
Synthesizer Breath: The Energizer

Sit calmly in the special area you've chosen for your exercises and perform the synthesizer breathing technique for at least five minutes before you exercise.

Synthesizer Warm-Up Exercises

SHOULDER LIFTS

Stretches the shoulders and neck

Comfortably standing erect, place your feet about 1 foot apart, weight evenly distributed. Breathing *normally* throughout this exercise, lift your right shoulder up to your right ear and hold for a count of two, then lift your left shoulder up to your left ear and hold for a count of two. Repeat the exercise ten times.

WAIST STRETCH

Continuing in your same stance, inhale and bring your left arm over your head; then exhale, pulling outward and over as far as you can go. Inhale and gently "bounce" for six counts as you exhale. Inhale coming up to the beginning position; then exhale. Repeat the exercise on the right side. Alternate each side for a count of ten.

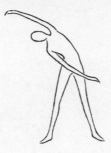

SPINE STRETCH

Opens your spine

From your standing position, inhale as you bring your arms up over your head. Exhale as you bend forward at your waist, stopping when your body is parallel to the floor, and slightly bend your knees. Inhale as you "dive" through your legs, swinging your arms through your legs, and return to the parallel position; then exhale. Repeat the swing for a count of six.

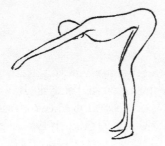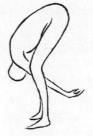

WAIST TWIST

Begins to increase your metabolism

Again, stand comfortably, arms at your sides. Inhale and jump up, twisting your body to the right and swinging your arms up to the left. Exhale. Inhale and jump up, twisting your body to the left and swinging your arms up to the right. Repeat for a count of ten.

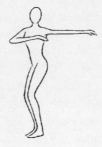

Jogging in Place

Helps to increase your pulse rate

Standing erect, place your feet together and begin to jog in place for twenty counts. Both the right and left foot should touch down in each count. Breathe at a normal rate throughout this exercise. Repeat three times.

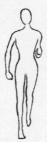

Synthesizer Reducing Exercises

Waist Tightener

Standing erect, separate your feet about 2 feet and slightly bend your knees. Inhale and bring your arms up in front of your chest, crossing them over each other with the right hand grasping the left elbow and the left hand grasping the right elbow. Exhale as you twist to the right six times looking over your right shoulder. Inhale and repeat six times on the left side.

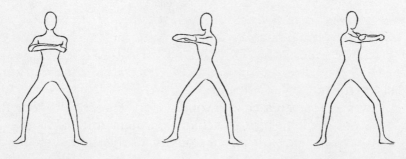

Inhale, letting go of your elbows, and let your arms swing to the right, then swing to the left, six times. Repeat the exercise three times.

STOMACH TIGHTENER

Gently lying down with your back on the floor, inhale as you raise both legs toward the ceiling—knees slightly bent and hands clasped behind your head. Exhale as you lift your upper body using your stomach muscles. *Don't* pull with your arms. Inhale as you release, going back toward the floor but *not* touching it. Repeat twenty times.

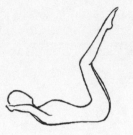 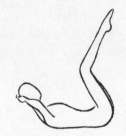

SCISSORS
Strengthens the abdomen
Still lying on your back, raise your legs straight up in the air, with your toes pointed, hands behind your head, and elbows as flat to the floor as possible. Inhale while lifting your head up off the floor as far as possible, crossing your right leg over your left. Exhale while crossing your left leg over your right. Inhale and exhale as you repeat these movements in rapid succession for a count of twenty.

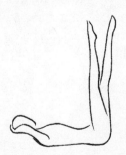

HIP TIGHTENER
Roll over on your stomach with your hips and chest on the floor. Raise your body on your left elbow, stretching your right arm and hand out in front of you. Straighten each leg out as far as possible, knees straight, toes

pointed. Inhale while crossing your right leg over your left and exhale while raising it as high as you can; hold for a count of one, then release it slightly. Lift and release for a count of ten. Then change over to the left leg and repeat the exercise.

23 Success at Last!

How does it feel to be a winner? My guess is, wonderful! I have one more gift to offer—the advice you need to stay slim, gorgeous, and healthy for good.

I have a few secrets to help you maintain your beautiful new figure and radiant health. First of all, you've learned to eat the *right foods* for your specific metabolism at the *right times* of day. If you make these two principles the cornerstone of your new lifestyle, I promise you, you will never have a weight problem again.

Next there are three important keys to keep you in balance, forever thin, and in resplendent health:

1. Maintaining your weight when you dine out, whether you're eating at dinner parties or restaurants
2. Maintaining your weight once you've reached your goal
3. And most important, keeping yourself forever young by cultivating and maintaining your regeneration from year to year

Eating Out with Ease

To get through even the most sumptuous occasion without losing your hard-earned balance, try this advice:

- Let your hosts know in advance that you may need to control your eating. That way they will not be insulted if you turn down a high-fat or sugar-filled specialty.
- Explain that you'd like to bring along a little of your cheat food, so that you can munch along with the other guests.
- As appetizers, try to fill up on *raw vegetables*—without the dip. It will help you feel a part of the party.
- Limit your alcohol intake to one glass of white wine, followed by a lot of water.
- Avoid fatty and salty foods and cream sauces.
- If necessary, eat a little bit of everything, but do *not* stuff yourself until you feel full. The operative word here is *little*, meaning a tiny portion.
- Take plenty of time to *chew your foods slowly*, and intersperse dinner conversations throughout your meal. That way you'll be able to eat smaller portions spaced over a longer period of time.
- Don't be tempted by the breads or rolls. Instead, reach for a *breadstick*, if provided by your hosts, and nibble it *slowly*.
- If you have a choice of desserts, reach for the *sorbet*, *fruit ice*, or *fruit* and eat it *slowly*. Otherwise, take just a tiny taste of the dessert provided for you, then drink plenty of water.
- Get right back on your diet the next day.

Here are some strategies for dining in restaurants without sabotaging your weight-loss program:

- If possible, pick a restaurant that you know is flexible about allowing you to order your meals the way you want them.
- Scan the menus for healthy dishes that contain foods best suited to your specific meta-type.
- Avoid saturated fats, cream sauces, and fried and sugar-filled foods.
- Avoid drinking alcohol. It will add calories and induce sugar cravings.
- Order à la carte. This gives you a greater variety of foods from which to pick and makes it easier to follow the food choice guidelines for your meta-type.
- Avoid *salt* and *salty foods* at all costs.
- Ask for oil and vinegar or lemon juice *on the side* as dressing for your salad. Use only the amount allotted for your meta-type dinner.
- No desserts. You don't need them.
- Try to limit your restaurant visits to only once or twice a week.
- Get right back on your diet the next day.

Maintaining Your Weight

The basic principles you've learned about your meta-type and weight loss include the specific foods that are right for your meta-type; what percentages of your foods should consist of proteins, carbohydrates, and fats; the best times of the day or evening for you to eat; and the proper way to combine your foods. Another key to making your program work is how many calories you take in per day.

Other than the amino acids in proteins and the vitamins and minerals in carbohydrates and fats used for the cellular regeneration of your body, your extra adipose tissue comes from eating more calories than you burn up in your daily activity. Remember, all the foods you eat—whether proteins, carbohydrates, or fats—will turn into stored body fat unless they are burned up as energy or used for your cellular regeneration. A *calorie* is a unit that represents the energy value of your foods after they have been broken down and are ready to be burned off.

Now I'm not asking you to count all your calories for your weight-loss diet. I've already done that for you in your specific meta-type diet. I've calculated the diets for women to have 1,000 to 1,200 calories per day and those for men to have 1,500 to 1,700 calories. But I *am* asking you to acquire some basic understanding of what it will take to maintain your desired weight. Since different people feel better at different weights, everyone has a different idea of what his or her own weight maintenance level should be. The idea here is for you to figure your ideal weight. You will then need some working knowledge of how to maintain that desired weight once you've accomplished your goal.

The most traditional way of determining the *total calories of energy* and *nutrients* needed per day for your specific metabolism is shown in the accompanying box. These calculations will give you the number of calories you need to support the maintenance of your desired weight.

Let's do an example. Suppose a woman regarded her ideal body weight as 135 pounds. We'll divide it by 2.2, giving us 61.36 kilograms, then multiply it by 22, leaving us with a total of 1,349.92. We'll round it off to 1,350, which is her basal metabolic rate.

In other words, she needs 1,350 calories per day just to stay alive at 135 pounds. Then we'll add her level of activity. Let's say this woman is a receptionist and has fairly light activity, so we take ½ of her metabolic rate $(1,350 \div 2 = 675)$, which we add to 1,350, giving us a total of 2,025. Then we add 6 percent energy: $2,025 \times .06 = 121.50 + 2,025 = 2,146.5$, which we'll round off to 2,146. Now the question is, what is her age? This woman has just turned 51, so we will subtract 10 percent: $2,146 - 214.6 =$

Calories Needed per Day to Maintain Your Desired Weight

Take what you feel to be your ideal body weight in pounds and divide it by 2.2 to get your weight in kilograms.

Then multiply it by 22 for women or 24 for men.

This result represents your basal metabolic rate.

Then *add* your daily level of activity:

Bed rest	Basal metabolic rate
Very light activity	Basal metabolic rate × $1\frac{1}{3}$
Light activity	Basal metabolic rate × $1\frac{1}{2}$
Moderate activity	Basal metabolic rate × $1\frac{2}{3}$
Heavy activity	Basal metabolic rate + 1
Pregnancy	Basal metabolic rate + 300
Lactating mother	Basal metabolic rate + 500

This gives you the initial amount of calories needed to maintain your desired weight.

Then you have to *add* an extra *energy* need of 6 percent (the preceding total multiplied by .06), which gives you the daily caloric needs for your specific meta-type to maintain your desired weight.

One last thing: If you're between 51 and 75 years old, subtract 10 percent of the preceding total. If you're more than 75 years old, subtract 20 percent.

1,931.4 calories, which we'll round off to 1,931. So this woman needs 1,931 calories per day to maintain her weight at 135 pounds.

You can use the accompanying worksheet to determine the total caloric intake you need in order to maintain your desired weight level based on your specific profile.

As an alternative to the preceding formula, you can use this "super-quick" method given to me by one of my teachers in Chinese medicine to determine the calories needed to maintain your specific ideal weight. First, pick your desired weight, then multiply it by the number from the following list that corresponds to your activity level:

Very light activity	13
Moderate activity	15
Strenuous activity	20

Worksheet: Caloric Intake Needed for Weight Maintenance

Your ideal body weight   _____

Divide by 2.2   _____

Multiply by 22 for women or 24 for men   _____

                                               (Your individual basal metabolic rate)

Add your daily level of activity   _____

Add 6% energy (.06 × the sum total)   _____

Subtract 10% for ages 51–75

    or 20% for ages 76 and older   _____

GRAND TOTAL   _____

                                               (Number of calories needed
to maintain your weight goal)

If your ideal weight is 135 pounds and you are a moderately active individual, you would multiply 135 × 15 = 2,025, which is the number we reached earlier before factoring in the added 6 percent energy and the older age. If you maintain a very heavy work schedule, are over 50, or are pregnant or lactating, then you need to take other factors into account in your calculations. Otherwise, the short formula will work for you.

For a *woman*, if your weight-loss diet was based on 1,000 to 1,200 calories, you will need to add enough extra calories to raise your total daily caloric intake to the amount needed to maintain your desired weight. For instance, if your weight-loss diet were based on 1,000 calories, and you needed 2,025 calories to *maintain* your weight, then you could *add* an extra 1,025 calories per day.

For a *man*, if your weight-loss diet was based on 1,500 calories, you will need to add enough extra calories to raise your caloric intake to the amount needed to maintain your desired weight. For instance, if your weight-loss diet were based on 1,500 calories, and you needed 3,000 calories to *maintain* your weight, then you would *add* an extra 1,500 calories per day.

Based on your own individual metabolic predisposition, those extra calories should be apportioned according to the needs of your meta-type. For instance, the accelerator would need 60 percent carbohydrates, 20 percent proteins, and 20 percent fats. So you would apportion the extra calories based on the percentages required for your metabolic type, as shown in the accompanying worksheets.

Accelerator: Allocation of Extra Calories

Desired weight _____

Number of extra calories needed
  to maintain desired weight _____

Amount of additional *carbohydrates* per day:
  60% of the total caloric addition _____

Amount of additional *proteins* per day:
  20% of the total caloric addition _____

Amount of additional *fats* per day:
  20% of the total caloric addition _____

Balanced Accelerator: Allocation of Extra Calories

Desired weight _____

Number of extra calories needed
  to maintain desired weight _____

Amount of additional *carbohydrates* per day:
  50% of the total caloric addition _____

Amount of additional *proteins* per day:
  30% of the total caloric addition _____

Amount of additional *fats* per day:
  20% of the total caloric addition _____

Mixed Accelerator: Allocation of Extra Calories

Desired weight _____

Number of extra calories needed
  to maintain desired weight _____

Amount of additional *carbohydrates* per day:
  45% of the total caloric addition _____

Amount of additional *proteins* per day:
  40% of the total caloric addition _____

Amount of additional *fats* per day:
  15% of the total caloric addition _____

Synthesizer: Allocation of Extra Calories

Desired weight _____

Number of extra calories needed
  to maintain desired weight _____

Amount of additional *proteins* per day:
  55% of the total caloric addition _____

Amount of additional *carbohydrates* per day:
  30% of the total caloric addition _____

Amount of additional *fats* per day:
  15% of the total caloric addition _____

Balanced Synthesizer: Allocation of Extra Calories

Desired weight _____

Number of extra calories needed
  to maintain desired weight _____

Amount of additional *proteins* per day:
  50% of the total caloric addition _____

Amount of additional *carbohydrates* per day:
  30% of the total caloric addition _____

Amount of additional *fats* per day:
  20% of the total caloric addition _____

Mixed Synthesizer: Allocation of Extra Calories

Desired weight _____

Number of extra calories needed
  to maintain desired weight _____

Amount of additional *proteins* per day:
  45% of the total caloric addition _____

Amount of additional *carbohydrates* per day:
  40% of the total caloric addition _____

Amount of additional *fats* per day:
  15% of the total caloric addition _____

Now turn to appendix 5, "General Food Choices and Their Calorie Content for Each Meta-Type," and you'll find all the acid and alkaline foods listed with their caloric value, similar to your own meta-type food choices. Just pick out the food categories listed in your specific metabolic diet and begin adding in the extra caloric values from each group. In this way you'll easily maintain your desired weight goal.

Let's say I'm a synthesizer and I've been on a weight-loss diet of 1,000 calories. I've reached my goal and want to stay at a maintenance weight of 135 pounds. This means that I should consume about 2,025 calories per day. Therefore, I can add 1,025 calories to my diet each day. Since my percentages should be 55 percent proteins, 30 percent carbohydrates, and 15 percent fats, I would divide up my extra caloric intake as follows:

55% protein (.55 × 1,025)   = 564 additional calories of proteins
30% carbohydrates (.30 × 1,025) = 307 additional calories of carbohydrates
15% fat (.15 × 1,025)   = 154 additional calories of fats

In this way I'm able to maintain my desired weight, play around with weight loss or gain, and ultimately be in control of my own destiny.

Staying Forever Young

We are all an intrinsic part of the universe, and like the animals and plants, we're subject to universal laws and the cyclical movements of nature. As each season changes, we watch nature reveal itself. Springtime emerges as a tree's sap rises from the darkest realms of its buried roots, pushing itself upward and outward with tremendous energy, finally exposing itself in new green growth and flowers. Summer brings forth great bursts of growth as the foliage matures and the fruit begins to ripen. Then the sap's slow descent to its roots is heralded by a blazing show of autumnal colors, signifying "a job well done," as the fruit is harvested. Everything then quiets down, a time for rest and repair as the sap is reenergized and renewed in its deep inner roots during the winter months, gathering again the intense energy needed for its next burst of growth.

Did you know that we also go through exactly the same cycles? Most of us are unaware of how greatly our lives are influenced by the seasonal cycles. We undergo a birth and death each year, whether it's in our body, mind, emotions, or spirit. This is how we evolve, grow, change, mature, and gain wisdom.

According to Chinese medicine, our "sap" or "spiritual energy" rises within us each year. Ideas, behavior patterns, and emotions that are found deep within us during the winter months surface as our consciousness bursts forth with new concepts in the spring. These ideas are nurtured by the summer months' heat and activity, bringing forth the fruits of that labor in autumn. Then our intense physical activity begins to quiet as our consciousness again starts its descent into our inner selves—"our roots"—during the winter months to be renewed and reenergized. Within our inner levels, we discover, through the experiences in our outer world, what parts of ourselves need to be changed, realigned, transformed, or developed to resurface for springtime birth or renewal.

This cyclical existence is based on the movement of our planet in relationship to the sun, our star. Spring is proclaimed at the spring equinox, when day and night are of equal length and we start a movement back toward the warmth and energy of the sun. In Chinese medicine this is called the beginning of the yang time of year. As we proceed closer to the sun, we become infused with its radiant energy, and vibrant growth is stimulated as the days grow longer. The autumn equinox signals the beginning of the movement away from the sun, when our days will become shorter and our nights longer as we journey out into our universe during the winter months. This time of year is called the beginning of the yin season.

Our physical body—which houses our emotional, mental, and spiritual natures—is bound by the same cyclical universal laws and acts as our shelter as we go through our changes and growth. It's literally the "field of action" or garden where our conscious levels sprout, grow, and are harvested. And like every good garden, it needs to be cultivated, fertilized, weeded, cleaned out, then turned over for winter. By utilizing the individual seasonal energies, we can constantly renew ourselves and rid ourselves of the debris of emotional clutter; mental overwork; rigid, outdated views; environmental toxins and pollutants; and overindulgence in foods.

In Chinese medicine *spring* corresponds to renewal and rebirth, expressed physically by the liver and gallbladder systems, called the organs of transformation. Utilizing spring to cleanse and detoxify your liver and gallbladder systems enables anger, rage, and resentment to be uprooted from your body while cleaning out the debris from winter. Mental clarity, focus, and concentration are enhanced as you prepare to integrate new ideas and patterns into your life. Vitality is renewed, immune function strengthened, and aging regressed, and your body's metabolism becomes balanced, harmonizing your parasympathetic nervous system. The mental clarity stimulates insight and intuition as your conscious and subconscious minds meld. In Chinese medicine the Liver meridian is the only energy pathway into the brain.

Summer is activated through the heart and small intestine organ systems, stimulating and increasing growth and maturation, which balance the whole energetic system of your body. By cleansing and regenerating these organ systems, the efficiency of digestion and assimilation is increased and your heart strengthened. This in turn balances the energy centers in your body (called chakras), their corresponding organ meridians, and your whole body's endocrine system. Shyness, overseriousness, overeating, and gloom are eliminated as playfulness is encouraged, which releases joy and calmness of your mind and spirit while supporting your individual growth and regeneration.

Late summer is a short season but a time of great transition and preparation for winter. The stomach and spleen organ systems are activated in this season. Gently cleaning out your lymphatic system (associated with the spleen and immunity) and augmenting your digestion with the right foods will easily prepare your body for the transitional journey into the darkness of winter. Adaptability, relaxation, and balance are encouraged through subconscious awareness and insight as resistance to change and apprehension are discarded.

Fall reveals the fruition of all your growth and renewal, what you have exhibited throughout the year, and helps prepare you for your body's rest and spiritual journey into your inner self. The lung and large intestine are fall's organ systems. Rejuvenating these systems gives your body the ability to strengthen your immune system and helps to prepare your body for the heavier foods of winter. Grief and sadness are released as well as any held-in emotions. This supports muscle strength and balance and strengthens your hair and skin while preparing you for the descent into winter. Indecision, confusion, obscurity, and fatigue are released, while consolidation, communication, and clarity of the self ensue.

Winter brings you face-to-face with your inner self, especially your fears. It represents a time when you must dig into yourself to identify and release negative habit patterns. It's a time of your subconscious voice speaking to you through your dreams and insights. Cleansing and rejuvenating your kidney and bladder organ systems allow for the speedy release of toxic emotions, especially hidden fears, while invoking the courage needed to make the required changes. This balances the adrenal glands, thereby balancing the sympathetic nervous system. Your ears and bones are strengthened, and adrenal energy is regenerated and stored in the body to support the new growth needed for springtime renewal.

Taking a few days out of each season to gently cleanse and regenerate each of your organ systems with fresh foods, vegetable juices, herbs, exercises, meditations, and writing down your dreams will help to rid your body of the accumulated physical and emotional wastes while removing any blocks that impede the flow of your life-giving energy.

With each new season, you prepare yourself physically, emotionally, mentally, and spiritually to meet life's special challenges, reinforcing a healthy, self-aware way of living. You won't have to wait for a health or emotional crisis to "bring you to the brink" and force you to reevaluate or "save" your life.

You'll be able to release life's continual stresses in nondestructive ways, gaining helpful insight into yourself and your surroundings. This automatically opens the doorway into your unconscious or subconscious mind, the conductor of your body's behavior, moods, emotions, perceptions, and motivations.

Seasonal regenerating programs will give you a fresh start and keep you on a healthy life track. They will help you replenish your energy reserves and increase your stamina and awareness, thereby allowing you to cope with many of life's potential stresses and keeping you eternally young.

Well, this is it—the end of your weight problems and the beginning of your new slender, healthy way of life!

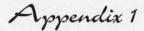

Meta-Type Advance Food Preparation
and Recipes

Equipment List for All Meta-Type Diets

Oven
Stovetop
Microwave
Juicer
Salad spinner
Food processor
Handheld blender
Cutting board
8-in. or 10-in. chef's knife
8-in. cast-iron skillet (or frying pan with metal handle)

Small, medium, and large saucepans
Small roasting pan or bread-baking pan
Half sheet pan
Oil mister
Plastic storage containers
Gallon-size resealable plastic food-storage bags

Accelerator

Larger quantities for men are shown in **boldface**.
Buy fish the day you prepare it or, at most, 1 day in advance.
Keep sprouted grain bread in the freezer.
The following recipes appear in the "General Recipes for All Meta-Types" section, which starts on page 417:

- Jicama Sticks
- Roasted Hazelnuts
- Roasted Onions
- Seaweed

Advance Food Preparation

This subsection presents dishes that you can make up ahead of time and keep on hand for use as needed. Investing a little time at the start of the week will enable you to prepare all the meals on your diet with minimal work during the week.

Fava Beans and Red Kidney Beans

Rinse and soak 2 cups fava beans in cold water for 2 hours. Rinse and soak ½ cup red kidney beans for 2 hours. Keep beans separate.

When beans have soaked, rinse again; then cover with fresh water in a medium saucepan. Bring to a boil; then lower heat and simmer for 1 hour or until beans are tender.

Drain off water and refrigerate beans.

Quinoa, Basmati Brown Rice, and Wild Rice

Cook the following grains according to the directions on the packages:

½ **(1)** cup quinoa
¾ **(1)** cup basmati brown rice
½ cup wild rice

The volume of the grains will triple after cooking and will yield enough for each of the recipes that follow. Refrigerate cooked grains separately in airtight plastic containers.

Accelerator Raw Vegetables

Cleaning and trimming raw vegetables in advance make it easy to prepare various salads during the week. Store each vegetable separately in an airtight plastic container or a resealable plastic bag. Yield is approximately 12 **(19)** cups.

2 lb. carrots, cleaned, trimmed, and cut into 2-in. sticks
2 bunches broccoli, cut into florets
1 **(2)** head cauliflower, cut into florets
1 **(2)** lg. yellow squashes, cut into ¼-in.-thick half-moons
1 **(2)** lg. zucchini, cut into ¼-in.-thick half-moons
½ red pepper, cut into 1-in. squares

Add more carrots and squash if necessary.

Hard-Boiled Eggs

Place 2 eggs in a small saucepan, cover with water, and bring to a boil. Cook at a rolling boil for 8 min.; then rinse under cold water and refrigerate.

Raw Veggie Slaw

In the bowl of a food processor, grate ½ lb. peeled carrots and 6 radishes. Combine with 1 thinly sliced sm. red onion, 1 **(lg.)** fennel bulb, and 1 **(lg.)** zucchini. Add 1 cup finely chopped celery, ½ cup chopped parsley, 1 tbs. fat-free mayonnaise, 1 tsp. cracked black pepper, and the juice from 1 lemon. Toss well and refrigerate. You can also add ¼ cup apple juice if on your diet.

Accelerator Elixirs

Having clean vegetables on hand makes juicing a lot easier and a lot less time-consuming. You will need the following vegetables to make the Accelerator Elixirs three times in the coming week:

2 lb. carrots
½ lb. beets
2 bunches parsley
1 head romaine lettuce
2 bunches alfalfa sprouts

Marinated Tofu

Marinade
Mix together the following ingredients: 1 tsp. curry powder, 1 cup freshly squeezed grapefruit juice, ¼ tsp. black pepper, and 1 tsp. honey dissolved in ¼ cup hot water.

Tofu
Slice 1 **(1½)** lb. tofu through the middle; then cut each piece into 4 **(6)** triangles. Place on a plate on paper towels and cover again with paper towels and another plate. Add a few cans or something heavy to the top plate to press the tofu. You want to squeeze as much water as possible out of the tofu so it will absorb the marinade. After pressing for 1 hour, transfer 4 **(6)** pieces of the tofu to a shallow container and cover with the marinade. It can sit in the marinade for up to 2 days. The remaining pieces can be frozen for future use.

Accelerator Salad Greens

1 **(2)** head romaine lettuce
1 **(2)** head red leaf lettuce
2 heads Boston lettuce
3 heads Belgian endive
1 head radicchio
1 lb. spinach

Cut or tear all greens into 2-in. or bite-size pieces. Rinse in cold water to remove all dirt; then spin dry. Wrap greens in portion-size amounts (2–3 cups) in paper towels; then store in gallon-size resealable plastic bags from which all the air has been squeezed out.

If greens are dried and stored properly, they can last for up to 4 to 7 days in the refrigerator. Not all greens will stand up to this kind of treatment. One option is to clean half your salad greens twice a week.

Add other greens as recipes indicate.

Dane's Enzyme Fruit Medley

Combine the following:

3 **(5)** cups cleaned green grapes
2 fresh pineapples, peeled and sliced
2 papayas, peeled, seeded, and cut into cubes
2 **(3)** pints strawberries, cleaned, destemmed, and sliced
2 **(3)** kiwifruits, peeled and sliced

Add the juice of 3 lemons and any juice released from the pineapples and papayas while slicing. Refrigerate in a large plastic container. Yield should be approximately 10 **(14)** cups.

Citrus Fruit Salad

Peel, section, and combine the following:

5 **(6)** pink grapefruits
4 **(5)** blood oranges
4 **(5)** navel oranges
4 **(6)** clementines
4 **(6)** tangerines

Squeeze out any juice left after sectioning and add it to the salad. Refrigerate in an airtight container.

Accelerator Salad Dressing

Blend together 1 cup olive or safflower oil, ½ cup lemon juice, 6 cloves crushed garlic, 2 tsp. cayenne pepper (or 4 tsp. black pepper), and 2 tbs. tarragon or other herbs. Mix well, cover, and refrigerate.

Black Bean Soup

Rinse 1½ cups black beans and soak for 2 hours. Rinse again; then place in a large saucepan and cover with three times as much water. Add 1 lg. yellow onion, chopped small; 2 tbs. roughly chopped peeled ginger; ½ cup cilantro leaves (yield from 1 bunch); 2 carrots, cleaned and diced; and ¼ cup balsamic vinegar. Bring to a boil, reduce to a simmer, and cook, stirring occasionally, for 2 hours or until beans are soft. Using a handheld blender, puree the soup in the pot and then transfer to 8-oz. portion-size containers. What is not going to be used in the next week can be frozen.

Recipes

Notes: Since the energy of microwave ovens varies, you may need to adjust the indicated microwave cooking times according to your own microwave's power.

When your daily menu instructs you to prepare your Accelerator Elixir, see page 380 for the proper combination of juices.

Vege Rejuvenation Dinner

Preheat broiler. Place Marinated Tofu on a sheet pan, lightly sprayed with oil (olive or canola). Place 4 in. from the flame and broil tofu for 5 min. on each side or until it begins to turn a golden brown and become firm on the surface.

Place 2 cups combined Accelerator Raw Vegetables in a microwavable container. Toss with 1 tsp. **(1 tbs.)** curry powder. Microwave for 7 min.

Microwave ¾ **(1½)** cup cooked basmati brown rice for 2 min. **(2 min. 30 seconds)** on HIGH. Top with grated ginger.

Serve with combined Accelerator Salad Greens topped with scallions and ½ cup cold or reheated Seaweed.

Egg-alicious Dinner

Egg Frittata

Preheat oven to 400°. Microwave 2 cups broccoli florets. Beat 3 eggs together in a mixing bowl with 1 tbs. dried oregano. Lightly spray the bottom of an 8-in. cast-iron skillet. Over a medium flame pour eggs into skillet and gently roll eggs around the bottom and halfway up the sides of the pan. When about half the egg mixture is cooked, place cooked broccoli and ½ cup Roasted Onions mixed with ½ cup grated carrots in center of pan.

Top with sliced tomato (optional) and place pan in oven for 10–15 min. until the eggs puff up around the vegetables, turn a golden brown, and are cooked through. Garnish with chopped scallions. Use any leftover Roasted Onions in any salad during the week.

Arugula Salad

Clean and dry 1 bunch arugula. Slice ½ red pepper and ½ sm. red onion paper-thin. Toss with ½ tsp. olive or walnut oil until completely covered. Sprinkle with balsamic vinegar to taste. Top with 1 **(2)** oz. crumbled goat cheese **(and 1 tbs. Roasted Hazelnuts)**.

Vitality Vegetarian Dinner

Reheat or microwave 1 **(2)** cup Black Bean Soup. Top with chopped cilantro leaves and ½ **(1)** piece toasted sprouted grain bread cut into bite-size croutons. Microwave or steam 1½ **(2)** cups combined Accelerator Raw Vegetables tossed with 1 tsp. cumin.

Microwave 1 **(2)** cup basmati brown rice tossed with ½ **(1)** tsp. turmeric and 1 **(2)** oz. Roasted Hazelnuts.

Serve with combined Accelerator Salad Greens to which watercress is added.

Jump for Joy Carbo Dinner

Preheat oven to 400°. Peel and slice 2 **(3)** parsnips and 2 **(3)** carrots into 2-in. sticks. Peel ½ **(1)** med. red onion and cut into fourths **(eighths)**. Slice ½ lg. fennel bulb into 6 or 8 pieces. Mix together with 1 cup cauliflower florets and ¼ cup fresh rosemary, roughly chopped. Place on a lightly sprayed sheet pan and roast for 20–25 min. or until vegetables feel soft. Transfer immediately to an airtight container and let sit for about 5 min.

Peel and cube 2 **(3)** med. beets. You can cook these at the same time as the other vegetables but do not mix together until just before eating; otherwise, they will color everything purple.

Slice an acorn squash in half lengthwise and remove all seeds. Rinse squash and sprinkle with cinnamon. Place facedown on a sheet pan lightly sprayed with oil and roast for 25 min. or until a fork slides in and out easily.

Spinach Salad

Mix 1½ **(2)** cups freshly washed spinach leaves with 1 **(2)** cups Accelerator Salad Greens. Dress with 1 **(2)** tsp. Accelerator Salad Dressing.

Hearty Vegetarian Salad Dinner

Mix together ¾ **(2)** cup cooked wild rice, 2 cups combined Accelerator Raw Vegetables, and ½ **(¾)** cup cooked Red Kidney Beans and toss with ½ tbs. Accelerator Salad Dressing. Place mixture on top of 2 cups Accelerator Salad Greens tossed with ½ tbs. Accelerator Salad Dressing. Top salad with chopped parsley, watercress, leftover Roasted Onions, chopped scallions, and sprouts **(and 1 slice sprouted grain bread, toasted and cut up into sm. croutons)**.

Fabulous Fish Dinner

You can cook two pieces of yellowtail tuna at dinnertime. The larger 6-oz. **(7-oz.)** piece is for dinner, and the smaller 4-oz. **(6-oz.)** piece will be served cold with tomorrow's lunch.

Preheat oven to 400°. Rinse both pieces of tuna. Heat a cast-iron skillet on top of the stove. When the pan is hot, place both pieces of tuna in the pan and sear on both sides, approximately 2 min. per side. Transfer tuna to the oven, baste with Dijon mustard and 1 tsp. chopped rosemary, and finish baking for about 3 min. more for medium rare. Cook longer if desired.

Steam or microwave ½ **(1)** cup turnips and ½ **(1)** cup carrots until very soft. Puree in the bowl of a food processor or in a mixing bowl with a handheld blender.

French Green Beans
Steam or microwave 1 cup French green beans (haricots verts) and serve with ¼ **(½)** tsp. Accelerator Salad Dressing.

Fennel Salad
Slice ½ bulb fennel paper-thin. Mix with 1 red onion, peeled and sliced very thin. Sprinkle with 1 tsp. Accelerator Salad Dressing and the feathery, dill-like top of the fennel bulb.

Vege-dairian Delight Dinner

Vegetable Lasagna
Vegetables can be cleaned and precooked earlier in the day or the day before. Preheat oven to 325°.

Steam 2 bunches Swiss chard. Clean and steam 3 med. leeks. Peel and grate 1 **(3)** carrot. Chop 3 scallions. Thinly slice ½ **(1)** fennel bulb.

Lightly spray a small roasting or bread pan. Cover bottom of pan with half the cooked Swiss chard. Top with half the cooked leeks, grated carrots, and sliced fennel. Cover vegetables with ½ (¾) cup low-fat ricotta cheese mixed with 1 tbs. oregano. Top cheese with remaining vegetables and cover everything with remaining Swiss chard. (*Option:* Top with sliced tomatoes if on your diet.) Cover and bake at 325° for about 30 min. Remove cover and top with 2 oz. grated low-fat mozzarella and any leftover Roasted Onions. Cook until cheese has melted. Serve immediately.

Cucumber Salad
Peel 1 cucumber. Slice into thin circles or half-moons. Mix with ¼ (½) cup fat-free yogurt and 2 tbs. chopped dill. This can be made 1 to 2 days in advance and refrigerated.

Balanced Accelerator

Larger quantities for men are shown in **boldface**.
Buy fish the day you prepare it or, at most, 1 day in advance.
The following recipes appear in the "General Recipes for All Meta-Types" section, which starts on page 417:

- Vegetable Stock
- Roasted Onions
- Roasted Hazelnuts
- Curried Tofu
- Tofu Scramble
- Seaweed
- Jicama Sticks
- Roasted Garlic

Advance Food Preparation

This subsection presents dishes that you can make up ahead of time and keep on hand for use as needed. Investing a little time at the start of the week will enable you to prepare all the meals on your diet with minimal work during the week.

Balanced Accelerator Raw Vegetables

Cleaning and trimming raw vegetables in advance make it easy to prepare various salads and vegetable dishes during the week. Store each vegetable separately in an airtight plastic container or a resealable plastic bag.

4 lb. carrots, cleaned, trimmed, and cut into 2-in. sticks
3 bunches broccoli, cut into florets
1 head cauliflower, cut into florets
1½ lg. yellow squashes, cut into ¼-in.-thick half-moons
½ lg. zucchini, cut into ¼-in.-thick half-moons
1 lb. turnips or rutabagas, trimmed and cut into 2-in. sticks
3 parsnips, trimmed and cut into 2-in. sticks
3 sticks celery, cleaned and diced
2 leeks, well cleaned and chopped into 1-in. pieces
2 fennel bulbs, trimmed, quartered, and thinly sliced
1 bunch scallions, trimmed and chopped small
1 lb. beets, trimmed, cleaned, and cut into 1-in. pieces

Balanced Accelerator Elixirs

Having clean vegetables on hand makes juicing a lot easier and a lot less time-consuming. You will need the following vegetables to make all four of the elixirs in the coming week:

4 lb. carrots
1 bunch celery
5 bunches parsley
1 head romaine lettuce
1 lb. spinach
2 boxes alfalfa sprouts

Balanced Accelerator Salad Greens

See "Accelerator Salad Greens," on page 380.

Dane's Delight Prep

You can prepare the following fruits, store them separately, and mix them as you need them:

3 **(6)** pineapples, peeled, cored, and sliced (approximate yield: 7⅓ **[14]** cups)
3 **(6)** papayas, peeled, seeded, and sliced (approximate yield: 6⅓ **[11]** cups)
4 **(6)** pints strawberries, cleaned and destemmed; slice as you use them
   (approximate yield: 6 **[7]** cups)
2 **(4)** bunches green grapes, cleaned and destemmed (approximate
   yield: 4 **[6]** cups)

Other fruit can be prepared as needed.

Tabouli

Place ½ **(1)** cup bulgur wheat in a large bowl and cover with 2 **(3½)** cups boiling water. Cover tightly and let sit for about 2 hours. Pressing the grain, squeeze out any excess water. Add the following ingredients: 1 bunch finely chopped parsley, ½ cup chopped scallions, ¼ **(½)** cup chopped mint leaves, and ¼ **(½)** cup fresh lemon juice. (Add 2 chopped plum tomatoes if on your diet.) Refrigerate in an airtight container.

Balanced Accelerator Salad Dressing

Combine 1½ cups safflower oil, ¾ cup lemon juice, 6 cloves crushed garlic, 2 tsp. cayenne or black pepper, and 1½ tbs. herbs (such as tarragon, oregano, or thyme). Mix well, cover, and refrigerate.

Recipes

Notes: Since the energy of microwave ovens varies, you may need to adjust the indicated microwave cooking times according to your own microwave's power.

When your daily menu instructs you to prepare your Balanced Accelerator Elixir, see page 166 for the proper combination of juices.

Dane's Delight

Combine ½ **(1)** cup fresh pineapple, ½ **(1)** cup fresh papaya, ½ **(1)** cup green grapes, and ¾ cup fresh strawberries. Sprinkle with chopped mint leaves and the juice of 1 lemon.

Fish Fiesta Dinner

You can cook the whole piece **(both pieces)** of yellowfin tuna at dinner-time. Slice off 2 oz. **(use second piece)** to be served cold with tomorrow's lunch.

Preheat oven to 400°. Rinse tuna. Heat a cast-iron skillet on top of the stove. When the pan is hot, place tuna in the pan and sear on both sides, approximately 2 min. per side. Transfer tuna to the oven and finish baking for about 3 min. more for medium rare. Cook longer if desired. Serve with Dijon mustard as a condiment.

Steam or microwave ½ **(1)** cup turnips and ½ **(1)** cup carrots until very soft. Puree in the bowl of a food processor or in a mixing bowl with a hand-held blender.

Fiesta Vegetables

Steam or microwave 1 cup haricots verts (green beans) and serve with 2 cups combined Balanced Accelerator Salad Greens with watercress added. Toss with 2 tsp. Balanced Accelerator Salad Dressing.

Protein Power Dinner

Hearty Vegetable Soup

Heat 2 cups Vegetable Stock and add the following ingredients:

½ head Roasted Garlic paste
1 tbs. oregano
½ **(1)** cup carrots, diced
½ **(1)** cup turnips, diced
2 leeks, cleaned and chopped
½ bunch kale, cleaned and chopped into 2-in. pieces

Simmer soup for ½ hour until carrots and turnips are tender.

Mustard Thyme Chicken

While soup is cooking, preheat broiler and prepare the chicken. After the chicken is cooked, you can slice off the 2-oz. **(6-oz.)** piece for Tuesday's lunch. Rinse chicken breast and cover the top with Dijon mustard and a generous sprinkling of dried thyme. Place under the broiler and cook for 8–10 min. until chicken is done. Cooking time will vary according to the thickness of the chicken. It is done when no pink shows inside the meat.

Power Salad

Add watercress, radishes, scallions, celery, and alfalfa sprouts to 2 cups Balanced Accelerator Salad Greens and toss with 2 tsp. Balanced Accelerator Salad Dressing.

Longevity Dinner

You will roast twice as many vegetables as needed. Half will be for dinner and the other half for Friday's Tofu-Amaranth Vegetarian Dinner.

Preheat oven to 400°. Lightly spray a baking pan with safflower oil. Combine ½ **(1¾)** cup extrafirm tofu cut into cubes, 1 cup carrots, 1 cup parsnips, ½ cup yellow squash, ½ cup zucchini, and 1 red onion peeled and cut into eighths. Toss with 3 tbs. chopped fresh rosemary and arrange on baking pan. Lightly spray with safflower oil and bake for 25–30 min. Vegetables are done when a fork slides easily in and out of the carrots and parsnips.

Prepare ½ **(1)** cup amaranth grain and top with grated ginger. Serve with roasted vegetables and tofu.

Seaweed Health Salad

Top Balanced Accelerator Salad Greens with scallions and combine with 2 tsp. Balanced Accelerator Salad Dressing and ½ cup cold or reheated Seaweed.

Pasta Party Vegetarian Dinner

Egg Pastina and Artichoke with Dijon Beets and Lemon Pepper Kale

Steam or microwave 1 artichoke. Heat 1 cup Vegetable Stock in a medium saucepan and add 1 head Roasted Garlic paste, ¼ tsp. black pepper, and 1 tsp. oregano. Prepare ⅓ **(⅔)** cup egg pastina (or angel-hair pasta) according to directions on the box (it will double in volume).

Add the pastina to the Vegetable Stock mixture.

While the artichoke is steaming, microwave ½ **(1)** cup beets tossed with fresh chopped rosemary and ½ tsp. Dijon mustard. Steam or microwave ½ bunch kale with ¼ cup cubed tofu. Top with juice of 1 lemon and black pepper to taste.

Arugula Fennel Salad
Clean and dry 1 bunch arugula. Slice ½ bulb fennel and ½ small red onion paper-thin. Toss with 1 tsp. Balanced Accelerator Salad Dressing.

Calypso Fish Dinner

Fill a small frying pan halfway with water and add the juice of 1 lemon. Bring to a simmer on medium heat.

Add 3 **(6)** oz. cleaned calamari cut into ½-in. rings. Simmer for approximately 3–4 min. Drain and, while still warm, add the juice of 1 lime, a pinch cayenne pepper, and chopped cilantro leaves.

Mixed Vegetables with Cumin
Steam or microwave ¼ **(½)** cup turnips or parsnips and ¼ **(½)** cup carrots or beets until very soft. Puree with ¼ cup Roasted Onions and ½ tsp. cumin in the bowl of a food processor or in a mixing bowl with a handheld blender.

Haricots Verts Salad
Steam or microwave 1 cup haricots verts and serve with 2 cups combined Balanced Accelerator Salad Greens with watercress added. Toss with 2 tsp. Balanced Accelerator Salad Dressing. Serve with marinated Jicama Sticks.

Veggie Delight Dinner

Preheat oven to 400°. Slice acorn squash in half lengthways and remove all seeds. Rinse squash and rub cavities with cinnamon. Place facedown on a sheet pan lightly sprayed with safflower oil and roast for 25 min. or until a fork slides in and out easily.

Combine ½ **(1)** cup parsnips, ½ **(1)** cup carrots, 1¼ **(2)** cups cauliflower, ½ red onion cut into fourths, and ½ cup fennel and toss with ½ cup chopped fresh rosemary. Place on a lightly sprayed sheet pan and roast for 20–25 min. or until vegetables feel soft. Transfer immediately to an airtight container and let sit for about 5 min.

Spinach Fennel Salad

Mix freshly washed spinach leaves with Balanced Accelerator Salad Greens and ¼ (½) chopped fennel bulb; then toss with 2 tsp. (1 tbs.) Balanced Accelerator Salad Dressing and 1 glass Balanced Accelerator Elixir.

Tofu-Amaranth Vegetarian Dinner

Mix together 2 (3) cups Balanced Accelerator Salad Greens with 1 sliced red onion and 1 tsp. Balanced Accelerator Salad Dressing. Combine ½ (1) cup cooked amaranth grain with 2 cups remaining roasted vegetables from Monday night's dinner, ½ cup Roasted Onions, and ¼ (¾) cup cold Curried Tofu with 1 (2) tsp. Balanced Accelerator Salad Dressing.

Mixed Accelerator

Larger quantities for men are shown in **boldface**.

Buy fish the day you prepare it or, at most, 1 day in advance.

The following recipes appear in the "General Recipes for All Meta-Types" section, which starts on page 417:

- Vegetable Stock
- Roasted Garlic (Use 3 heads of garlic instead of the 2 specified in the instructions.)
- Seaweed
- Curried Tofu
- Tofu Scramble (Use 1½ [2½] lb. extrafirm tofu instead of the 1 [2] lb. specified in the instructions and eliminate the Roasted Onions.)

Advance Food Preparation

This subsection presents dishes that you can make up ahead of time and keep on hand for use as needed. Investing a little time at the start of the week will enable you to prepare all the meals on your diet with minimal work during the week.

Roasted Peanuts

Preheat oven to 375°. Place ¼ (¾) cup peanuts on a cookie sheet or half sheet pan. Place in the oven and roast for 10 min., shaking the nuts every

2 or 3 min. Remove from oven and allow to cool; then refrigerate in an air-tight container.

Mixed Accelerator Elixirs

Having clean vegetables on hand makes juicing a lot easier and a lot less time-consuming. You will need the following vegetables to make all four of the elixirs in the coming week:

2 lb. carrots
2 bunches celery
7 bunches parsley
2 lb. spinach

Mixed Accelerator Raw Vegetables

Cleaning and trimming raw vegetables in advance make it easy to prepare various salads and vegetable dishes during the week. Store each vegetable separately in an airtight plastic container or a resealable plastic bag.

9 lb. carrots, cleaned, trimmed, and cut into 2-in. sticks
½ med. yellow squash, cut into ¼-in.-thick half-moons
½ med. zucchini, cut into ¼-in.-thick half-moons
2 lb. turnips or rutabagas, trimmed and cut into 2-in. sticks
1 bunch celery, cleaned and cut into sticks—minus what is used in
    Vegetable Stock. Use what you need of these sticks when recipes call
    for diced celery.
2 fennel bulbs, trimmed, quartered, and thinly sliced
2 bunches scallions, trimmed and chopped small
4 packages of mushrooms, cleaned and dried—minus what you use in
    Vegetable Stock

Mixed Accelerator Salad Greens

1 **(2)** head romaine lettuce
1 **(2)** head red leaf lettuce
1 **(2)** head green leaf lettuce
1 **(2)** head chicory

Cut or tear all greens into 2-in. or bite-size pieces. Rinse in cold water to re-move all dirt; then spin dry. Wrap greens in portion-size amounts (2–3 cups) in paper towels; then store in gallon-size resealable plastic bags from which all the air has been squeezed out. If greens are dried and stored properly, they can last for up to 4 to 7 days in the refrigerator. Not all greens will stand up to this kind of treatment. One option is to clean half your salad greens twice a week.

Add other greens as recipes indicate. At this time you can also clean and dry 2 bunches of kale and 2 lb. spinach for use in other recipes during the week.

Dane's Sunshine Fruit Bowl and After-Meal Fruit

You can prepare the following fruits, store them separately, and mix them as you need them:

3 **(6)** oranges, peeled and sectioned
3 **(6)** tangerines, peeled and sectioned
3 **(6)** kiwifruits, peeled and sliced
1 med. bunch green grapes, cleaned and destemmed
2 pineapples, peeled and sliced
2 papayas, peeled and sliced

Other fruit can be prepared as needed.

Mixed Accelerator Salad Dressing

Combine 1½ cups safflower oil, ¾ cup lemon juice, 6 cloves crushed garlic, 2 tsp. cayenne or black pepper, 1½ tbs. herbs (such as tarragon, oregano, or thyme). Mix well, cover, and refrigerate.

Recipes

Notes: Since the energy of microwave ovens varies, you may need to adjust the indicated microwave cooking times according to your own microwave's power.

When your daily menu instructs you to prepare your Mixed Accelerator Elixir, see page 197 for the proper combination of juices.

Option: Prepare enough of your morning drink, Miraculous Thin and Trim Cocktail, for the entire week and refrigerate.

Miraculous Thin and Trim Cocktail

Blend the following ingredients: 4 oz. pineapple juice (or 2 thin slices fresh pineapple liquefied in a blender), 1 tsp. blackstrap molasses, ½ tsp. wheat germ, ½ tsp. cod-liver oil (optional), and ½ tsp. kelp powder or blue-green algae.

Mushroom and Egg Frittata

Preheat oven to 400°. Beat 2 eggs or 3 egg whites together in a mixing bowl with ½ bunch cleaned and shredded basil. Lightly spray the bottom of an 8-in. cast-iron skillet. Over a medium flame pour eggs into skillet and gently roll eggs around the bottom and halfway up the sides of the pan. When about half the egg mixture is cooked, place ½ cup sliced mushrooms, **(½ cup low-fat cottage cheese)**, and ½ cup scallions in center of pan. Top with sliced tomato (optional) and place pan in oven for 10–15 min. until eggs puff up around vegetables, turn a golden brown, and are cooked through.

Spinach and Egg Surprise

Steam or microwave 1 lb. spinach. Top with 2 poached eggs and a generous sprinkling of freshly cracked pepper. **(Serve with 4 oz. fat-free yogurt to which a few drops of vanilla or almond extract have been added.)**

Sunrise Special

Combine 1 **(2)** orange, 1 **(2)** tangerine, 1 **(2)** kiwifruit, ½ cup strawberries, and ½ cup raspberries. Sprinkle with chopped mint leaves and the juice of 1 lemon.

Power Punch Morning Drink

Blend 4 oz. **(1 cup)** low-fat milk, 1 **(1½)** scoop whey protein powder, and ½ cap vanilla or almond extract. You may also add cinnamon and/or nutmeg to taste.

Or you may have 4 **(8)** oz. fat-free yogurt mixed with 3 drops vanilla or almond extract. You may also add cinnamon and/or nutmeg to taste.

Tropical Delight

Combine 2 oranges, 2 tangerines, 2 kiwifruits, ½ **(1)** cup papaya, and ¼ **(½)** cup green grapes. Sprinkle with chopped mint leaves and the juice of 1 lemon.

Fruit Frolic

Combine 1 **(2)** orange, 1 **(2)** tangerine, 1 **(2)** kiwifruit, ½ cup blueberries, and ½ nectarine. Sprinkle with chopped mint leaves and the juice of 1 lemon.

ThinFin Dinner

You can cook both pieces of yellowfin tuna at dinnertime. The 3-oz. **(6-oz.)** piece will be for dinner; the 8-oz. **(12-oz.)** piece will be sliced and served cold at two different lunches.

Preheat oven to 400°. Rinse both pieces of tuna. Heat a cast-iron skillet on top of the stove. When the pan is hot, place both pieces of tuna in the pan and sear on both sides, approximately 2 min. per side. Transfer tuna to the oven and finish baking for about 3 min. more for medium rare. Cook longer if desired. Serve with ½ tsp. mustard. Wrap the larger piece intended for lunches tightly in plastic and refrigerate.

Steam or microwave ½ **(1)** cup rutabagas and ½ **(1)** cup carrots until very soft. Puree in the bowl of a food processor or in a mixing bowl with a handheld blender.

Steam or microwave 2 cups asparagus. Top with the juice of ½ lemon. Serve with 2 cups Mixed Accelerator Salad Greens with watercress added. Toss with 1 tsp. Mixed Accelerator Salad Dressing.

Chicken Surprise

Hearty Vegetable Soup
Heat 2 cups Vegetable Stock and add the following ingredients: ½ head Roasted Garlic paste, 1 tbs. oregano, 1 cup carrots (diced), 1 **(2)** lb. chopped spinach, 1 cup sliced mushrooms, and ¼ cup scallions. Simmer soup for ½ hour until carrots are tender.

Mustard, Thyme, and Roasted Garlic Chicken
While soup is cooking, preheat broiler and prepare the chicken. Some 4

(7) oz. will be for dinner; the rest 4 **(7)** oz. will be served cold with Monday's lunch. Rinse chicken breast, cover top with mixture of ½ head Roasted Garlic puree, ½ **(1)** tsp. Dijon mustard, and ¼ tsp. dried thyme. Place under the broiler and cook for 8–10 min. until chicken is done. Cooking time will vary according to the thickness of the chicken. It is done when no pink shows inside the meat.

Health Salad
Combine 2 cups Mixed Accelerator Salad Greens with watercress and alfalfa sprouts. Toss with 1 tsp. Mixed Accelerator Salad Dressing.

Couscous Supreme

Cover ¼ **(½)** cup couscous with ½ **(1)** cup boiling water, cover tightly, and let stand for 20–30 min. Drain any excess water and fluff grains with a fork. While couscous is sitting, combine ½ cup carrots and ½ cup rutabagas with 2 tsp. curry powder and microwave for 7 min. **(7 min. 30 sec.)**. Add ½ **(1)** cup yellow squash, ½ **(1)** cup zucchini, and 1 **(2)** plum tomato (diced) to the root vegetables; toss well; and microwave for another 3 min. Top cooked couscous with Roasted Peanuts and curried vegetables.

Savory Salad
Serve with Mixed Accelerator Salad Greens topped with scallions and 2 tsp. Mixed Accelerator Salad Dressing and ½ cup cold or reheated Seaweed.

Carrot and Rutabaga Pasta Delight

Preheat oven to 400°. Combine ¼ **(½)** cup carrots, ¼ **(½)** rutabagas, 1 cup mushrooms, and ¼ **(¾)** cup tofu cut into 1-in. cubes. Toss with 1 tbs. freshly chopped rosemary leaves. Spray a baking sheet with safflower oil and arrange vegetables on sheet. Lightly spray vegetables. Bake for 20–30 min. until a fork slides easily in and out of the rutabagas.

While vegetables are roasting, heat 1 cup Vegetable Stock in a medium saucepan, add 1 head Roasted Garlic paste, ¼ tsp. black pepper, and ½ cup shredded basil leaves. Prepare ¾ **(1)** cup egg pastina (or angel-hair pasta) according to directions on the box. (It will double in volume.) When pasta is cooked, add it to the Vegetable Stock mixture.

Radicchio Fennel Salad

Shred 1 sm. head radicchio and mix with ½ cup sliced fennel sticks. Toss with 1 tsp. Mixed Accelerator Salad Dressing.

Simply Veggies

Preheat oven to 400°. Slice an acorn squash in half lengthways and remove all seeds. Rub cavities with cinnamon. Place facedown on a sheet pan lightly sprayed with safflower oil. Roast for 25 min. or until a fork slides in and out easily. *Or* scrub 1 lg. yam or potato and roast in oven until done.

Steam or microwave ½ bunch kale; then top with the juice of 1 lemon and black pepper to taste. Steam or microwave 1 **(1½)** cup carrots and 1 cup yellow squash tossed with 1 tsp. tarragon.

Spinach Salad

Serve vegetables with Mixed Accelerator Salad Greens and freshly washed spinach leaves tossed with 1 tsp. Mixed Accelerator Salad Dressing.

Seafood Supreme

Fill a large frying pan halfway with water. Add the juice of 1 lemon and bring to a boil. Add 4 **(6)** oz. scallops and lower heat to simmer. Poach for approximately 5 min. (Large sea scallops may take a few minutes longer.) Fish is done when it is no longer translucent inside. Drain and immediately toss with the juice of 1 lime, a dash of cayenne pepper, and chopped cilantro leaves.

Steam or microwave ½ **(1)** cup rutabagas, ½ **(1)** cup carrots, 1¾ cups yellow beans, and ¼ **(½)** cup red pepper tossed with 1 tbs. cumin.

Watercress Salad

Serve with 1½ cups Mixed Accelerator Salad Greens with 1 cup watercress added. Toss with 1 tsp. Mixed Accelerator Salad Dressing.

Tabouli, Tofu, and Veggie Health Salad

Combine 2 cups Mixed Accelerator Salad Greens and 1 cup grated carrots with 1 tsp. Mixed Accelerator Salad Dressing. Serve with ½ **(1)** cup tabouli.

Steam or microwave ½ bunch kale and ¼ **(½)** cup tofu with 1 head Roasted Garlic puree. Top with the juice of 1 lemon.

Synthesizer

Larger quantities for men are shown in **boldface**.

Buy fish the day you prepare it or, at most, 1 day in advance.

The following recipes appear in the "General Recipes for All Meta-Types" section, which starts on page 417:

- Roasted Garlic
- Roasted Onions (Use 2 lb. onions instead of the 3 lb. specified in the instructions.)
- Seaweed
- Couscous
- Moroccan-Style Vegetables for Couscous

Advance Food Preparation

This subsection presents dishes that you can make up ahead of time and keep on hand for use as needed. Investing a little time at the start of the week will enable you to prepare all the meals on your diet with minimal work during the week.

Synthesizer Salad Dressing

Combine 1½ cups safflower oil, ¾ cup lemon juice, 6 cloves crushed garlic, 2 tsp. cayenne or black pepper, and 1½ tbs. herbs (such as tarragon, oregano, or thyme). Mix well, cover, and refrigerate.

Synthesizer Elixirs

Having clean vegetables on hand makes juicing a lot easier and a lot less time-consuming. You will need the following vegetables to make all four of the elixirs in the coming week:

4 lb. carrots
1 bunch celery
5 bunches parsley
2 lb. spinach
2 beets
1 cucumber
1 bunch dandelion greens (optional)

Synthesizer Salad Greens

1 head red leaf lettuce
1 head chicory
1 head escarole
1 head radicchio
1 lb. spinach
1 head Boston lettuce

Cut or tear all greens into 2-in. or bite-size pieces. Rinse in cold water to remove all dirt; then spin dry. Wrap greens in portion-size amounts (2–3 cups) in paper towels; then store in gallon-size resealable plastic bags from which all the air has been squeezed out. If greens are dried and stored properly, they can last for up to 4 to 7 days in the refrigerator. Not all greens will stand up to this kind of treatment. One option is to clean half your salad greens twice a week.

Add other greens as recipes indicate. At this time you can also clean and dry 2 lb. spinach for use in other recipes during the week.

Roasted Garlic Mashed Potatoes

Steam or microwave 1 (1½) cup Yukon gold potatoes. Mash with ½ head Roasted Garlic and ¼ cup shredded basil leaves. Add ½ cup Roasted Onions. Refrigerate in an airtight container.

Balsamic Strawberries

Slice 1 (2) cup strawberries. Mix ½ tsp. honey with ¼ tsp. balsamic vinegar. (This will be easier to do if you microwave the mixture for 20 sec.) Pour over the strawberries and mix well.

Recipes

Notes: Since the energy of microwave ovens varies, you may need to adjust the indicated microwave cooking times according to your own microwave's power.

When your daily menu instructs you to prepare your Synthesizer Elixir, see page 226 for the proper combination of juices.

Option: Prepare enough of your morning drink, Call-to-Arms Weight-Buster Morning Drink, for the entire week and refrigerate.

Call-to-Arms Weight-Buster Morning Drink

Combine 4–6 oz. spring water with ½ tsp. grated or powdered ginger, 1 tbs. apple cider vinegar, 1 flat tsp. Tupelo honey, ½ tsp. kelp powder or blue-green algae, ½ tsp. cayenne pepper, and ½ tsp. flaxseed oil.

Salmon Surprise

Fill a small skillet three-quarters of the way with water and bring to a simmer. Poach 4 **(6)** oz. salmon for approximately 5 min. Cooking time will vary according to the thickness of the fish. Remove fish to a heated plate. Empty skillet; then refill it and bring water to a simmer. Poach 2 eggs.

Microwave 2 lb. spinach for 3 min. Drain water and toss spinach with a combination of 1 tsp. safflower oil, 1 tsp. Roasted Garlic, and the juice of 1 lemon.

Assemble meal with spinach on bottom, flaked salmon spread over the spinach, and poached eggs on top. Sprinkle with 1 **(2)** oz. sesame seeds.

Protein-Power Breakfast

Scramble 2 eggs in a skillet with 1 tsp. safflower oil. Serve with 3 **(5)** oz. sliced cold beef from the previous day's lunch and 2 cups steamed or microwaved asparagus. Sprinkle cooked asparagus with the juice of ½ lemon.

Slim and Thin Protein Drink

In a blender, mix 1½ **(2)** cups soy milk with 1½ **(2)** scoops soy-based protein powder and 1 cap almond extract. You may also add cinnamon or nutmeg to taste.

Spanish Supreme

Preheat oven to 400°. In a cast-iron skillet, sauté ½ **(1)** cup tomatoes, ½ **(1)** cup mushrooms, and ½ **(1)** cup red peppers in 1 tsp. safflower oil. When vegetables are soft, add ½ cup Roasted Onions and 1 **(2)** oz. pine nuts.

Beat 2 **(3)** eggs with 1 tsp. water and ¼ cup shredded basil. Pour over the vegetables and roll eggs around the pan. When about half the egg mixture is cooked, place skillet in oven for approximately 5 min. and continue cooking until eggs are cooked through and turn a golden brown.

Chicken Delight

Sauté ½ cup mushrooms, ½ cup thinly sliced fennel, and ½ cup thinly sliced red onion in 1 tsp. safflower oil. When vegetables are soft, add ½ **(¾)** cup peas and 4 **(6)** oz. cooked chicken from Tuesday's lunch, cut into cubes. Toss well. Beat 2 eggs with 1 tsp. water and add to the pan. Toss vegetables, chicken, and eggs until eggs are cooked through. Top with 1 **(2)** oz. pine nuts.

Skinny-Minnie Regeneration Lunch

Preheat oven to 400°. Lightly spray a cast-iron skillet and heat on top of the stove. Place a 9-oz. **(15-oz.)** piece of beef filet in the pan. Sear on both sides for 2 min. Transfer skillet to oven and continue cooking for 5 min. more for medium rare. Remove the meat from the pan. Cut off one-third to be used the next day. Return the pan to the stove top. Add ¼ cup balsamic vinegar to the pan. Scrape the bottom of the pan until half the vinegar has evaporated. Pour over the larger piece of beef.

Microwave ½ cup prepared Roasted Garlic Mashed Potatoes.

Super Salad
Combine 2–3 cups Synthesizer Salad Greens with ½ cup raw zucchini, ½ cup yellow squash, ½ cup mushrooms, **(½ cup grated carrots)**, and ½ cup tomatoes. Toss with 1½ tsp. Synthesizer Salad Dressing. Top salad with 1 **(2)** oz. cashews.

Moroccan Makeover

Reheat or prepare ¾ **(1)** cup Couscous. Reheat 1½ **(2¾)** cups Moroccan-Style Vegetables mixture, making sure that it contains ½ **(¾)** cup chickpeas. Serve with ½ cup hot or cold Seaweed sprinkled with a little rice vinegar.

Red Onion and Sprout Salad
Toss 2–3 cups Synthesizer Salad Greens with 1 tsp. Synthesizer Salad Dressing. You may add radish sprouts and sliced red onion.

Egg-a-licious Lunch

In a small skillet sauté ¼ (**½**) cup chopped red peppers and ¼ (**½**) cup mushrooms with ½ (**1**) tsp. safflower oil. When vegetables are soft, add ¼ (**½**) cup peas, ¼ (**½**) cup Roasted Onions, and ¼ (**½**) cup shredded basil. Remove vegetables and wipe pan. Beat 3 eggs with 1 tsp. water. Using ½ tsp. safflower oil, make an omelet and fill with cooked vegetables.

Microwave ½ (**¾**) cup Roasted Garlic Mashed Potatoes.

Fennel and Carrot Salad
Mix 2–3 cups Synthesizer Salad Greens with ½ cup sliced fennel, ½ cup grated carrots, (**2 oz. cashews**), and ½ cup radishes. Toss with ½ tsp. Synthesizer Salad Dressing.

Chicken Dijon

Preheat oven to 375°. Mix 1 tbs. Dijon mustard with 1 tsp. Roasted Garlic, ¼ tsp. dried thyme, and the juice of 1 lemon. Spread mixture on top of 10-oz. (**1-lb.**) cleaned skinless chicken breast. Bake for 20–25 min. Cooking time will vary according to the thickness of the meat. Meat is done when no pink shows inside. Reserve 4 oz. cooked chicken for another meal.

Reheat ½ (**1**) cup Roasted Garlic Mashed Potatoes.

Sunshine Salad
Mix 2–3 cups Synthesizer Salad Greens with ½ cup raw zucchini, ½ cup yellow squash, ½ cup sliced mushrooms, ½ cup grated carrots, and ½ cup sliced tomatoes. Toss with 1½ tsp. Synthesizer Salad Dressing.

Fabulous Fish Fiesta

Preheat oven to 375°. Rub 6-oz. (**8-oz.**) salmon filet with 1½ tsp. freshly grated ginger mixed with ½ tsp. soy sauce. Bake for approximately 8 min. Cooking time will vary according to the thickness of the fish.

Microwave ½ (**1**) cup fresh corn mixed with ½ cup carrots and 1 cup sugar snap peas. (**Top with 2 oz. sesame seeds.** To toast seeds, heat a small skillet, add seeds, and cook on high heat, tossing all the while, for 1 min. or so until seeds turn brown.)

Cucumber Salad
Mix 2–3 cups Synthesizer Salad Greens with 1 (**1½**) cup cucumbers. Toss with 1½ tsp. Synthesizer Salad Dressing.

Hearty Vegetarian Lunch

Reheat or prepare ¾ cup couscous. Reheat 2½ cups Moroccan-Style Vegetables mixture, making sure that there is ½ cup chickpeas.

Toss 2–3 cups Synthesizer Salad Greens with 1 tsp. Synthesizer Salad Dressing. You may add radish sprouts and sliced red onion.

Enjoy with 1 glass Synthesizer Elixir.

Outrageous Omelet

Fill a small skillet three-quarters of the way with cold water and the juice of 1 lemon. Bring to a boil and poach 4 **(6)** oz. cleaned shrimp for 3 min. Drain the shrimp and set them aside.

Beat 3 eggs with 1 tsp. water and ½ tsp. dried thyme. Using 1 tsp. safflower oil, make an omelet and fill with the cooked shrimp and 1 oz. pine nuts.

Tomato and Onion Salad

Mix 2–3 cups Synthesizer Salad Greens with ½ cup sliced tomatoes, ½ cup red onion, ½ cup sliced mushrooms, and ½ cup peas. Toss with 1 tsp. Synthesizer Salad Dressing. Top with 1 **(2)** oz. cashews.

Burdock, Sassafras, and Hops Relaxer

Mix together equal quantities of burdock root, sassafras bark, and hops flower and store the mixture in an airtight plastic container or a resealable plastic bag.

To prepare tea, boil 1 cup water; then steep 1 tbs. of the herbal mix in it for 20 min.

Great Grapefruit

Preheat broiler. Slice 1 grapefruit in half. Reserve half for another meal. Spread ¼ tsp. honey over the top of the grapefruit. Broil for 5 min. until surface begins to brown. Top with ½ cup Balsamic Strawberries. Sprinkle with 2 oz. pecans.

Balanced Synthesizer

Larger quantities for men are shown in **boldface**.

Buy fish the day you prepare it or, at most, 1 day in advance.

The following recipes appear in the "General Recipes for All Meta-Types" section, which starts on page 417:

- Roasted Garlic (Use 4 heads of garlic instead of the 2 specified in the instructions.)
- Roasted Red Pepper Puree
- Couscous
- Red Kidney Beans
- Seaweed

Advance Food Preparation

This subsection presents dishes that you can make up ahead of time and keep on hand for use as needed. Investing a little time at the start of the week will enable you to prepare all the meals on your diet with minimal work during the week.

Exotic-Style Vegetables

This vegetable mixture can be prepared in advance and used two times during the coming week. Combine the following in a large saucepan:

1 cup nonsalted tomato juice
2 cups eggplant, cut into 1-in. pieces
2 cups mushrooms, left whole
3 cups plum tomatoes, seeded and cut into eighths
1 lg. onion, peeled and cut into eighths
3 cloves minced garlic
1½ cups cooked red beans

Add a pinch of saffron, ¼ tsp. turmeric, and ½ tsp. cardamom seed. (*Option:* Add harissa—a hot Moroccan spice—to taste.) Cook on low heat for approximately 20 min. until eggplant is al dente. Vegetables will finish cooking when reheated during the week. Refrigerate in an airtight container.

Balanced Synthesizer Salad Dressing

Combine 1 **(1½)** cup safflower oil, ⅓ **(¾)** cup lemon juice, 3 **(6)** cloves crushed garlic, 1 tsp. cayenne or black pepper, and 1 **(2)** tbs. herbs (such as tarragon, oregano, or thyme). Mix well, cover, and refrigerate.

Balanced Synthesizer Elixirs

Having clean vegetables on hand makes juicing a lot easier and a lot less time-consuming. You will need the following vegetables to make all five of the elixirs in the coming week:

4 lb. carrots
1 bunch celery
5 bunches parsley
2 lb. spinach
2 beets
1 head romaine lettuce
1 lb. string beans
1 lb. Brussels sprouts
1 bunch dandelion greens (optional)
3 cucumbers

Balanced Synthesizer Salad Greens

1 **(2)** head red leaf lettuce
1 sm. **(lg.)** bunch kale
1 **(3)** bunch parsley
1 bunch chicory

Cut or tear all greens into 2-in. or bite-size pieces. Remove woody stems from parsley. Rinse in cold water to remove all dirt; then spin dry. Wrap greens in portion-size amounts (2–3 cups) in paper towels; then store in gallon-size resealable plastic bags from which all the air has been squeezed out. If greens are dried and stored properly, they can last for up to 4 to 7 days in the refrigerator. Not all greens will stand up to this kind of treatment. One option is to clean half your greens twice a week.

Add other greens as recipes indicate. At this time you can also clean and store 3 lb. spinach and 1 bunch arugula for other recipes.

Fennel, Dill, and Cucumber Salad

Clean and peel 3 lg. cucumbers. Cut them in half lengthways and remove all seeds. Slice cucumbers into thin half-moons. Slice ¼ (½) bulb fennel. Combine with the cucumber. Toss with ¼ cup chopped fresh dill and 1 tbs. vinegar. Yield should be approximately 2½ cups.

Balanced Synthesizer Vegetable Sticks

Slice 1 lg. jicama into sticks and toss with the juice of 1 lime. Peel 2–3 carrots and cut them into sticks. Cut 2–3 stalks celery into sticks. Pack separately and refrigerate for midafternoon snacks during the week.

Recipes

Notes: Since the energy of microwave ovens varies, you may need to adjust the indicated microwave cooking times according to your own microwave's power.

When your daily menu instructs you to prepare your Balanced Synthesizer Elixir, see page 258 for the proper combination of juices.

Option: Prepare enough of your morning drink, Hot Tomato Energizer, for the entire week and refrigerate.

Hot Tomato Energizer

Combine 4–6 oz. nonsalted tomato juice with 1 tbs. apple cider vinegar, ½ tsp. kelp powder or blue-green algae, ½ tsp. wheat germ oil, and ½ tsp. cayenne pepper.

Poached Salmon and Egg Delight

(Heat 1 oz. sesame seeds in a small skillet until they begin to turn brown [approximately 1–2 min.]. Remove to a small bowl.) Cook 1 8-oz. **(12-oz.)** piece salmon; divide in half and save half for a lunch. Fill skillet three-quarters of the way with water and bring to a simmer. Poach salmon for about 3–5 min. Cooking time will vary according to the thickness of the salmon and how well you like it cooked. Remove the cooked salmon to a warm plate and, in the same water, poach 2 eggs. Serve eggs with poached salmon. **(Sprinkle with toasted sesame seeds.)**

Chipper Chicken Omelet

Preheat oven to 400°. Beat 2 eggs together in a mixing bowl with ¼ cup cleaned and shredded basil. Lightly spray the bottom of an 8-in. cast-iron skillet. Over a medium flame pour eggs into skillet and gently roll eggs around the bottom and halfway up the sides of the pan. When about half the egg mixture is cooked, place 2 oz. cubed poached chicken **(and 1 oz. sunflower seeds)** in center of pan. Place pan in oven for 10–15 min. until eggs puff up around chicken, turn a golden brown, and are cooked through.

Whole-Grain Cereal Breakfast

Cover 1 cup whole-grain cereal—your choice—**(and 1 oz. pecans)** with 4 oz. soy milk. If desired, toast 1 slice sprouted grain bread and top with 1 *flat* tsp. *sugar-free* fruit spread. (*Note:* Keep sprouted grain bread in the freezer.)

Slim-and-Thin Protein Drink

Combine 1 **(1½)** cup soy milk with 1 **(2)** scoop protein powder in a blender. You can add ¼ **(½)** cap of vanilla or almond extract with cinnamon, nutmeg, or mace.

Exotic Vegetables and Couscous

Prepare or reheat ½ **(¾)** cup Couscous. Reheat 1½ **(2¼)** cups Exotic-Style Vegetables mixture, and add ¼ **(½)** cup red beans.

Salad Greens
Serve vegetables with 1 cup Balanced Synthesizer Salad Greens tossed with 1 tsp. Balanced Synthesizer Salad Dressing.

Health Salad with Ricotta Cheese

Toss 1 **(2–3)** cup cleaned Balanced Synthesizer Salad Greens with 1 **(2)** tsp. Balanced Synthesizer Salad Dressing. Top with radish sprouts. Serve with 6 **(8)** oz. low-fat ricotta cheese mixed with ⅓ cup chopped scallions, ⅓ cup grated carrots, and ⅓ cup grated radishes.

Health Salad with Beef

Add ½ cup sliced tomatoes and ½ cup raw mushrooms instead of the vegetables indicated in the Health Salad with Ricotta Cheese recipe. Serve with 4 **(6)** oz. sliced cold beef with mustard and ½ cup Fennel, Dill, and Cucumber Salad.

Health Salad with Salmon

Add ½ cup yellow squash to the vegetables indicated in the Health Salad with Beef recipe. Serve with 4 **(6)** oz. cold salmon topped with ½ cup Fennel, Dill, and Cucumber Salad.

Poached Chicken Lunch

Toss 2 **(3)** oz. cold cubed poached chicken breast in Roasted Red Pepper Puree, and serve with 1½ cups cold steamed green beans tossed with a little lemon juice.

Salad Greens with Sprouts

Mix 1 cup Balanced Synthesizer Salad Greens with radish sprouts. Toss with 1 tsp. Balanced Synthesizer Salad Dressing.

Mineral Makeover Dinner

Preheat broiler. Steam or microwave 1 **(2)** cup sugar snap peas tossed with ½ **(1)** tsp. grated fresh ginger. Broil 4 **(6)** oz. shrimp or sea scallops. Mix peas and seafood together and sprinkle with a little soy sauce.

Tomato, Pepper, and Mushroom Salad

Combine ½ cup diced tomato, ½ cup diced green pepper, and ½ cup sliced raw mushrooms. Add ¼ cup sliced red onion, ½ tsp. dried thyme, and 1 tsp. Balanced Synthesizer Salad Dressing.

Think Thin Dinner

Lightly spray a small skillet. Add 1 cup thinly sliced onion and cook on medium heat, stirring, until onions begin to brown. Add 1 cup sliced mushrooms and ½ tsp. dried thyme. Continue cooking until mushrooms are soft and have released their juice. Save for beef.

Preheat oven to 400°. Heat an ungreased cast-iron skillet and place

8-oz. **(12-oz.)** piece of beef tenderloin in the pan (½ will be served cold for tomorrow's lunch). Sear for 2 min. on both sides. Transfer pan to oven and continue cooking for 5 min. more for rare beef. Cook longer if desired. Top with mushroom/onion mixture, and serve with Dijon mustard.

Steam 1 cup asparagus.

Fennel, Radicchio, and Spinach Salad

Shred 1 sm. head radicchio and combine with ½ fennel bulb, thinly sliced, and 2 cups raw spinach. Toss with 1 tsp. Balanced Synthesizer Salad Dressing.

Tasty Tangier Dinner

Prepare ½ **(¾)** cup Couscous or grain of your choice. Reheat 1¼ **(2)** cups Exotic-Style Vegetables mixture, and add an additional ¼ **(½)** cup red beans.

Serve with cooked Seaweed (warm or cold) sprinkled with a little soy sauce.

Celery and Cucumber Salad

Combine ½ cup diced celery and ½ cup scallions with 1 cucumber, peeled, seeded, and sliced. Toss with 1 tsp. Balanced Synthesizer Salad Dressing.

Saucy Salmon Dinner

Preheat broiler for 5 min. Sprinkle 4-oz. **(6-oz.)** piece of salmon with soy sauce or a light coating of Dijon mustard and dried thyme. Place salmon filet under the broiler and cook for approximately 8–10 min. Cooking time will vary according to the thickness of the fish.

Roast Garlic Mashed Potatoes with Basil

Steam or microwave 1 cup Yukon gold potatoes. Mash with ½ head Roasted Garlic, ¼ cup shredded basil, and 1 tsp. Balanced Synthesizer Salad Dressing.

Sauteed Tomatoes

Lightly spray a small skillet. Add ½ cup cherry tomatoes and toss over medium heat until the skins start to split. Pour over the salmon when done.

Steam 1 cup green beans or a green vegetable of your choice.

Spinach and Mushroom Salad

Mix 1–2 cups raw spinach (or more) with ½ cup sliced mushrooms and radish sprouts. Toss with 1 tsp. Balanced Synthesizer Salad Dressing.

Cheerful Chicken Dinner

Fill a small skillet three-quarters of the way with water. Bring to a simmer. Poach 8-oz. **(2 5-oz. pieces)** chicken cutlet for approximately 8 min. Cooking time will vary according to the thickness of the chicken. Top ½ **(1 5-oz. piece)** the chicken with half the reheated Roasted Red Pepper Puree. Save the poaching liquid and refrigerate. (When the other half **[other 5-oz. piece]** of the chicken cools, cut into cubes, toss with the remaining Roasted Red Pepper Puree, and refrigerate.)

Steam or microwave 3½ cups green beans. Save 1½ cups for next day's lunch and serve the other 2 cups with dinner.

Endive and Watercress Salad

Mix 1 lg. Belgian endive, cut into thirds and separated, with 1 bunch watercress. Toss with 1 tsp. Balanced Synthesizer Salad Dressing.

Pasta Parade with Artichoke

Steam or microwave 1 artichoke. Heat 1 cup reserved poaching liquid from Wednesday's chicken in a medium saucepan, and add 1 head Roasted Garlic paste, ¼ tsp. black pepper, and 1 tsp. oregano. Two min. before serving, add ½ cup peas. Prepare a *little* less than ½ **(¾)** cup egg pastina or angel-hair pasta according to the directions on the box (it will double in volume). When pasta is cooked, add it to the chicken stock mixture. Eat pastina and peas with the artichoke.

While the artichoke is steaming, microwave ¼ cup tofu cut into small cubes. (*Note:* Unused tofu can be cut into portions and frozen.) Mix with ½ cup diced tomatoes and ¼ cup shredded basil. Toss with ½ tsp. Balanced Synthesizer Salad Dressing.

Arugula, Onion, and Watercress Salad

Mix 1 bunch arugula with 1 bunch watercress and ½ cup red peppers, thinly sliced. Toss with 1 tsp. Balanced Synthesizer Salad Dressing, and top with thinly sliced red onion.

Dijon-Garlic Chicken Dinner

Preheat broiler. Combine ½ tsp. Dijon mustard with 1 tsp. Roasted Garlic and a little lemon juice. Rinse 4-oz. **(6-oz.)** piece of chicken breast and cover with mustard/garlic mixture. Place under the broiler for approximately 8 min. Cooking time will vary according to the thickness of the breast. Chicken is done when no pink shows in the meat.

Steam or microwave 2 cups asparagus. Sprinkle with a little lemon juice.

Boston Lettuce Salad with Red Onion

Toss 1 sm. head Boston lettuce with 1 tsp. Balanced Synthesizer Salad Dressing. Top with thinly sliced red onion.

Mixed Synthesizer

Larger quantities for men are shown in **boldface**.

Buy fish the day you prepare it or, at most, 1 day in advance.

The following recipes appear in the "General Recipes for All Meta-Types" section, which starts on page 417:

- Roasted Garlic
- Roasted Red Pepper Puree (Use all the peppers in the Roasted Red Pepper Puree.)
- Couscous
- Red Kidney Beans (Use 1½ **[1¾]** cups beans.)
- Moroccan-Style Vegetables for Couscous
- Seaweed

Advance Food Preparation

This subsection presents dishes that you can make up ahead of time and keep on hand for use as needed. Investing a little time at the start of the week will enable you to prepare all the meals on your diet with minimal work during the week.

Mixed Synthesizer Salad Dressing

Combine 1 cup safflower oil, ½ cup lemon juice, 3 cloves crushed garlic, 1 tsp. cayenne or black pepper, and 1 tbs. herbs (such as tarragon, oregano, or thyme). Mix well, cover, and refrigerate.

Mexican-Style Brown Rice Salad

Cook ¾ cup brown rice (it will double in volume). While rice is cooking, prepare the following vegetables: ½ cup diced red pepper, ½ cup peas, ½ cup plum tomatoes (seeded and diced), ¼ cup chopped fresh cilantro, and 1 tbs. minced garlic. Combine cooked rice with vegetables, 1 tsp. cumin, ½ **(1)** cup cooked Red Kidney Beans, and 1 tsp. Mixed Synthesizer Salad Dressing. Refrigerate in an airtight container.

Mixed Synthesizer Elixirs

Having clean vegetables on hand makes juicing a lot easier and a lot less time-consuming. You will need the following vegetables to make all four of the elixirs in the coming week:

4 lb. carrots
1 bunch celery
5 bunches parsley
2 lb. spinach
2 beets
1 cucumber

Mixed Synthesizer Salad Greens

1 head romaine lettuce
1 head red leaf lettuce
1 bunch kale
1 bunch Swiss chard

Cut or tear all greens into 2-in. or bite-size pieces. Rinse in cold water to remove all dirt; then spin dry. Wrap greens in portion-size amounts (2–3 cups) in paper towels; then store in gallon-size resealable plastic bags from which all the air has been squeezed out. If greens are dried and stored properly, they can last for up to 4 to 7 days in the refrigerator. Not all greens will stand up to this kind of treatment. One option is to clean half your salad greens twice a week.

Add other greens as recipes indicate. At this time you can also clean and dry 1 bunch kale for use in other recipes during the week.

Recipes

Notes: Since the energy of microwave ovens varies, you may need to adjust the indicated microwave cooking times according to your own microwave's power.

When your daily menu instructs you to prepare your Mixed Synthesizer Elixir, see page 289 for the proper combination of juices.

Option: Prepare enough of your morning drink, Fat-Buster Tonic, for the entire week and refrigerate.

Fat-Buster Tonic

Combine 4–6 oz. warm spring water with 1 tbs. apple cider vinegar, 1 flat tsp. Tupelo honey, and ½ tsp. cayenne pepper.

Slim and Thin Protein Drink

In a blender mix 8 oz. nonfat (**regular**) soy milk or 4 oz. regular soy milk, 1 (**2**) scoop protein powder, and 1 flat tsp. kelp powder or blue-green algae. (*Option:* Add 1 flat tsp. bone-meal powder.)

Spicy Vegetables and Couscous

Prepare (or reheat) ¾ (**1**) cup Couscous. Top with half the Moroccan-Style Vegetables reheated in the microwave.

Seaweed Salad

Toss 2 cups assorted Mixed Synthesizer Salad Greens with ½ cup Seaweed (warm or cold); then toss with 1½ tsp. Mixed Synthesizer Salad Dressing.

Mushroom and Tomato Omelet

Preheat oven to 400°. Beat 3 eggs together in a mixing bowl with ½ bunch cleaned and shredded basil. Lightly spray the bottom of an 8-in. cast-iron skillet. Over a medium flame pour eggs into skillet and gently roll eggs around the bottom and halfway up the sides of the pan. When about half the egg mixture is cooked, place 1 cup sliced mushrooms and 1 cup diced plum tomatoes in the center of the pan. Place pan in oven for 10–15 min. until eggs puff up around vegetables, turn a golden brown, and are cooked through.

Salad Greens

Toss 2–3 cups cleaned Mixed Synthesizer Salad Greens with 1½ tsp. Mixed Synthesizer Salad Dressing.

Turkey Delight

Bake or microwave 1 sm. **(med.)** sweet potato. Steam or microwave 1 bunch kale. Serve with 4 **(6)** oz. sliced roast turkey from the night before. (*Options:* Sprinkle sweet potato with a little cinnamon or top kale with the juice of ½ lemon.)

Watercress and Sprout Salad

Toss 2 cups Mixed Synthesizer Salad Greens with ½ bunch watercress, alfalfa sprouts, and 1½ tsp. Mixed Synthesizer Salad Dressing.

Moroccan Salad

Prepare (or reheat) ¾ **(1)** cup Couscous. Top with half the Moroccan-Style Vegetables reheated in the microwave. Serve with 2 cups assorted Mixed Synthesizer Salad Greens tossed with 1½ tsp. Mixed Synthesizer Salad Dressing.

Fabulous Fish Fiesta

Preheat broiler for 5 min. Place 4-oz. **(5-oz.)** salmon filet under broiler and cook for approximately 8–10 min. Cooking time will vary according to the thickness of the fish. Lightly spray a small frying pan with oil. Add 1 pint cleaned cherry tomatoes and ¼ tsp. dried thyme. Cook on a low flame until skins start to split. Pour over the cooked salmon.

Steam or microwave 1 lb. spinach.

Red Pepper and Onion Salad

Mix 1 bunch arugula with thinly sliced red pepper and red onion. Toss with 1½ tsp. Mixed Synthesizer Salad Dressing.

Chicken with Red Pepper Puree

Reheat the remaining cubed 6 oz. poached chicken breast in Roasted Red Pepper Puree from Monday's dinner.

Steam or microwave 1 cup sugar snap peas.

Radish Sprouts and Watercress Salad
Combine 1–2 **(2–3)** cups cleaned Mixed Synthesizer Salad Greens with radish sprouts, ½ bunch watercress, and ¼ cup parsley. Toss with 1½ tsp. Mixed Synthesizer Salad Dressing.

Seared Tuna Lunch

Serve 5 **(6)** oz. sliced cold seared tuna with 2 cups cold or warm steamed asparagus.

Arugula and Cucumber Salad
Combine 2 cups cleaned Mixed Synthesizer Salad Greens with ½ bunch arugula and 1 chopped cucumber. Toss with 1½ tsp. Mixed Synthesizer Salad Dressing.

Mexican-Style Brown Rice Health Salad

Add ½ bunch watercress and ½ cup sprouts to 2 **(3)** cups Mixed Synthesizer Salad Greens and toss with ½ tsp. Mixed Synthesizer Salad Dressing. Top with ½ **(1)** slice toasted sprouted grain bread cut into croutons. (*Note:* Keep sprouted grain bread in the freezer.) Serve with half the prepared Mexican-Style Brown Rice Salad.

Turkey Jamboree

Preheat oven to 350°. Place both turkey breasts (the other 4-oz. **[6-oz.]** piece will be for tomorrow's lunch) in the bottom of a lightly sprayed shallow roasting pan. Surround with ½ cup water and sprinkle with dried thyme and paprika. Roast for about 15 min. Cooking time will vary according to the thickness of the breasts. They are done when a thermometer reads 145° or when no pink is showing in the meat.

Steam or microwave 1 lb. spinach.

Cauliflower and Tomato Salad

Toss 1 **(2–3)** cup Mixed Synthesizer Salad Greens with 1 cup raw cauliflower, 1 cup tomatoes, and 1 tsp. Mixed Synthesizer Salad Dressing.

Simple Chicken

Fill a small frying pan two-thirds of the way with water and bring to a boil. Add both chicken breasts (the larger one will be for another meal) and poach for approximately 10 min. Cooking time will vary according to the thickness of the chicken. Top one 4-oz. **(6-oz.)** piece with half the reheated Roasted Red Pepper Puree.

After the remaining 4-oz. **(6-oz.)** piece of chicken has cooled, dice it into 1-in. cubes and toss with remaining Roasted Red Pepper Puree. Refrigerate for another meal.

Steam or microwave ½ cup string beans and ½ cup zucchini. Serve with the chicken.

Tomato and Mushroom Salad

Combine 1–2 cups Mixed Synthesizer Salad Greens with 1 cup tomatoes and 1 cup sliced raw mushrooms and toss with 1 tsp. Mixed Synthesizer Salad Dressing.

Simple Simon Salmon

Preheat broiler for 5 min. Place 5-oz. **(6-oz.)** salmon filet under broiler and cook for approximately 8–10 min. Cooking time will vary according to the thickness of the fish. (*Option:* You can cook both pieces of salmon now and eat the smaller piece cold for tomorrow's lunch.)

Steam or microwave 1 cup asparagus.

Raw Veggie Salad

Combine 1–2 **(2–3)** cups Mixed Synthesizer Salad Greens with 1 cup raw zucchini and 1 cup yellow squash and toss with 1½ tsp. Mixed Synthesizer Salad Dressing.

Tasty Delight Tuna

You can cook both pieces of tuna at dinnertime. The larger piece will be served cold with Friday's lunch.

Preheat oven to 400°. Rinse the tuna. Heat a cast-iron skillet on top of the stove. When the pan is hot, place both pieces of tuna in the pan and sear on both sides, approximately 2 min. per side. Transfer tuna to the oven and finish baking for about 3 min. for medium rare. Cook longer if desired. Wrap the piece intended for lunch tightly in plastic and refrigerate.

Steam or microwave ½ (¾) cup carrots, ½ (¾) cup celery, and ½ (¾) cup parsnips.

Cauliflower and Red Onion Salad

Combine 2 cups Mixed Synthesizer Salad Greens with 1 cup cauliflower, ¾ cup tomatoes, ¼ cup sliced red onion, and ½ bunch watercress. Toss with 1½ tsp. Mixed Synthesizer Salad Dressing.

Easy Egg Salad

Mix 2 (2–3) cups Mixed Synthesizer Salad Greens with 2 (3) hard-boiled eggs, 1 cup sliced raw mushrooms, and 1 cup diced tomatoes. Toss with 1½ tsp. Mixed Synthesizer Salad Dressing.

General Recipes for All Meta-Types

Roasted Hazelnuts

Preheat oven to 400°. Place 2 oz. hazelnuts on a cookie sheet or half sheet pan. Place in the oven and roast for 10 min., shaking the nuts every 2 or 3 min. Remove from oven and allow to cool before roughly chopping nuts in a food processor using the pulse button. Refrigerate in an airtight container.

Roasted Onions

Preheat oven to 375°. Peel and slice 3 lb. yellow onions and cut into half-moons (any size will do). Separate onions on a sheet pan and roast for 10–15 min. until they begin to blacken around the edges. Transfer cooked onions to an airtight container, cover immediately, and refrigerate.

Seaweed

Rinse the seaweed two to three times before cooking to remove any salt. Steam or boil the seaweed per the instructions on the package. Refrigerate in an airtight container. Serve warm or use as a cold salad.

You may also get prepared "seaweed salad" to take out at many Japanese restaurants.

Roasted Garlic

Preheat oven to 375°. Place 2 heads garlic on a piece of aluminum foil, reduce heat to 325°, and bake for 25–40 min., depending on the size of the heads. The garlic is done when it begins to bubble up out of the top and is soft to the touch. Wrap in the same piece of aluminum foil and refrigerate.

Jicama Sticks

Peel 1 jicama, cut it into ½-in. strips, and cover it with the juice of 2 limes. This will last for 3–4 days in the refrigerator.

Vegetable Stock

This stock is used as the base for hearty vegetable soups and for reheating grains and vegetables.

Combine the following vegetables in a large (8- to 10-qt.) stockpot:

2 leeks, cleaned and chopped
4 oz. mushrooms, cleaned and chopped
½ zucchini
½ yellow squash
3 carrots, cleaned but not peeled
2 sticks celery, cleaned and chopped into 3-in. pieces

Cover with water and bring to a boil; then lower heat and simmer until reduced by half.

Curried Tofu

Preheat oven to 375°. Slice 1½ **(2)** pounds tofu through the middle; then cut each piece into eight squares. Toss with 1 tbs. curry powder. Spray a baking sheet with misted safflower oil (or Pam). Arrange all the pieces on the sheet and spray the top of the tofu again. Bake for 20 min. Allow to cool and refrigerate in an airtight container.

Tofu Scramble

Shred 1 **(2)** pound extra firm tofu by hand in a food processor using the grating blade. Squeeze out as much liquid as possible from the grated tofu (save the liquid), add ½ **(1)** tsp. turmeric and ½ **(1)** tsp. cumin powder, and toss well. Lightly spray a nonstick skillet with safflower oil. Heat ¼ cup minced scallions and ¼ **(⅓)** cup grated carrots in the pan; then add the seasoned tofu and cook for 15 min., tossing tofu frequently. Add a little of the liquid you saved if it begins to stick. Add ¼ **(½)** cup Roasted Onions. Allow to cool and refrigerate in an airtight container.

Couscous

Couscous can be cooked in advance and served at room temperature or reheated before use. In a large mixing bowl or plastic container, cover ¾ **(1)** cup couscous with 1½ **(2)** cups boiling water. Cover container and let sit for approximately 25 min. Drain any excess water and refrigerate.

Roasted Red Pepper Puree

Preheat broiler for 5 min. Slice 2 red peppers in half and remove seeds. Place 1½ pieces (save ½ piece for another recipe)—skin up—on broiler pan and roast until skin blackens and chars. Remove immediately to an airtight container and allow to cool. After peppers have cooled, remove skin and any leftover seeds and place peppers in the bowl of a food processor or blender. Add 1 sm. head Roasted Garlic and puree. Refrigerate until needed.

Red Kidney Beans

Cover 1 **(2)** cup red kidney beans with water and soak for several hours. Drain water. Cover with fresh water, bring to a boil, lower to simmer, and cook for approximately 1 hour until beans are soft. Drain and refrigerate and add to other recipes as needed.

Moroccan-Style Vegetables
for Couscous

This recipe can be prepared in advance.
    Combine the following in a large saucepan:

¾ cup water
¾ **(1)** cup zucchini, cut into 1-in. pieces
¾ **(1)** cup yellow squash, cut into 1-in. pieces
¾ **(1)** cup eggplant, cut into 1-in. pieces
2 cups mushrooms, left whole
2 cups plum tomatoes, seeded and cut into eighths
1 lg. yellow onion, peeled and cut into eighths
3 cloves minced garlic
1 **(1½)** cup cooked chickpeas

Add a pinch of saffron, ¼ tsp. turmeric, and ½ tsp. cardamom seed. (*Option:* Add ½ tsp. or more of harissa, a hot Moroccan spice.) Cook on low heat for approximately 30 min. until vegetables are al dente. They will finish cooking when reheated during the week. Refrigerate in an airtight container.

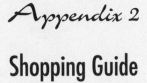

Appendix 2

Shopping Guide

Aromatherapy

Essentially Yours
P.O. Box 38
Romford
Essex RMI DN
England

Elizabeth Dane, Inc.
2472 Broadway, Suite 290
New York, NY 10025
(212) 866-3807
Fax: (212) 866-2349
E-mail: edane@nyc.rr.com
www.elizabethdane.com

Aroma Vera Inc.
P.O. Box 3609
Culver City, CA 90231

Bach Flower Remedies

The Bach flower remedies are available from most health-food stores and some pharmacies. For further information contact:

The Dr. Edward Bach Center
Mount Vernon
Sorwell
Wallingford
Oxon OX10 0PZ
England

Herbs and Herbal Teas

Lin Sisters
4 Bowery
New York, NY 10013

Elizabeth Dane, Inc.
2472 Broadway, Suite 290
New York, NY 10025
(212) 866-3807
Fax: (212) 866-2349
E-mail: edane@nyc.rr.com
www.elizabethdane.com

Herb Products
11012 Magnolia Blvd.
North Hollywood, CA 91601

Juicers

Champion Juicers and Braun Juicers are extremely good and can be purchased from your local health-food stores.

Amino Acids, Vitamins, and Minerals Formulas

American Biologics
P.O. Box 1880
San Ysidro, CA 92073

Elizabeth Dane, Inc.
2472 Broadway, Suite 290
New York, NY 10025
(212) 866-3807
Fax: (212) 866-2349
E-mail: edane@nyc.rr.com
www.elizabethdane.com

Allergy Research Group
400 Preda St.
San Leandro, CA 94577

Karuna
42 Digital Dr., Suite 7
Novato, CA 94949

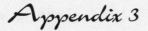

Appendix 3

Actions of Calming (Yin) and Energizing (Yang) Vitamins, Minerals, and Foods

Calming Nutrients (Anabolic/Alkaline)

Vitamins

Vitamin A (Retinol/Beta-Carotene)

A fat-soluble nutrient that helps the body resist infection and repair and maintain its tissue. Maintains the acid-base balance if fat consumption is high. Essential for body growth and for bones, eyes, hair, skin, soft tissue, and teeth. Also essential in reproductive disorders. Key points:

- Plays a coenzyme role in glycoprotein synthesis.
- Functions like steroid hormone, leading to tissue differentiation.
- Necessary for thyroxine formation, the synthesis of corticosterone from cholesterol, and the synthesis of glycogen, protein, and some hormones.
- Important for resisting infections.
- Important for the repair and maintenance of body tissue.
- Important for visual purple production.
- The herb mugwort contains vitamin A.
- Daily intake: 10,000 IU (especially if taking vitamin E).

Best food sources: carrots, cod-liver oil, liver, dark green leafy vegetables (dandelion greens, beet greens, chard, collard, kale, mustard greens, and spinach), yellow foods (pumpkins, sweet potatoes, winter squashes, apricots, peaches, papayas, and mangoes), and some seafood (oysters, salmon, and swordfish).

Vitamin D (Calciferol, Ergosterol, Viosterol)

Fat-soluble vitamin absorbed from the sun through the skin or ingested in the diet. Essential for calcium and phosphorus regulation; maintaining the nervous system; normal blood clotting; skin respiration; health and action of the bones, skin, teeth, and heart; and assimilating vitamin A. Can prevent colds when taken with vitamins C and A. Key points:

- Increases the absorption of calcium from the small intestine.
- Important for growth and mineralization of teeth and bones.
- Increases the absorption of phosphorus through the intestinal wall.
- Increases the reabsorption of phosphates from the kidney tubules.
- Maintains normal levels of blood citrate.
- Protects against loss of amino acids from the kidneys.
- An active compound of D functions as a hormone.
- Daily intake: 400 IU to 1,000 IU.

Best food sources: fatty fish (herring, kipper, mackerel, salmon, sardines, and tuna), fish roe, liver, egg yolk, cream, and cheese.

B-Complex Vitamins
Vitamin B$_5$ (Pantothenic Acid)
See page 437.

Vitamin B$_6$ (Pyridoxine Hydrochloride)
See page 437.

Vitamin B$_{12}$ (Cobalamin/Cyanocobalamin)
For DNA metabolism (red blood cell production). The largest and most complex of the vitamin molecules, B$_{12}$ functions in two coenzyme forms—coenzyme B$_{12}$ and methyl B$_{12}$—in the cellular level of the body, especially in the bone marrow, nerve tissue, and gastrointestinal tract. Essential for body regeneration. Produces and regenerates red blood cells; stimulates appetite and growth; regenerates brain cells and nerves; stimulates concentration and memory; reduces irritability; stimulates energy and reduces fatigue. Needs a properly functioning thyroid gland for proper utilization. Requires the gastrointestinal "intrinsic factor" for its absorption, which takes about three hours compared to seconds for the other water-soluble vitamins. Key points:

- Important for RNA/DNA cell formation and nucleic acid synthesis.
- Important for protein, carbohydrate, and fatty acid metabolism.
- Supplies and maintains nerve tissue.
- Forms red blood cells and controls pernicious anemia.
- Important for the synthesis or transfer of single carbon units.
- Acts as a revitalizer when combined with folic acid.
- Stimulates the metabolism.
- Alleviates irritability, mental depression, apathy, and nervous abnormalities.
- Daily intake: 50 mcg to 2,000 mcg.

Best food sources: liver, organ meats (heart and kidney), muscle meats, fish, shellfish, eggs, and cheese.

Vitamin B$_{13}$ (Orotic Acid)
Metabolizes folic acid and vitamin B$_{12}$; may prevent premature aging and liver problems. A good source is calcium orotate.

Best food sources: whey, sour or curdled milk, and root vegetables.

- Daily intake has not been established.

Vitamin B$_{17}$ (Amygdalin/Amygdalic Acid)

The one B vitamin not found in brewer's yeast. Made from apricot pits and purported to have cancer-preventive properties. Also found in the whole kernels of apples, cherries, peaches, plums, and nectarines. (Careful: Ingesting an overabundance could be toxic.)

Choline

For fat emulsification, transport, metabolism, and brain health. Works with inositol. Manufactured from methionine (an amino acid), vitamin B$_{12}$, and folacin. Essential for improving the memory. Penetrating the blood-brain barrier, it binds with acetate to form acetylcholine (a neurotransmitter), needed to "bridge" nerve cells transmitting nerve impulses in the brain. Forms lecithin, regulates the gallbladder and liver, and reduces cholesterol. Key points:

- Important for transporting lipids in the body.
- Important for the emulsification of fats; prevents fatty livers.
- Important for the synthesis of phosphatidylcholine (lecithin).
- Works with inositol to utilize fats and emulsify cholesterol. (Inositol and choline should be taken in equal amounts.)
- Essential for liver and gallbladder regulation.
- Facilitates metabolism by transmethylation.
- Has a calming effect and soothes nervousness.
- An important neurotransmitter.
- Daily intake: 500 mg to 1,000 mg.

Best food sources: egg yolk, eggs, liver, soybeans, cabbage, wheat bran, navy beans, alfalfa leaf meal, rice polishings, rice bran, whole grains, hominy, turnips, and blackstrap molasses.

Folic Acid (Folacin)

For DNA metabolism and protein metabolism. A vital group of at least five active enzymes essential for body growth, regeneration, and reproduction; hydrochloric acid production; red blood cell formation; protein metabolism; RNA/DNA production; healthy skin; division of body cells; and sugar and amino acid utilization. Inhibits anemia, prevents canker sores, acts as a pain reliever, and stimulates lactation. Key points:

- Important for the formation of purines/pyrimidines, which are needed for the synthesis of nucleic acid (RNA/DNA).
- Important for DNA cell division.
- Important for amino acid metabolism, including:
  —Conversion of serine to glycine
  —Formation of tyrosine from phenylalanine and glutamic acid from histidine
  —Formation of methionine from homocysteine
  —Synthesis of choline from ethanolamine
- Important for the formation of heme, the iron-containing protein in hemoglobin.
- Prevents macrocytic anemia.
- Needs vitamins C, B_{12}, and B_6 to work.
- Together with para-aminobenzoic acid (PABA) and vitamin B_5 (pantothenic acid), restores color to gray hair.
- Daily intake: 400 mcg to 5 mg. (Strengths higher than 800 mcg can be obtained only by prescription.)

Best food sources: liver, kidney, avocados, beans, beets, celery, chickpeas, eggs, fish, green leafy vegetables, nuts, oranges, soybeans, and whole wheat.

Inositol

For emulsification and metabolism of fatty acids. Works with choline. Essential for the formation of lecithin and the reduction of cholesterol. Retards hardening of the arteries, stimulates hair growth and prevents hair loss, inhibits eczema, redistributes body fat, and nourishes brain cells. Key points:

- Important for fat and cholesterol metabolism and emulsification.
- Combines with choline to form lecithin.
- Important for brain function/memory (together with choline).
- Protects the heart.
- Prevents hardening of the arteries.
- Precursor of phosphoinosities—especially found in the brain, among other places.
- Transports lipids.
- Use with choline, methionine, and betaine hydrochloride (lipotropic factors).
- Daily intake: 250 mg to 1,000 mg.

Best food sources: organ meats (liver, brain, heart, kidney), wheat germ, citrus fruits, blackstrap molasses, muscle meats, fruits, whole grains, brans, nuts, legumes, milk, and vegetables. (In meat inositol is found as part of the phospholipids; in plants it's found in the form of phytic acid binding zinc, calcium, and iron in an insoluble complex that interferes with their absorption.)

PABA (Para-aminobenzoic Acid)

For protein metabolism. Functions as an essential part of the folacin molecule. Essential for blood cell formation; restores color to gray hair (use with vitamin B_5 [pantothenic acid] and folic acid); stimulates intestinal flora; protects against sunburn; inhibits skin wrinkling; stimulates healthy skin; and prevents eczema. Sometimes used in the treatment of parasitic diseases such as typhus and Rocky Mountain spotted fever. Key points:

* Helps form folic acid and helps the assimilation of B_5.
* Delays wrinkles.
* Prevents gray hair.
* Daily intake has not been established.

Best food sources: torula yeast, fish, soybeans, peanuts, beef liver, eggs, wheat germ, lecithin, and molasses.

Vitamin K (Menadione)

Essential for blood clotting (needed for synthesis of the four blood-clotting factors) and detoxification. Has an antibacterial function; reduces excess menstrual flow; prevents internal bleeding and hemorrhages; and helps to prevent diarrhea. Chlorophyll—a potent source of vitamin K—occurs only in green plants. Key points:

* Important for raising calcium ions in the blood serum and liver, causing a more alkaline condition.
* Important for synthesis of the four blood-clotting factors, especially prothrombin, from precursor proteins.
* Prevents infections.
* Daily intake: 300 mcg to 400 mcg.

Best food sources: green tea, turnip greens, broccoli, lettuce, cabbage, liver, spinach, asparagus, watercress, and oats.

Minerals: Macronutrients

Calcium (Ca)

Calcium is an inorganic enzymatic cofactor, whose primary function is building bones and teeth. Essential as a regenerator for repair of the blood, bones, heart, skin, soft tissue, and teeth. Is the most abundant mineral in the body. The calcium to phosphorus ratio is usually two to one, although two to one or one to two can also be considered satisfactory. Key points:

- Fundamental to clotting of the blood.
- Fundamental to regulation of the heart rhythm.
- Fundamental to muscle contraction and relaxation, especially the heartbeat.
- Fundamental to nerve transmission and tranquilization.
- Fundamental to cell wall permeability: controls fluid passage through cell walls.
- Calcium and phosphorus work together for healthy bones and teeth; calcium and magnesium work together for cardiovascular health.
- Most commonly felt to have a two-to-one relationship with phosphorus (2 Ca to 1 P) as well as magnesium (2 Ca to 1 Mg).
- Activates certain enzymes.
- Helps metabolize the body's iron.
- Responsible for muscle growth and contraction.
- Secretes a number of hormones and hormone-releasing factors.
- Parathyroid hormone keeps blood calcium at normal levels.
- Needs the vitamins A, C, D, and F along with the minerals iron, magnesium, manganese, and phosphorus.
- Excessive stress and lack of exercise greatly reduce blood calcium levels.
- Large quantities of fat, oxalic acid (found as oxalates in chocolate, rhubarb, and spinach), and phytic acid in grains can prevent proper calcium absorption.
- Alleviates aging, arthritis, foot and leg cramps, insomnia, menstrual cramps, menopausal problems, nervousness, and premenstrual tension.
- Increased blood calcium levels may indicate poor emulsification of fats, faulty protein digestion in the liver, or poor gallbladder function; decreased calcium levels may indicate poor fatty acid metabolism and poor protein digestion in the liver.
- The herb horsetail grass is rich in calcium.
- Daily intake: 500 mg to 1,600 mg.

Best food sources: cheese, wheat flour, blackstrap molasses, almonds, Brazil nuts, caviar, cottonseed flour, dried figs, fish with soft edible bones, green leafy vegetables, hazelnuts, milk, oysters, soybean flour, and yogurt.

Potassium (K)

A trace element needed to maintain water, acids, and bases in the fluid *inside* the cells. Transfers nutrients. Needed for the blood, heart, kidneys, muscles, nerves, and skin. Potassium is the third most abundant mineral in the body and should be in a balance of twice as much potassium as sodium (2 K to 1 Na). Required for the regulation of the heartbeat, proper muscle contraction, and nerve tranquilization and growth. Hypoglycemia causes potassium loss. Key points:

- Essential in maintaining the proper acid-base balance inside the cells as well as transferring nutrients into and out of individual cells.
- Relaxes the heart muscle; works with calcium, which stimulates the heart muscle.
- Required for secretion of insulin by the pancreas.
- Aids in reducing allergic reactions.
- Hypoglycemia and mental or physical stress can cause potassium loss.
- Sends oxygen to the brain, thereby aiding clear thinking.
- Required by enzyme reactions involving phosphorylation of creatine.
- Disposes of body wastes.
- Essential for carbohydrate metabolism and protein synthesis.
- Inhibits heart rhythm irregularities, irritability, and muscle weakness.
- Reduces blood pressure.
- Coffee drinkers, smokers, and sugarholics lose potassium.
- The concentration of potassium needs to be twice that of sodium (2 K to 1 Na). Potassium also needs vitamin B_6.
- Increased blood levels of potassium may indicate congestion of tissues, possibly the heart if accompanied by a slow heartbeat; decreased potassium levels may indicate hyperoxidation, with a possibly weak heart muscle. (Potassium levels can be seriously lowered by the use of diuretics.)
- Daily intake: 900 mg or twice the concentration of sodium.

Best food sources: dehydrated fruits, molasses, potato flour, rice bran, seaweed, soybean flour, spices, sunflower seeds, wheat bran, avocados, beef, dates, guavas, most raw vegetables, nectarines, nuts, poultry, sardines, and veal.

Magnesium (Mg)

Essential for maintaining the acid-alkaline balance in the body and for enzyme activation. Needed for the arteries, bones, heart, muscles, nerves, and teeth. Essential for nerve and muscle functioning. Key points:

- Required for cellular metabolism: activates the enzymes involved in the transfer of adenosine diphosphate (ADP) and adenosine triphosphate (ATP).
- Required for protein digestion: activates certain peptidases.
- Relaxes nerve impulses: works antagonistically to calcium (similar to potassium).
- Required for the metabolism of calcium and vitamin C along with phosphorus, sodium, and potassium.
- Maintains the acid-alkaline balance.
- Regulates blood sugar metabolism by converting blood sugar to energy.
- Is the "antistress" mineral.
- Helps prevent heart attacks and supports a healthy cardiovascular system.
- Along with potassium, helps to prevent kidney stones and gall-stones as well as calcium deposits.
- Has a direct relationship to cortisone production.
- Is an essential part of all molecules and needed for growth and repair.
- Serves as a catalyst for some chemical reactions in the body.
- Requires the vitamins B_6, C, and D and the minerals calcium and phosphorus.
- Inhibits easily aroused anger, confusion, disorientation, nervousness, rapid pulse, and depression.
- Low blood levels of magnesium are associated with heightened nervous irritability, dilation of the peripheral blood vessels, and cardiac arrhythmia. High blood levels of magnesium are associated with suppression of nervous system activity.
- Daily intake: 300 mg to 400 mg.

Best food sources: cottonseed flour, peanut flour, sesame seeds, soybean flour, spices, wheat bran and germ, blackstrap molasses, nuts, peanut butter, whole grains, and torula yeast.

Minerals: Microminerals, Trace Elements

Copper (Cu)

Required to convert the body's iron into hemoglobin; heightens energy by ensuring effective oxygen absorption. Part of several enzyme systems. Key points:

- Essential for liberating iron from the liver and reticuloendothelial system.
- Essential for facilitating the absorption of iron from the intestinal tract.
- Helps in the formation of hemoglobin.
- Is a component of several enzyme systems and the copper-containing amino acids.
- Essential for the development and maintenance of the blood vessels, tendons, and bones.
- Essential for the structure and functioning of the central nervous system.
- Facilitates availability of the amino acid tyrosine to work as the pigmenting factor for hair color.
- Essential for reproduction and fertility.
- Required for the utilization of vitamin C.
- Copper's utilization can be hampered by high levels of calcium, iron, zinc, lead, molybdenum, sulfur, cadmium, and silver.
- Excess copper lowers zinc blood levels and may produce hair loss, insomnia, irregular menses, and depression.
- Only 2 mg daily is needed, and usually enough is taken into the body through green leafy vegetables or liver. Some people wear copper bracelets.

Best food sources: black pepper, blackstrap molasses, liver, raw oysters, lobster, nuts and seeds, green olives, soybean flour, and wheat bran and germ (roasted).

Chromium (Cr)

Needed for burning fat and producing energy. Forms part of the glucose tolerance factor. Essential for enzyme activation and fatty acid synthesis. Works with insulin in the metabolism of sugar and is a protein carrier. Key points:

- Essential as a component of the glucose tolerance factor in the pancreas, which enhances the effect of insulin in the metabolism of blood sugar. Essential for diabetes, hypoglycemia, or carbohydrate intolerance.

- Activates certain enzymes in the pancreas involved in the release of energy from proteins, carbohydrates, and fats.
- Stabilizes nucleic acids (RNA/DNA) and transports protein molecules to where they're needed.
- Stimulates the synthesis of fatty acids and is therefore a "fat burner."
- Helps synthesize cholesterol in the liver.
- Stimulates growth.
- Lowers high blood pressure.
- Chromium levels in the body decline with age.
- Daily intake: 50 mcg to 200 mcg.

Best food sources: blackstrap molasses, cheese, eggs, liver, apple peels, bananas, beef, chicken, cornmeal, oysters, vegetable oils, and wheat bran.

Zinc (Zn)

Needed for the synthesis and metabolism of proteins and nucleic acid (RNA/DNA) as well as for insulin function. Responsible for the maintenance of enzyme systems and cells, protein synthesis, and the formation of insulin. Directs muscle contractions, maintains the acid-alkaline balance of the body, and supports all reproductive organs. Important in brain function. Meats and seafood are the best sources of zinc. Key points:

- Essential for skin, bones, and hair.
- Required as a component in several enzyme systems in digestion and respiration, especially by the pancreas's enzyme-producing system.
- Required for synthesis and metabolism of proteins and nucleic acids.
- Essential for the proper functioning of insulin.
- Transfers carbon dioxide in red blood cells.
- Needed to work with calcium for the proper calcification of bone—important in preventing osteoporosis.
- Essential for the development and functioning of all reproductive organs. Aids in infertility problems as well as menopausal or prostate problems.
- Accelerates the healing of wounds and burns.
- Eliminates loss of taste.
- Stimulates brain function and mental alertness.

- Reduces cholesterol.
- Zinc's accessibility is inhibited by phytates (in grains and beans), high calcium intake, oxalates (in spinach and rhubarb), high fiber intake, copper (drinking water carried in copper pipes), and certain food additives.
- If taking higher amounts of B_6, you need additional zinc; if taking higher amounts of zinc, you need vitamin A.
- Daily intake: 15 mg to 50 mg.

Best food sources: beef, liver, oysters, spices, wheat bran, crab, lamb, peanuts, popcorn, and poultry.

Trace Minerals in Very Small Amounts

Cobalt (Co)
An integral part of vitamin B_{12} that is essential in the formation of red blood cells and must be obtained from food. Usually no more than 8 mcg is needed. The best food sources are those listed for vitamin B_{12} (see page 425).

Fluorine (F)
Needed for sound teeth and bones. Large amounts of calcium or aluminum can reduce the absorption of fluorine. Usually 1 mg per day is needed; 20 to 80 mg per day can be toxic. The best food sources are dried seaweed, tea, mackerel, sardines, salmon, and shrimp.

Molybdenum (Mo)
Needed for the metabolism of carbohydrates, fats, proteins, RNA/DNA, and iron. Also a component of tooth enamel. Excess copper can cause a molybdenum deficiency. Helps prevent anemia. Intake should be about 45 mcg to 500 mcg daily. Dark green leafy vegetables, organ meats, whole grains, and legumes are the best sources.

Silicon (Si)
Necessary for normal growth and skeletal development as well as healthy skin and hair. Also helps to speed wound healing. Normally 1 gram per day is needed and can be ingested from food. Good sources include cucumbers, the fibrous parts of whole grains, organ meats, and meat connective tissue. The homeopathic remedy silicea can also be used.

Vanadium (V)

Inhibits the formation of cholesterol in blood vessels. Daily intake is not known. Fish is the best source.

Energizing Nutrients (Catabolic/Acid)

Vitamins

B-Complex Vitamins

Organic enzymatic cofactors. The B vitamins are water-soluble and maintain the body's acid-base balance if protein consumption is high. The herb burdock contains B vitamins.

Vitamin B_1 (Thiamine)

Used in energy production (is a coenzyme in energy metabolism). Benefits the nervous system, muscles, and mind. Heat, sugar consumption, and smoking destroy B_1. Key points:

- Converts glucose to energy (adenosine triphosphate, or ATP).
- Converts nucleic acids to energy.
- Synthesizes lipids.
- Maintains peripheral nerve function.
- Preserves normal appetite.
- Sustains muscle tone.
- Helps in upholding a healthy mental attitude.
- Needed for production of hydrochloric acid (HCl).
- Binds pyrarate dehydrogenase enzyme, which needs the five coenzymes: B_1, B_2, B_3, B_5, and lipoic acid.
- B_1 needs B_2 and B_6 in equal amounts.
- Daily intake: 100 mg to 500 mg.

Best food sources: torula yeast, sunflower seeds, rice bran, wheat germ, pine nuts, dried coriander leaf, safflower seeds, soybeans, alfalfa seeds, peanuts, sesame seeds, Canadian bacon, beef kidneys, and rye flour (dark).

Vitamin B_2 (Riboflavin)

Used in energy production. Forms FAD (flavin adenine dinucleotide) coenzyme, which transports hydrogen ions and other coenzymes. Benefits skin, hair, nails, and vision. Involved in the functioning of the adrenal gland. Eliminates mouth sores and lip cracks. Is not destroyed by heat but is destroyed by ultraviolet light and alcohol. Key points:

- Converts glucose, amino acids, carbohydrates, and fatty acids to energy.
- Produces flavoprotein for adenosine triphosphate (ATP) production.
- Plays an essential role in reducing oxidation in all body cells, thereby increasing the production and release of energy.
- Activates vitamin B_6 for the formation of B_3 (niacin) from the amino acid tryptophan.
- Required for corticosteroid production in the adrenal cortex.
- May be a component of the eyes' retinal pigment.
- Needed for antibody and red blood cell production.
- Required for cell respiration.
- Daily intake: 100 mg to 300 mg.

Best food sources: organ meats (liver, heart, kidneys), almonds, cheese, lean beef, pork or lamb, raw mushrooms, turnip greens, wheat bran, soybeans, and Canadian bacon.

Vitamin B_3 (Niacin/Niacinamide)

Niacin (animal source—flushing) and niacinamide (plant source—nonflushing) have equal niacin activity. For glucose production and the conversion of proteins and fatty acids to energy. An essential constituent of the coenzymes nicotinamide adenine dinucleotide (NAD) and nicotinamide adenine dinucleotide phosphate (NADP), which are necessary for cell respiration. Essential for production of the hormones estrogen, progesterone, and testosterone; healthy nervous system and brain function; healthy skin; immune function; adrenal function; and circulation. Helps to reduce cholesterol and migraine headaches. Lack of B_3 can cause negative personality shifts. Key points:

- Converts glucose, carbohydrates, fatty acids (steroid hormones), and protein to energy.
- Essential for hormone production and adrenal function.
- Necessary for the oxidation retardation reaction (cell respiration).
- Synthesized from tryptophan.
- Stimulates growth and regeneration in the body.
- Reduces cholesterol.
- Protects to a degree against myocardial infarction (heart attack).
- Reduces or eliminates irritability, anxiety, and depression.
- Daily intake: 100 mg to 1,000 mg.

Best food sources: liver, kidney, lean meats, poultry, fish, rabbit, nuts, peanut butter, milk, cheese, eggs, bran flakes, sesame seeds, and sunflower seeds.

Vitamin B₅ (Pantothenic Acid/Calcium Pantothenate/Panthenol—Coenzyme A)

Used in fat and energy production. Functions in the body as two enzymes: CoA (coenzyme A) and ACP (acyl carrier protein). One of the most important substances in body metabolism. Essential for burning fat, central nervous system development, adrenal function, healthy skin, cell building, antibody synthesis, and utilization of PABA (para-aminobenzoic acid) and choline. Key points:

- Needed for metabolism of cholesterol to hormones.
- Converts fat, glucose, carbohydrates, and proteins to energy.
- Essential for the formation of acetylcholine, a neurotransmitter (with choline and PABA) that transmits messages to the brain.
- Synthesizes prophyrin, a precursor of heme necessary for hemoglobin synthesis.
- Synthesizes cholesterol and other lipids.
- Metabolizes lipids and steroid hormones formed by the adrenals and sex glands.
- Essential for maintenance of normal blood sugar.
- Together with vitamin C, needed by the body during and after a stress response.
- Necessary for the health of the adrenal glands.
- Reduces irritability, restlessness, mental depression, fatigue, and weakness.
- Helps the body excrete sulfonamide drugs.
- Daily intake: 10 mg to 500 mg.

Best food sources: organ meats (liver, heart and kidney), cottonseed flour, wheat bran, rice bran, rice polishings, nuts, mushrooms, soybean flour, salmon, blue cheese, eggs, buckwheat flour, lobster, sunflower seeds, and brown rice.

Vitamin B₆ (Pyridoxine, Pyridoxal)

For protein metabolism. Essential for nerves and skin disorders as well as immune function in the production of antibodies and red blood cells. Activates amino acids; assimilates amino acids (protein) and fat; regulates adrenal function; necessary for the absorption of vitamin B₁₂; helps to remember dreams; aids in HCl production and magnesium utilization; needed for body regeneration; acts as a natural diuretic; reduces muscle spasms; combats neuritis in the extremities; alleviates nausea; and maintains sodium to potassium balance. Has been used to treat autism in children as well as to counter the antagonistic drug used in tuberculosis. Key points:

- Important for amino acid metabolism—transamination, decarboxylation, deamination, transsulfuration, and absorption of proteins.
- Converts tryptophan to niacin.
- Essential in hemoglobin production.
- Important for the metabolism of carbohydrates and fats to energy—glycogen to glucose and linoleic acid to arachidonic acid.
- Important for the formation of gamma-aminobutyric acid (GABA) from glutamic acid.
- Reduces or eliminates seborrheic dermatitis (skin, nose, mouth, and eyes).
- Calms central nervous system disturbances, such as irritability and mental depression.
- Helpful in eliminating kidney stones and nonresistant anemia.
- Important for liver and heart function.
- Daily intake: 50 mg to 500 mg.

Best food sources: rice bran, wheat bran, sunflower seeds, avocados, bananas, corn, fish, kidney, lean meat, liver, nuts, poultry, brown rice, soybeans, and whole grains.

Vitamin B_{15} (Pangamic Acid)

For oxygen utilization. Essential for cell oxidation and respiration, extending cell life, as well as for gland and nerve stimulation. Inhibits fatigue; aids protein synthesis; stimulates immune responses; stops alcohol cravings; protects the liver; lowers cholesterol; inhibits damage done to the body from pollutant exposure; great for athletes. Key points:

- Important for stimulating transmethylation reactions.
- Important for stimulating oxygen uptake.
- Important for inhibiting the formation of a fatty liver.
- Controls blood cholesterol.
- Important for improving muscle performance.
- Stimulates energy reserve and reduces "hypoxia" (low supply of oxygen to the cells).

- In Russia, used in the treatment of cardiovascular, liver, and skin diseases.
- Daily intake: 50 mg to 300 mg.

Best food sources: grains, cereals, rice, apricot kernels, and torula yeast.

Biotin (Coenzyme R/Vitamin H)

For fat and energy metabolism. Metabolically related to folacin, B_5, and B_{12}. Removes carbon dioxide from carbohydrate, fat, and protein during metabolism. Forms purines and urea. Essential in the first step of the Krebs cycle in the deamination of amino acids. Essential for cell growth, fatty acid production, and B-vitamin utilization. Restores color to gray hair; alleviates eczema and dermatitis; relieves muscle pain; helps prevent baldness; needs B_2, B_6, niacin, and A for healthy skin; stimulates immunity by antibody formation; and regenerates the body. Egg whites and antibiotics inhibit the production of biotin. Key points:

- Converts amino acids (protein) and carbohydrates to energy.
- Needed for the synthesis of fatty acids to energy.
- Formulates antibodies.
- Forms alpha-amylase (starch-digestion enzyme) in the pancreas.
- Stimulates cell growth.
- Necessary in the utilization of vitamins B and C.
- Essential in immune function, fat metabolism impairment, and regeneration of the body.
- Daily intake: 25 mcg to 300 mcg.

Best food sources: kidney, liver, soybean flour, cauliflower, eggs, mushrooms, nuts, peanut butter, sardines, salmon, wheat bran, and chocolate.

Lipoic Acid (Thiotic Acid)

For the production of energy from carbohydrates, fats, and proteins. Functions in the same manner as many of the other B-complex vitamins. Acts as a coenzyme and is essential in the conversion of nutrients to energy. Key points:

- Together with the B_1 (thiamine) enzyme, is essential in carbohydrate metabolism, converting pyruvic acid to acetyl coenzyme A, sending it into the final energy cycle.
- Joins the intermediary products of protein and fat metabolism in the Krebs cycle, producing energy from these nutrients.

- Lipoic acid also requires magnesium or calcium, B_1, B_5 (pantothenic acid), B_3 (niacin), and B_2 (riboflavin) for this oxidative decarboxylation.

Best food sources: liver and torula yeast.

Vitamin C (Ascorbic Acid)

Maintains the acid-base balance if carbohydrate and sugar consumption is high. For the synthesis and metabolism of tryptophan and tyrosine. For energy and body healing and repair. Essential for adrenal gland health; building blood capillary walls; connective tissue formation; formation and health of the skin, teeth, ligaments, bones, gums, and heart; collagen production; proper digestion; iodine conservation; red blood cell formation; and resistance to infection. Stimulates digestion and vitamin oxidation; accelerates healing; decreases blood cholesterol; acts as a natural laxative; reduces blood clots; holds protein cells together; and reduces allergens. Key points:

- Releases iron for hemoglobin synthesis.
- Important for the metabolism of tryptophan and tyrosine.
- Metabolizes fats and lipids; controls cholesterol.
- Is used more rapidly by the body under stress.
- Daily intake: 500 mg to 6,000 mg.

Best food sources: acerola cherries, rose hips, citrus fruit, guavas, hot green peppers, black currants, parsley, turnip greens, poke greens, and mustard greens.

Vitamin E (Tocopherol)

Also known as alpha-tocopherol; the most effective of the eight tocopherols. Used in DNA synthesis. Acts as an anticoagulant, a vasodilator, and an antioxidant. Essential for preventing the oxidation of fat, vitamin A, selenium, and vitamin C. Enhances the activity of vitamin A; retards cellular aging due to oxidation; dissolves blood clots; inhibits fatigue; helps to prevent miscarriages; strengthens fertility and male potency; provides lung protection with vitamin A; needed for muscle and nerve maintenance; boosts blood flow to the heart; accelerates healing; helps to prevent scarring and the formation of scar tissue; can lower blood pressure; and enhances the supply of oxygen to the body. Key points:

- Important for the health of the hormonal and reproductive systems.
- Retards the rancidification of fats.

- Protects body cells from toxic substances formed from the oxidation of unsaturated fats.
- A powerful antioxidant, in that it oxidizes itself.
- Essential for red blood cell integrity.
- Essential to cellular respiration, especially in heart and muscle tissues.
- Regulates the synthesis of DNA, vitamin C, and coenzyme Q10.
- Protects lung tissue from pollution.
- Important in combating aging.
- Strengthens muscles.
- Important for the restoration of red blood cells.
- Daily intake: 200 IU to 1,200 IU.

Best food sources: oils (except coconut), alfalfa seeds, nuts, sunflower-seed kernels, asparagus, avocados, beef, organ meats, blackberries, eggs, green leafy vegetables, oatmeal, rye, seafoods (lobster, salmon, shrimp, and tuna), and tomatoes.

Vitamin F (Unsaturated Fatty Acids/Linoleic and Arachidonic)

Used in energy production. Essential for preventing arterial cholesterol deposits. Protects against X rays, liberates calcium for the cells, strengthens the heart, and stimulates growth. Key points:

- Burns saturated fat.
- Stimulates glandular action (thyroid and adrenals).
- Feeds skin and hair and stimulates their health.
- High consumption of carbohydrates increases the need for unsaturated fatty acids.
- Important for blood coagulation.
- Destroys gallstones.
- Normalizes blood pressure.
- Intake should be included in the percentage of fat consumed in your diet. An excess can lead to unwanted pounds.

Best food sources: oils (safflower, sunflower-seed, wheat germ, corn, soy, cottonseed, peanut, palm, and olive), cod-liver oil, walnuts, Brazil nuts, peanuts, almonds, and wheat germ.

Vitamin P (Citrus Bioflavonoids, Rutin, Hesperidin)

For proper absorption and functioning of vitamin C and capillary strength. Essential for increasing the strength of capillaries and regulating their permeability, enhancing vitamin C absorption. With vitamin C strengthens connective tissue; prevents bruising hemorrhages and ruptures; fights and builds resistance to infection; inhibits bleeding of gums; and increases the effectiveness of vitamin C. Key points:

- Important for blood vessel wall maintenance.
- Important for minimization of bruising.
- Has a synergistic effect with vitamin C.
- Stabilizes vitamin C within the tissues.
- Has an active antioxidant effect.
- Possesses metal-chelating capacity.
- Affects the activity of enzymes and membranes.
- Has a bacteriostatic or an antibiotic effect, preventing infections.
- Possesses anticarcinogenic properties.
- Daily intake: 300 mg to 3,000 mg.

Best food sources: citrus peels, white pulp of citrus fruits, tangerine juice, rose hips, buckwheat leaves, leafy vegetables, red or yellow onions, fruit, and tea.

Minerals: Macronutrients

Phosphorus (P)

Essential for energy utilization. Comprises one-quarter of the body's total mineral composition, with 80 percent of phosphorus combined with calcium in the bones and teeth. Necessary for cellular growth and repair; energy production; heart muscle contraction; kidney function; calcium and sugar metabolism; and nerve and muscle activity. Takes part in the chemical reactions with proteins, carbohydrates, and fats. Key points:

- Essential for bone formation and maintenance and tooth development—promotes healthy gums and teeth.
- Needs to be balanced in a two-to-one ratio with calcium (2 Ca to 1 P).
- Requires vitamin D and calcium to function.
- Involved in all physiological chemical reactions.
- Essential for kidney functioning.
- Needed for transference of nerve impulses.
- Essential for the synthesis of RNA/DNA—as a component of the nu-

cleic acids important in genetic transmission and control of cellular metabolism.

- Essential for normal milk secretion.
- A must in building muscle tissue.
- Maintains the osmotic and acid-base balance.
- Mandatory in:
  —Energy metabolism and utilization (formation of adenosine triphosphate, or ATP)
  —Phospholipid formation
  —Amino acid metabolism
  —Starch metabolization
  —Enzyme systems and activation
- Lessens arthritic pain.
- Requires the vitamins A, D, and F and the minerals calcium, iron, and manganese.
- Increased blood levels of phosphorus may indicate underactive hydrochloric acid production, with an alkaline stomach environment that inhibits digestion. Decreased blood levels of phosphorus may indicate overactive hydrochloric acid production, with an overacid stomach environment that inhibits proper digestion.
- Excessive intake of magnesium or refined carbohydrates (especially white sugar) decreased phosphorus blood levels.
- Daily intake: 500 mg to 1,500 mg.

Best food sources: cocoa powder, cottonseed flour, fish flour, pumpkin and squash seeds, rice bran and polishings, soybean flour, sunflower seeds, wheat bran, beef, cheese, fish and seafood, lamb, liver, nuts, poultry, and whole-grain flours.

Sodium (Na)

Needed to maintain water, acids, and bases in the fluid *outside* the cells. Needed for the absorption of sugars as well as for blood, lymph, muscles, and nerves. Generally the need for sodium in our diets is low, since most of our foods contain such high levels of sodium chloride (NaCl) and table salt is used extensively. Excess sodium leads to high blood pressure and edema. Deficiencies usually occur only if there has been prolonged sweating, diarrhea, vomiting, or adrenal cortical insufficiency. Key points:

- Essential for maintaining the water, bases, and acids in the fluids outside the cells.

- Must be balanced with potassium at twice the amount of sodium (1 Na to 2 K).
- Is a constituent of pancreatic juice, bile, sweat, and tears.
- Supports proper muscle contraction.
- Facilitates the travel of nerve pulses to muscle.
- Helps nerves respond to stimulation.
- Plays an important role in carbohydrate absorption.
- Increased blood sodium levels may indicate an alkaline kidney membrane, with a need for potassium; fluid retention is often seen. Decreased blood sodium levels may indicate an acid kidney membrane, with a need for calcium or sodium.
- Daily intake: 500 mg to 1,500 mg.

Best food sources: anchovy paste, bacon, bologna, bran cereal, butter, Canadian bacon, corned beef, cucumber pickles, cured ham, dehydrated cod, dried squid, frankfurters, green olives, luncheon meats, oat cereal, parmesan cheese, pasteurized process cheese, potato chips, pretzels, sausages, seaweed, shrimp, smoked meats and fish, soda crackers, soy sauce, tomato ketchup, and most packaged or canned foods.

Sulfur (S)

Essential for regulating energy metabolism and protein synthesis. Found in every cell of the body and essential for life itself. Constitutes 10 percent of the mineral content of the body. Is a component of the vitamins biotin and B_1 (thiamine) as well as coenzyme A. Essential for healthy skin, nails, and hair. Works with the B-complex vitamins for the body's metabolism. Key points:

- Important in fat metabolism as a component of biotin.
- Is the major component in the sulfur-containing amino acids: methionine, cystine, and cysteine.
- Important in carbohydrate metabolism as a component of vitamin B_1 and insulin.
- Important in energy metabolism as a component of coenzyme A.
- Regulates energy metabolism as a component of glutathione, selenium, and insulin.
- Detoxifies the body by converting toxic substances to nontoxic forms.
- Aids the liver in bile secretion.
- Maintains oxygen balance for brain function.
- Essential for collagen synthesis—important in various connective tissues as a component of certain complex carbohydrates.

- Helps fight bacterial infections.
- Tones skin and helps hair to shine.
- No dietary recommendations have been made. The rule of thumb is that if you're getting enough protein in your diet, you're getting enough sulfur.

Best food sources: cheese, grains, eggs, fish, legumes, meat, nuts, and poultry.

Chloride (Cl; Chloride)

Needed for osmotic pressure regulation, water and acid-base balance, and the formation of all gastric juices. Essential for regulating the blood's alkaline-acid balance. Works with sodium and potassium in combination. Key points:

- Plays a major role in the regulation of osmotic pressure, water balance, and acid-base balance.
- Required for the production of hydrochloric acid (HCl) in the stomach. HCl is necessary for the absorption of B_{12} and iron, activation of the starch enzyme, and suppressing microorganisms entering the stomach with food.
- Aids in cleaning the body of waste by helping the liver to function.
- Increased blood levels of chloride may indicate improper membrane lubrication, while decreased blood levels of chloride could mean tissue breakdown in the large intestine, bladder, or elsewhere in the body.
- If your daily sodium (or salt) intake is sufficient, you're getting enough chloride.

Best food sources: those listed for sodium (see page 444).

Minerals: Microminerals, Trace Elements

Iron (Fe)

Essential for oxidation within cells, hemoglobin production, and energy metabolism. Required for life. Roughly 70 percent of iron is present in the red pigment of the blood cells as hemoglobin; 30 percent is stored in the spleen, liver, and bone marrow as ferretin (iron bound to protein) and in the tissues as myoglobin (red pigment in skin and muscles); 4 grams are found in the hair. Stimulates growth and healthy skin color. Needed for bones, nails, teeth, and blood. Prevents fatigue and iron deficiency anemia and encourages resistance to infections and disease. Key points:

- Essential for combining with protein to make hemoglobin.
- Essential for transporting oxygen within the cells, thereby maintaining cellular oxygenation.
- A key component of enzymes involved in energy metabolism.
- Prevents anemia.
- Requires copper, cobalt, manganese, calcium, phosphorus, vitamin C, and folic acid for proper assimilation.
- Increased blood levels of iron may indicate that more exercise or exposure to sunlight might be needed, while decreased blood levels of iron may mean lowered bone cell production and/or anemia.
- If iron intake is too high, a phosphorus deficiency could result.
- Iron's availability can be inhibited by phytates (in grains and beans) and the phosphoproteins in eggs.
- Ferrous gluconate, ferrous fumerate, ferrous citrate, or ferrous peptonate (organic irons) do not neutralize vitamin E and should be taken if iron supplementation is needed. Ferrous sulfate (an inorganic iron found in most formulas) destroys vitamin E.
- Supplements up to 300 mg are available. Doses of 200 mg per kilogram of body weight are usually toxic.

Best food sources: beef kidneys, blackstrap molasses, caviar, chicken giblets, fish flour, liver, oysters, potato flour, rice polishings, soybean flour, spices, sunflower-seed flour, wheat bran and germ, and orange pekoe tea.

Iodine (I; Iodide)

Essential for producing thyroxine, regulating metabolism, and burning fat. Two-thirds of the body's iodine is in the thyroid gland, which controls the metabolism. If an iodine deficiency exists, the thyroid gland enlarges in an attempt to make sufficient thyroxine. Key points:

- An essential constituent of thyroxine and the iodine-containing hormones secreted by the thyroid gland.
- Regulates the rate of oxidation within the cells.
- Influences physical, mental, and hormonal growth.
- Essential for the functioning of the nervous system as well as for muscle tissue and circulation.
- Essential for the metabolism of all nutrients.
- Burns excess fat.
- Stimulates energy.
- Improves brain function.
- Essential for healthy hair, skin, nails, and teeth.

- Raw vegetables of the cabbage family inhibit iodine's effectiveness.
- Iodine-poor soil is common in the Midwest.
- Natural kelp is the best source of iodine, but supplements can be taken in doses of 0.15 mg (150 mcg) per day.

Best food sources: kelp, seafood, and vegetables grown on iodine-rich soil.

Manganese (Mn)

Needed for enzyme activation and thyroxine formation. Alkaline soil may produce manganese-poor plants. Helps to eliminate fatigue, strengthens muscle reflexes, improves memory, and calms nerves. Key points:

- Essential for the formation of bone and connective tissue.
- Activator of various enzymes, especially thyroxine, in the metabolism of carbohydrates, fats, proteins, and RNA/DNA (nucleic acids).
- Important in the formation of thyroxine.
- Activates enzymes for the body's utilization of the vitamins biotin, B_1, and C.
- Necessary for proper digestion and food utilization.
- Synthesizes cholesterol.
- Along with choline and inositol, improves memory.
- Supports the action of insulin.
- Important in blood clotting along with vitamin K.
- Essential in situations of carbohydrate intolerance and abnormal metabolism of fats, choline, and cholesterol.
- Large intakes of calcium and phosphorus can inhibit the absorption of manganese.
- Daily intake: 1 mg to 9 mg.

Best food sources: brown rice, rice bran, spices, walnuts, wheat bran and germ, blackstrap molasses, blueberries, lettuce, dry beans (lima, navy, and soy), peanuts, potatoes, sunflower seeds, torula yeast, and whole grains.

Selenium (Se)

Essential for oxidation. The "man's mineral." The functions of selenium are closely related to vitamin E and the other sulfur-containing amino acids. Half the supply of selenium in a male is in the testicles and seminal ducts, with a loss of selenium occurring in the semen. Selenium-rich soils are found in the Rocky Mountains, the Dakotas, Wyoming, and the Great Plains. Key points:

- Essential for protection of tissues against damage due to the oxidation of polyunsaturated fatty acids (free-radical damage) as a component of the enzyme glutathione peroxidase.
- Protects tissues against other poisonous and toxic substances.
- May neutralize certain carcinogens, protecting tissues from some cancers.
- Helps alleviate prostate problems.
- Alleviates hot flashes and other menopausal problems.
- Synergistic with vitamin E and the other sulfur-containing amino acids.
- Daily intake: 50 mcg to 200 mcg.

Best food sources: Brazil nuts, butter, lobster, smelt, blackstrap molasses, cider vinegar, clams, crabs, eggs, lamb, mushrooms, oysters, pork kidneys, garlic, cinnamon, chili powder, nutmeg, Swiss chard, turnips, wheat bran, and whole grains.

Enzymes

Coenzyme Q10 (Ubiquinone)
Collective name for a number of ubiquinones somewhat similar to vitamin E. Provides the stimulus for body synthesis. Essential as a catalyst for respiration. Key points:

- *The* enzyme needed in the respiratory chain that liberates energy as adenosine triphosphate (ATP) from nutrients.
- May prevent some vitamin E deficiencies.

Best food sources: coenzyme Q10 occurs widely in aerobic organisms. Most ubiquinone supplements are prepared synthetically since coenzyme Q10 is synthesized only in the body.

- Daily intake has not been established.

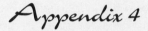

Appendix 4

Actions of Calming (Yin) and Energizing (Yang) Amino Acids

Amino acids, as you've already learned, are the building blocks—the essential structure—of our bodies. Out of the combinations of these amino acids are constructed the proteins that make up our own unique cells. Some eighty or more amino acids exist in nature, but it takes only twenty of these precious nutrients to energize or repair our bodies. Some of these amino acids can't be manufactured in our bodies, so we must get them from our food sources. These few are called essential amino acids. Current theory lists the following eleven as essential:

NEUTRAL ALIPHATIC
- Threonine (needs serine for metabolism)
- Isoleucine
- Leucine
- Valine

NEUTRAL CYCLIC
- Phenylalanine (produces tyrosine and synthesizes dopa, precursor to the neurotransmitters dopamine, norepinephrine, and epinephrine)
- Tyrosine (produces the thyroid hormones: T3 and T4)
- Tryptophan (produces the neurotransmitters serotonin and melatonin)

SULFUR-CONTAINING
- Methionine (produces cysteine and needs serine for metabolism)
- Cysteine (synthesized from methionine and produces taurine, needed for bile production)

BASIC (ALKALINE)
- Lysine (produces carnitine)
- Histidine

Then there are the following nonessential amino acids. They may or may not be necessary for survival but are fully or partially produced in our own bodies, using the essential amino acids as "building blocks."

NEUTRAL ALIPHATIC
- Glycine
- Alanine (Part of coenzyme A that is needed in metabolism and is synthesized by pantothenic acid—B_5.)
- Serine (needed for the metabolism of threonine [essential], aspartate, and methionine [essential])

NEUTRAL CYCLIC
- Proline
- Hydroxyproline

BASIC (ALKALINE)
- Arginine (synthesizes ornithine, citrulline, and arqininosuccinic acid—all needed for urea biosynthesis)

ACIDIC
- Aspartic acid (needs serine for metabolism)
- Glutamic acid (synthesizes to glutamine; synthesizes GABA [gamma-aminobutyric acid], an inhibitor neurotransmitter)

Milk, cheese, eggs, fish, fowl, and meat contain all the essential amino acids and are therefore called complete proteins, while vegetables and grains are deficient in some—especially lysine—and are called incomplete proteins. Amino acids pass unchanged through the digestive tract and are broken down to their smallest components in the liver. From there they go into general circulation to be absorbed by the cells according to the specific amino acid needed by each individual cell to make its own unique protein. The unused amino acids are converted into urea and excreted from the body.

Present theory suggests that because so much of our diet consists of processed foods, our bodies are being robbed of the nutrients that help us manufacture the nonessential amino acids. Therefore, some of the nonessential amino acids are now believed to be essential. I've indicated those amino acids as "conditionally essential" in the following paragraphs.

The rest of this appendix lists the actions and food sources of the various amino acids.

Essential Amino Acids: Regenerating and Calming

Neurotransmitters

Neutral Cyclic

Tryptophan ("The Parasympathetic Neurotransmitter Maker") (Essential)

Vital for stress-related problems. Produces a calming effect on the body and may even suppress pain. Key points:

- A precursor for the production of the "soothing" neurotransmitters: serotonin, tryptamine, and melatonin.
- Also a precursor for nicotinic acid (niacin), a component of the B-complex family of vitamins that may be useful in countering the effects of nicotine.
- Released by the parasympathetic nervous system but does compete with phenylalanine and tyrosine across the blood-brain barrier.
- Affects the hormone system.
- Produced in large quantities by the pineal gland. A deficiency may well cause insomnia, irritability, and restlessness.

Vital for: depression, insomnia, anxiety, premenstrual syndrome (PMS), obesity, bulimia, and pain.

Active with: vitamin B_6, the complete B-vitamin complex, magnesium, and niacin to produce serotonin. (For a sound sleep, take a 500-mg tablet of 5-hydroxytryptophan [a metabolite of tryptophan] with 100 mg of B_6, 100 mg of niacinamide, and 130 mg of magnesium before bed.)

Precautions: liver disease, bladder cancer, pregnancy, and diabetes.

Best food sources: beef, chicken, turkey (rich in tryptophan), fish, eggs, cottage cheese, milk, peanuts, dried dates, and bananas.

Glutamine ("The Muscle and Neurotransmitter Maker") (Conditionally essential)

Synthesized from glutamic acid and a precursor to gamma-aminobutyric acid (GABA). Converted to citrulline, alanine, and proline in the small intestine. Vital for stress-related problems. Key points:

- A powerful amino acid and the most abundant in muscle and plasma. Metabolized by the liver and kidneys.
- Crosses the blood-brain barrier more readily than glutamic acid.
- Regulates synthesis of muscle protein and nucleic acids.
- The recommended dosage is 1,000 mg to 4,000 mg. For depression, fatigue, or impotence, take 500 mg to 1,000 mg for the first week, then 1,200 mg to 1,500 mg for the next few weeks, and finally 2,000 mg daily after a month.

Vital for: stressful conditions, fatigue, cellular regeneration, alcoholism, and any gastrointestinal disorders.

Active with: vitamin B_6, folic acid, magnesium, and glycine.

Precautions: neuromuscular disorders, liver cancer, and encephalopathy.

Best food sources: beef, soy protein, chicken, turkey, fish, eggs, cottage cheese, milk, nuts, baked beans.

Building Amino Acids

Basic (Alkaline)

Lysine ("The Great Mother")
(Essential)

Precursor to carnitine, citrulline, and pipecolic acid (a neurotransmitter).

The building block of *all* protein, lysine is definitely essential—and if you're a strict vegetarian, this is the *one* amino acid you'll miss in your grains and vegetables. Wheat, rice, oats, corn, millet, and sesame seeds are some of the lysine-deficient foods. You'll be amazed at what this wonderful amino acid does:

- It's an essential component in the production of antibodies, hormones, and enzymes—the stuff of life itself.
- It aids in the repair of all cellular tissue as well as the production of collagen.
- It's essential for growth and development, especially in children, and also aids in the absorption of calcium into bones and teeth and the maintenance of a proper nitrogen balance in adults.
- It's essential for cholesterol metabolism and lowers high levels of fat or triglycerides in the blood.
- Lysine might best be known as an immune stimulant widely praised for its destruction of the herpes simplex virus. It not only protects the skin against viral infection but helps support the immune function as well.

Vital for: energy, inability to concentrate, irritability, anemia, growth retardation, reproductive disorders, hair loss, bloodshot eyes, cold sores, viruses, flus, sports injuries, and surgery.

Active with: vitamins B_6 and C, calcium, and iron.

Precaution: hyperammonemia.

Best food sources: fish, milk, lima beans, meat, cheese, yeast, eggs, soy products, chicken, beef, ham, pork, goat's milk, peanuts, and oatmeal.

Histidine ("The Daughter")
(Essential)

Precursor to histamine, glutamic acid, proline, and ornithine. Key points:

- Like its alkaline companion lysine, histidine is essential for the growth and repair of all body tissues and also aids in the production of red and white blood cells.
- A "heavy hitter," histidine also aids in general digestive problems, such as ulcers, hyperacidity of the stomach, and indigestion.
- Histamine is formed from histidine and is usually released under the gun of an immune response.

Vital for: rheumatoid arthritis, anemia, and allergies.
Active with: vitamins B_6 and C and calcium.
Precautions: manic-depression, premenstrual syndrome (PMS), and hypertension.
Best food sources: beef, chicken, fish, eggs, cottage cheese, nuts, wheat germ, oats.

Neutral Aliphatic

Threonine ("The Cell and Muscle Maker")
(Essential)

Precursor to glycine and serine. Key points:

- Can be converted to acetyl CoA that is needed in the energy-producing Krebs cycle.
- Essential in maintaining protein balance and in the formation of collagen and elastin. Present in the heart, central nervous system, and all skeletal muscles.
- When in combination with aspartic acid and methionine, it helps the liver and gallbladder to emulsify fats.
- Helps to keep your immune system strong.
- Helps to control epileptic seizures.

Vital for: muscle spasticity and ALS (amyotrophic lateral sclerosis).
Active with: serine.
Precautions: None known.

Best food sources: beef, chicken, fish, ham, pork, soy protein, soybeans, liver, eggs, and cottage cheese.

Isoleucine ("The Blood Maker")
(Essential)

Must be taken with the correct amounts of leucine and valine. Key points:

- Isoleucine occurs and is metabolized primarily in muscles—and is required for the formation of hemoglobin.
- It also helps to regulate blood sugar levels. A deficiency in this amino acid can lead to hypoglycemia (low blood sugar).

Vital for: muscle support, ALS (amyotrophic lateral sclerois), liver disease, anorexia, hyperthyroidism, and schizophrenia.

Active with: leucine and valine.

Precautions: None known.

Best food sources: beef, chicken, soybeans, soy protein, ham, pork, eggs, cottage cheese, liver, baked beans, and milk.

Leucine ("The Healer")
(Essential)

Must be taken with the correct amounts of isoleucine and valine. Key points:

- Similar to isoleucine, leucine is found primarily in the muscle tissue but is necessary for regulating muscle protein synthesis.
- Promotes wound healing as well as the healing of bones, skin, and muscles.
- Lowers elevated blood sugar levels—so it should be taken in a balanced amount with isoleucine and valine, or hypoglycemia could result.

Vital for: muscle support, ALS (amyotrophic lateral sclerois), liver disease, anorexia, hyperthyroidism, diabetes, and schizophrenia.

Active with: isoleucine and valine.

Precautions: None known.

Best food sources: The same as those listed for isoleucine (see above).

Valine ("An Aided Healer")
(Essential)

Must be taken with the correct amounts of isoleucine and leucine. Key points:

- Like both leucine and isoleucine, valine occurs primarily in the muscles.
- It enhances muscle metabolism, cellular repair, and nitrogen balance.
- It's been used to treat severe amino acid deficiencies caused by addictions.
- It has the effect of stimulating healing.

Vital for: muscle support, ALS (amyotrophic lateral sclerosis), liver disease, anorexia, hyperthyroidism, and schizophrenia.
Active with: leucine and isoleucine.
Precautions: None known.
Best food sources: beef, chicken, fish, soy protein, soybeans, ham, pork, eggs, liver, cottage cheese, baked beans, and milk.

Essential Amino Acids: Energizing

Neurotransmitters

Neutral Cyclic

Phenylalanine ("The Sympathetic Neurotransmitter Maker")
(Essential)

Precursor to tyrosine. Vital for stress-related problems. Key points:

- Literally feeds the sympathetic nervous system: produces the catecholamines needed by the adrenal glands both for daily activity and for the "flight-or-fight" response as well as the neurotransmitters dopamine, norepinephrine, and epinephrine.
- Can help to elevate moods and decrease pain from migraines, menstrual problems, and arthritis.
- Helps with memory, learning, and obesity.
- DL-phenylalanine (DLPA) is a mixture of equal parts of D (synthetic) and L (natural) phenylalanine that intensifies and prolongs the body's own natural painkilling response by producing endorphins.

Vital for: any stressful situation, depression, or appetite suppression.
Active with: vitamins B_6 and C, calcium, magnesium, and manganese. Needs vitamin C to work in the body.

Precautions: hypertension, monoamine oxidase (MAO) inhibitors, malignant melanoma, anxiety attacks, schizophrenia, and pregnancy.

Best food sources: soy protein, beef, chicken, soybeans, fish, eggs, cottage cheese, lima beans, almonds, milk, peanuts, pumpkin, and sesame seeds.

Tyrosine ("The Hormone and Neurotransmitter Maker") (Conditionally essential)

Synthesized from phenylalanine in the liver. Vital for stress-related problems as well as for neurotransmitter production of:

- Catecholamines: dopamine, norepinephrine, and epinephrine
- Thyroid hormones (produces thyroxine, raising the body's metabolic rate)
- Melanin

Key points:

- A deficiency of tyrosine causes depression.
- Tends to normalize blood pressure.

Vital for: stress, depression, withdrawals (smoking, drugs), appetite suppression, narcolepsy, and blood pressure abnormalities.

Active with: vitamins B_6 and C, calcium, magnesium, and manganese. Take with vitamins C, B_1, B_2, and niacinamide.

Precautions: monoamine oxidase (MAO) inhibitors, malignant melanoma, schizophrenia, and pregnancy.

Best food sources: soy protein, beef, chicken, soybeans, fish, eggs, cottage cheese, baked beans, almonds, milk, and peanuts.

Building Amino Acids

Sulfur-Containing

Methionine ("The Energizer, Stress Reliever, and Painkiller") (Essential)

Precursor for cysteine and taurine and converted in the liver.

A vitally important amino acid, methionine functions in several ways:

- It's involved in the synthesis of choline (part of the B-complex family) to make the parasympathetic nervous system's essential neurotransmitter acetylcholine.

- It may increase the sympathetic nervous system's essential neurotransmitters dopamine, epinephrine, and norepinephrine.
- Along with choline and folic acid, methionine has been found to break apart cholesterol deposits and inhibit tumors.
- It's involved in the synthesis of carnitine, creatine, and melatonin along with the breakdown of epinephrine, histamine, nicotinic acid, and pyridine derivatives used in the Krebs cycle: nicotinamide adenine dinucleotide (NAD) and nicotinamide adenine dinucleotide phosphate (NADP).
- Vital for the stress response and/or pain, methionine produces endorphins—normal brain peptides that bind some neurotransmitters that mimic opiates—and gives you a euphoric feeling if you're under the gun of pain or stress.

Along with being known as the antifatigue amino acid, methionine is also a powerful antioxidant. Interacting with other substances, it helps to neutralize toxins, heavy metals, and high histamine levels. It's used as an aid in toxemia during pregnancy as well as in the treatment of rheumatic fever.

Methionine's other claim to fame is that of being a fat emulsifier. Working with choline and inositol (part of the B-complex family), it assists in breaking down fats as well as preventing fatty buildup in the liver, arteries, and other organs—especially around the heart. It's a great aid to the digestive system.

Methionine helps to prevent brittle hair and osteoporosis, brings energy to weak muscles, and is extremely beneficial for allergic symptoms—especially in people who are sensitive to chemicals.

Vital for: antioxidant stimulation and free-radical inhibition, allergies, gallbladder problems, and depression.

Active with: vitamins B_6, B_{12}, and C; folic acid; and magnesium.

Precautions: None known.

Best food sources: chicken, beef, fish, ham, pork, eggs, cottage cheese, liver, soybeans, soy protein, sardines, milk, and yogurt.

Cysteine ("Mr. Clean")
(Conditionally essential)

Precursor for taurine (needed for bile production) and chondroitin sulfate (the main component of cartilage) and synthesized from methionine in the liver. Key points:

- Like its parent methionine, cysteine is a powerful antioxidant and minimizes the damaging effect of free radicals in the body. It's known as the free-radical scavenger. Helps rid the body of the harmful effect of free radicals formed from smoking and drinking.

- Helps combat copper toxicity.
- A powerful immune enhancer, cysteine activates white blood cells in an immune response, breaks down excess and damaging mucus, protects against the harmful effects of smoking and drinking, and promotes wound healing.
- Known as the "hangover remedy," cysteine is a "membrane stabilizer," which helps excess alcohol to pass out of the body quickly.
- Cysteine *is* the protein in hair—keratin—and can be very beneficial in any type of hair loss.

Vital for: antioxidant therapy, metal detoxification, cigarette smoking, hair loss, wound healing, liver or chronic disease, and skin disorders (such as psoriasis and eczema).

Active with: vitamins B_6, B_{12}, and C; folic acid; and magnesium. For protection from free radicals, take cysteine, vitamin C, and B_1.

Precautions: diabetes and kidney or liver stones. May cause stomach irritation. May negate the effectiveness of insulin.

Best food sources: The same as those listed for methionine (see page 458).

Nonessential Amino Acids: Regenerating and Calming

Neuromodulators/Neurotransmitters

Taurine ("The Quiet Fat Buster")
(Conditionally essential)

Synthesized from methionine and cysteine (both yang) in the liver. Key points:

- A neuroinhibitor whose power is equal to that of GABA (gamma-aminobutyric acid) and glycine, taurine calms the nervous system down. It also helps to increase the conversion of glutamine to GABA.
- As a heart protector, taurine helps to regulate the heart's contractions via calcium-regulating effects and also has a "hypotensive," or relaxing, effect on the circulation. It also has the highest concentration of any of the free amino acids in the heart.
- Since taurine is responsible for bile production as well, we could consider this amino acid the "fat buster." Without bile, triglycerides and cholesterol can't be broken down.

- Also known as a staunch immune supporter, taurine stimulates the white blood cell action of the neutrophils and keeps your blood platelets from clumping together.

Vital for: congestive heart failure, epilepsy, hyperactivity, vegetarianism, gallbladder dysfunction, and alcohol withdrawal.
Active with: vitamins B_6 and B_{12}, magnesium, and zinc.
Precaution: Stimulates stomach acid (hydrochloric acid, or HCl).
Best food sources: The same as those listed for methionine (see page 458).

GABA (Gamma-aminobutyric Acid; "Ms. Mellow Mood") (Nonessential)

Synthesized from glutamic acid (yang) in the brain and glutamine (yin). Key point:

- *The* neuroinhibitor, GABA is known as the "natural valium," since it has the ability to suppress anxiety.

Vital for: anxiety, schizophrenia, hypertension, diabetes, appetite suppression, and certain types of depression.
Active with: vitamin B_6, folic acid, magnesium, and glycine.
Precautions: None known.
Best food sources: The same as those listed for glutamine (see page 453).

Neutral Aliphatic

Glycine ("Ms. Brain Food") (Nonessential)

Synthesized from threonine in the brain and a precursor to glutathione and creatinine.

- Strengthens pituitary function.
- Helps in muscle function (great in muscular dystrophy).
- Helps in hypoglycemia by releasing glucogen, which liberates glycogen into the bloodstream.
- Helps to reduce gastric hyperacidity and acidemia of the blood.

A neuroinhibitor similar to GABA (gamma-aminobutyric acid), glycine helps to calm the body, as in cases of anxiety. It's also involved in the body's regeneration:

- It synthesizes heme to hemoglobin.
- It converts creatine, utilized in nucleic acid (RNA/DNA) construction (regenerating the body).
- It's involved along with taurine in bile acid metabolism—so it helps to fight fat.
- It retards muscle degeneration.
- It's essential for the functioning of the central nervous system.
- It's fundamental to a healthy prostate.
- It's required by the immune system to produce the nonessential amino acids.
- It can be used in some kinds of depression, such as that associated with bipolar disorder.

Vital for: hypoglycemia, spastic muscles, hysteria, and wound healing.
Active with: vitamin B_6, folic acid, niacin, and zinc.
Precaution: fatigue.
Best food sources: The same as those listed for threonine (see page 455).

Alanine ("Ms. Stability")
(Nonessential)
Synthesized from glutamine in the small intestine. Key points:

- A neuroinhibitor and readily converts to pyruvate in energy production.
- Helps to stabilize blood sugar levels.
- Along with arginine, acts as an immune stimulant by activating the thymus gland.

Vital for: hypoglycemia, immune deficiency, ketosis (from exercise or diabetes), and anxiety.
Precautions: None known.
Best food sources: The same as those listed for glutamine (see page 453).

Building Amino Acids

Carnitine ("A Powerful Fat Buster")
(Nonessential)
Synthesized from lysine and methionine in the liver. Key points:

- Essential for fatty acid utilization, carnitine transports the long-chain fatty acids into the cells' mitochondria, where they are utilized for energy.

- It therefore prevents fat buildup, aiding in weight loss and strengthening the heart.
- Enhances the effectiveness of antioxidants: vitamins E and C.
- Can increase athletic ability and endurance.
- If you're a vegetarian and lysine-deficient in your food intake, then you'll also be carnitine-deficient.

Vital for: ischemic heart disease, congestive heart failure, high triglycerides, liver disease, muscle weakness, endurance training, and reduction of body fat.

Active with: choline, inositol (part of the B-complex family), arginine, ornithine, and coenzyme Q10.

Precautions: uremia.

Best food sources: The same as those listed for lysine and methionine (see pages 453 and 458).

Glutathione ("Ms. Antiaging")
(Nonessential)

Synthesized from cysteine, glycine, and glutamic acid. Key points:

- Liver detoxifier: protects liver cells and maintains the integrity of red blood cells.
- Free-radical scavenger: helps to rid the body of free radicals and protects the cells from the damage they can cause.
- Immune protector: stimulates the white blood cells' bacteria-killing functions.
- A powerful antioxidant that assists the mineral selenium.

Vital for: immune function and combating aging.

Active with: selenium.

Precautions: None known.

Best food sources: The same as those listed for methionine and glutamine (see pages 458 and 453).

Neutral Aliphatic

Serine ("The Brain Builder")
(Nonessential)

Synthesized from threonine and can be used interchangeably with glycine. Key points:

- A precursor to phospholipids and can help to inhibit memory loss.

Vital for: antiaging and memory loss.
Active with: glycine.
Precautions: Can be immunosuppressive.
Best food sources: The same as those listed for threonine (see page 455).

Neutral Cyclic

Proline ("The Cement Maker")
(Nonessential)
Synthesized predominantly from glutamine and somewhat from histidine. Key points:

- An important constituent of collagen production.
- Strengthens the heart, joints, and tendons.
- Helps to heal cartilage and improves skin texture.

Vital for: all connective tissue injuries.
Precautions: When combined with cigarette smoking or dietary nitrates, procarcinogens can be formed.
Best food sources: The same as those listed for glutamine (see page 453).

Nonessential Amino Acids: Energizing

Neuromodulators/Neurotransmitters

Acidic

Aspartic Acid ("Mr. Energizer")
(Nonessential)
Converts with asparagine and oxaloacetate in the energy-producing Krebs cycle. Key points:
- Since its action is primarily excitatory in the body's nervous tissue, aspartic acid builds up resistance to fatigue.
- It's also fundamentally involved in RNA/DNA (nucleic acid) synthesis, the transportation of minerals in the bloodstream, and the detoxification of ammonia.
- The usual dose is 500 mg one to three times per day with juice or water.

Vital for: fatigue.
Active with: vitamins B_6 and B_{12} and calcium.
Precaution: neuromuscular disorders.
Best food sources: wheat germ, oats, cottage and ricotta cheese, chicken, turkey, wild game.

Glutamic Acid ("The Thinker")
(Nonessential)

Precursor to GABA (gamma-aminobutyric acid) and glutamine (yin). Key points:

- Like its cousin aspartic acid, glutamic acid is an energizer, which acts as an excitatory amino acid in the nervous system.
- It also helps to detoxify brain ammonia.
- Take the same amount as indicated for glutamine (see page 452).

Vital for: mental alertness.
Active with: vitamins B_6 and B_{12} and calcium.
Precaution: neuromuscular disorders.
Best food sources: The same as those listed for glutamine (see page 453).

Building Amino Acids

Basic (Alkaline)

Arginine ("The Regenerator")
(Conditionally essential)

The precursor of ornithine, arginine is synthesized from citrulline (originally from lysine and glutamine).

Necessary for pituitary function, along with ornithine and phenylalanine.

A powerful immune stimulant that has been shown to:

- Increase thymus gland activity by increasing T cell formation and action.
- Decrease tumor growth and development.
- Increase the size of the thymus.
- Speed wound-healing and cellular repair.

Acts as a hormone regulator:

- Speeds up the production of growth hormone.
- Helps to support and regulate insulin production.
- Is involved in stimulating sperm production.

Functions as a liver detoxifier, which detoxifies ammonia into urea and aids in protein synthesis.

Acts as a regenerator:

- Builds muscle mass and tones muscles.
- Reduces body fat.
- Helps in the production of collagen.

Best taken in a 2,000-mg dose on an empty stomach just before bed or one hour before doing a physical workout—for muscle toning.

Vital for: hyperammonemia, alcoholism, hepatitis, infertility, injury, surgery, or metabolism disorders.

Active with: vitamin B_6, magnesium, manganese, and zinc.

Precautions: herpes simplex, schizophrenia, severe liver disease, and moderate kidney failure.

Best food sources: nuts, popcorn, carob, gelatin desserts, chocolate, brown rice, oatmeal, raisins, sunflower and sesame seeds, whole wheat bread, beef, fowl, fish, and eggs.

Ornithine ("The Fat Fighter") (Nonessential)

Synthesized from arginine in the liver. Key points:

- With its parent arginine, ornithine stimulates and regenerates the immune system, especially the thymus gland.
- Stimulates insulin secretion.
- Stimulates the release of the growth hormone that metabolizes excess body fat, especially when combined with carnitine and arginine. Also helps to synthesize the production of sperm.
- Helps to detoxify ammonia from the liver, enhancing liver function.

Vital for: immune deficiency.

Active with: vitamin B_6, magnesium, manganese, and zinc.

Precautions: herpes simplex, schizophrenia, severe liver disease, and moderate kidney failure.

Best food sources: The same as those listed for arginine (see above).

Citrulline ("A Cleaner")
(Nonessential)

Synthesized from glutamine, lysine, and ornithine. Basically detoxifies ammonia from the liver.

Vital only if there is an ornithine deficiency—an inborn metabolic deficiency.

Active with: vitamin B_6, magnesium, manganese, and zinc.

Precautions: None known.

Best food sources: The same as those listed for glutamine and lysine (see page 453).

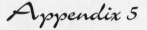

Appendix 5

General Food Choices and Their Calorie Content for Each Meta-Type

The higher the calcium content in foods, the more alkaline the food residue will be; conversely the higher the phosphorus content, the more acid the residue. *Residue* refers to the "ash," or the end products of foods after they've been broken down in the body and stored in the fat cells.

In the tables in appendix 5, rows 1–3 list alkaline foods—foods that are predominantly yin in nature and represent the synthesizer alkaline structure. These foods, whose structure is the opposite of the acid accelerator profiles, are exactly what accelerators require. Conversely rows 4–6 list acid foods—foods that are predominantly yang in nature and represent the accelerator acid structure. Since the structure of these foods is the opposite of the alkaline synthesizer profiles, they are exactly what synthesizers need.

Within each "Food Type" row in the tables, the foods in the "Food" column are listed in descending order according to the level of their acid or alkaline content—starting with those that have the highest acid or alkaline content and ending with those that have the lowest acid or alkaline content.

The accompanying table shows which food types are the most appropriate for each metabolic type. In general, you should avoid foods that form the same acid or alkaline structure as your own meta-type. The foods that "bookend" your meta-type may be eaten occasionally or once or twice a week. The foods whose acid or alkaline structure is the opposite of your own meta-type can be eaten often or on a daily basis. For instance, the very acid accelerators should stay away from the strong acid foods and only have the acid forming and weak acid foods once in a while, but they can eat the alkaline forming, strong alkaline, and weak alkaline foods every day.

Proteins

Meat

Combine with slightly starchy and nonstarchy vegetables. *Don't* combine with grains, starches, starchy vegetables, oils, or fats.

FOOD TYPE	FOOD	AMOUNT	CALORIES
1 Strong Alkaline pH: 8–7.5 (synthesizer)	—	—	—
2 Alkaline Forming pH: 7.4—blood (balanced synthesizer)	—	—	—
3 Weak Alkaline pH: 6.8 (mixed synthesizer)	—	—	—
4 Weak Acid pH: 6.2 (mixed accelerator)	—	—	—
5 Acid Forming pH: 5 (balanced accelerator)	—	—	—
6 Strong Acid pH: 4.5–4 (accelerator)	Venison	3½ oz.	140
	Veal	3 oz.	250
	Kidneys	3 oz.	120
	Liver	3 oz.	160
	Sweetbreads	2½ oz.	125

FOOD TYPE	FOOD	AMOUNT	CALORIES
	Ham		
	Baked	3 oz.	375
	Baked	1 slice, ¼ × 3½ × 2½	100
	Prosciutto	1½ oz.	170
	Beef		
	Pot roast	3 oz.	340
	Hamburger	3 oz.	185
	Steak hamburger	3 oz.	400
	London broil	4 oz.	200
	Filet mignon	3 oz.	248
	Porterhouse	4 oz.	290
	Sirloin	4 oz.	250
	T-bone	4 oz.	295
	Roast	3½ oz.	340
	Club	3½ oz.	190
	Rib steak	4 oz.	315
	Round steak	3 oz.	288
	Sirloin tips	4 oz.	200
	Oxtails	4 oz.	250
	Soup	1 cup	190
	Beef organs		
	Brains	3 oz.	106
	Heart	3 oz.	192
	Kidneys	3 oz.	120
	Liver	1 lb.	635
	Lamb		
	Breast	4 oz.	350
	Broiled chop	1" thick	250
	Leg roast	4 oz.	350
	Lean	4 oz.	160
	Roast	4 oz.	200
	Shoulder roast	4 oz.	350
	Liver	4 oz.	207
	Kidneys	4 oz.	120
	Rabbit	3½ oz.	175

Fowl

Combine with slightly starchy and nonstarchy vegetables. *Don't* combine with grains, starches, starchy vegetables, oils, or fats.

FOOD TYPE	FOOD	AMOUNT	CALORIES
1 Strong Alkaline pH: 8–7.5 (synthesizer)	—	—	—
2 Alkaline Forming pH: 7.4—blood (balanced synthesizer)	—	—	—
3 Weak Alkaline pH: 6.8 (mixed synthesizer)	—	—	—
4 Weak Acid pH: 6.2 (mixed accelerator)	—	—	—
5 Acid Forming pH: 5 (balanced accelerator)	Eggs		
	Boiled/poached	1	75
	Scrambled	1	125
	Omelet	2 eggs	185
	Yolk	1	62
	Yolks	1 cup	880
	Yolks, dried	1 oz.	200
	White	1	15
	Whites	1 cup	120
6 Strong Acid pH: 4.5–4 (accelerator)	Turkey		
	Roasted	4 oz. (2 slices: 4″ × 2½″ × ¼″)	304
	Smoked	2½ oz.	125
	Giblets	⅓ cup	160
	Goose		
	Meat without skin	3½ oz.	155
	Fat	1 tbs.	145
	Liver	6 oz.	150
	Squab		
	Roasted	Whole	200
	Chicken		
	Broth	1 cup	35
	Breast	½	200
	Leg or thigh	1	180
	Slices	3 (¼″ × 3½″ × 2½″)	175
	Giblets	⅓ cup	160
	Liver	1 med.	50
	Capon, roast	3 oz.	225
	Duck		
	Meat with skin	4 oz.	300
	Meat without skin	4 oz.	160

FOOD TYPE	FOOD	AMOUNT	CALORIES
	Roasted	4 oz.	200
	Egg	1	125
	Wild	3½ oz.	275
	Frog legs		
	Raw	4 oz.	80
	Fried	4 oz.	175
	Pheasant		
	Breast	½	145
	Thigh	1	145
	Quail	1 lb.	330

Fish

Combine with slightly starchy and nonstarchy vegetables. *Don't* combine with grains, starches, starchy vegetables, oils, or fats.

FOOD TYPE	FOOD	AMOUNT	CALORIES
1 Strong Alkaline pH: 8–7.5 (synthesizer)	—	—	—
2 Alkaline Forming pH: 7.4—blood (balanced synthesizer)	—	—	—
3 Weak Alkaline pH: 6.8 (mixed synthesizer)	—	—	—
4 Weak Acid pH: 6.2 (mixed accelerator)	Caviar	1 tbs.	50
	Anchovies	6 (1 oz.)	50
	Sardines, canned		
	Solids only	3 oz.	180
	Oil, liquid, and solids	3 oz.	290
	Natural pack	3 oz.	170
	In oil	1 (2½″)	40
	Herring		
	Atlantic	1 med.	217
	Lake	1 med.	140
	Kippered	1 oz.	60
	Pacific	1 sm.	94
	Pickled	2 sm.	223
	Smoked	½ fish	210
5 Acid Forming pH: 5 (balanced accelerator)	Carp	6 oz.	100

FOOD TYPE	FOOD	AMOUNT	CALORIES
	Yellowtail	4 oz.	200
	Hake, baked	4 oz.	125
	Salmon		
	Baked/broiled steak	1–6 oz.	294
	Steamed	4 oz.	140
	Nova	2 oz.	200
	Smoked	2 oz.	200
	Perch		
	Lake	4 oz.	75
	Ocean	4 oz.	85
	Bass, sea	4 oz.	105
	Trout, broiled	4 oz.	130
6 Strong Acid			
pH: 4.5–4 (accelerator)	Mackerel, broiled	3 oz.	200
	Roe	1 tbs.	17
	Halibut, broiled steak	4 oz.	225
	Red snapper	4 oz.	100
	Sole		
	Fillet, broiled	4 oz.	125
	Raw	4 oz.	80
	Tuna		
	Fresh	3 oz.	170
	Cooked	¾ cup	100
	Bluefish	4 oz.	195
	Eel		
	Raw	4 oz.	180
	Baked/broiled	4 oz.	180
	Swordfish, broiled steak	4 oz.	225
	Squid	4 oz.	125
	Cod		
	Steak	½ lb.	190
	Dried	3.5 oz.	122
	Liver oil	1 tbs.	150
	Roe	1 tbs.	130
	Mullet/haddock, baked/broiled	4 oz.	158
	Sturgeon	2 oz.	175
	Octopus (calamari)	4 oz.	85

Shellfish

Combine with slightly starchy and nonstarchy vegetables. *Don't* combine with grains, starches, starchy vegetables, oils, or fats.

FOOD TYPE	FOOD	AMOUNT	CALORIES
1 Strong Alkaline pH: 8–7.5 (synthesizer)	—	—	—
2 Alkaline Forming pH: 7.4—blood (balanced synthesizer)	—	—	—
3 Weak Alkaline pH: 6.8 (mixed synthesizer)	—	—	—
4 Weak Acid pH: 6.2 (mixed accelerator)	Oysters		
	Raw	12	100
	Cooked	12	85
	Stew	1 cup	200
	Scallops, raw	4 oz.	90
5 Acid Forming pH: 5 (balanced accelerator)	Crab		
	Hard-shell	3 oz.	90
	Meat	½ cup	65
	Soft-shell	1 med.	100
	Lobster		
	Boiled	4 oz.	90
	Boiled	1 whole	175
	Tails	4 oz.	100
	Scallops, cooked	4 oz.	100
	Clam		
	Cherrystone, raw/steamed	12 med.	125
	Broth	6 oz.	50
	Chowder, Manhattan	1 cup	100
	Chowder, Boston	1 cup	275
	Juice	6 oz.	50
	Mussels	12	125
	Shrimp/crayfish	10 av.	100
	Boiled	4 oz.	120
6 Strong Acid pH: 4.5–4 (accelerator)	Abalone	3.5 oz.	100
	Canned	½ cup	80

Dairy

Combine with slightly starchy and nonstarchy vegetables. *Don't* combine with grains, starches, starchy vegetables, oils, or fats.

FOOD TYPE	FOOD	AMOUNT	CALORIES
1 Strong Alkaline pH: 8–7.5 (synthesizer)	—	—	—
2 Alkaline Forming pH: 7.4—blood (balanced synthesizer)	—	—	—
3 Weak Alkaline pH: 6.8 (mixed synthesizer)	Whey, dried	1 tbs.	39
	Milk, goat's	1 cup	165
		1 qt.	655
	Yogurt		
	Whole	1 cup	166
	Low-fat	1 cup	123
	Milk, cow's		
	Whole	1 cup	159
	Low-fat	1 cup	145
	Skim	1 cup	88
	Cream		
	Heavy	1 tbs.	50
		½ pt.	780
	Light	1 tbs.	30
		½ pt.	490
	Whipped	1 tbs.	35
		½ pt.	390
	Sauce	1 tbs.	45
	Sour	¼ cup	200
	Buttermilk	1 cup	85
		1 qt.	350
	Cheese		
	Parmesan	1 oz.	112
		1 tbs.	30
	Limburger	1 oz.	95
	Cheddar	1 oz.	115
	Brick	1 oz.	100
	Swiss	1 oz.	105
4 Weak Acid pH: 6.2 (mixed accelerator)	Cheese		
	Camembert	1 oz.	85
	Brie	1 oz.	100
	Edam	1 oz.	88

FOOD TYPE	FOOD	AMOUNT	CALORIES
	Gruyère	1 oz.	115
	Cottage, whole	1 cup	240
		1 oz.	25
	Cottage, noncream	1 cup	125
	Farmer	½ cup	200
	Feta	1 oz.	88
	Ricotta	½ cup	200
	Muenster	1 oz.	100
	Monterey Jack	1 oz.	103
	Provolone	1 oz.	95
	Mozzarella	1 oz.	95
	Goat	1½ oz.	175
	Blue	1 oz.	105
	Gorgonzola	1 oz.	100
	Whey, liquid	1 cup	85
5 Acid Forming pH: 5 (balanced accelerator)	—	—	—
6 Strong Acid pH: 4.5–4 (accelerator)	—	—	—

Seeds

Combine with slightly starchy and nonstarchy vegetables. *Can* be combined with grains, starches, starchy vegetables, oils, and fats.

FOOD TYPE	FOOD	AMOUNT	CALORIES
1 Strong Alkaline pH: 8–7.5 (synthesizer)	—	—	—
2 Alkaline Forming pH: 7.4—blood (balanced synthesizer)	—	—	—
3 Weak Alkaline pH: 6.8 (mixed synthesizer)	—	—	—
4 Weak Acid pH: 6.2 (mixed accelerator)	—	—	—
5 Acid Forming pH: 5 (balanced accelerator)	—	—	—
6 Strong Acid pH: 4.5–4 (accelerator)	Pumpkin seeds		
	Whole	4 oz.	464
	Hulled	4 oz.	625

FOOD TYPE	FOOD	AMOUNT	CALORIES
	Sunflower seeds		
	Whole	1 oz.	86
	Hulled	1 oz.	159
	Sesame seeds		
	Whole	1 oz.	86
	Hulled	1 oz.	165
	Squash seeds, hulled	4 oz.	525
	Safflower seeds, hulled	1 oz.	165
	Flaxseeds, whole	1 oz.	86

Nuts

Combine with slightly starchy and nonstarchy vegetables. *Can* be combined with grains, starches, starchy vegetables, oils, and fats.

FOOD TYPE	FOOD	AMOUNT	CALORIES
1 Strong Alkaline pH: 8–7.5 (synthesizer)	—	—	—
2 Alkaline Forming pH: 7.4—blood (balanced synthesizer)	—	—	—
3 Weak Alkaline pH: 6.8 (mixed synthesizer)	Coconut milk	1 cup	60
4 Weak Acid pH: 6.2 (mixed accelerator)	Filberts (hazelnuts)	1 oz.	110
	Hickory nuts	1 oz.	110
5 Acid Forming pH: 5 (balanced accelerator)	Pecans, raw	1 oz.	190
	Pistachio nuts, raw	1 oz.	170
	Walnuts	1 oz.	150
	Brazil nuts	1 oz.	180
	Macadamia nuts	1 oz.	200
	Chestnuts	1 oz.	50
	Almonds	1 oz.	160
	Almond meal	1 oz.	116
6 Strong Acid pH: 4.5–4 (accelerator)	Pine nuts	1 oz.	160
	Water chestnuts	1 oz.	128
	Cashews	1 oz.	160
	Coconut meat	2″ × 2″ × ½″ piece	160
	Shredded	1 cup	350
	Dried shredded	1 cup	345

Legumes: Protein

Combine with slightly starchy and nonstarchy vegetables. *Can* be combined with grains, starches, starchy vegetables, oils, and fats.

FOOD TYPE	FOOD	AMOUNT	CALORIES
1 Strong Alkaline pH: 8–7.5 (synthesizer)	—	—	—
2 Alkaline Forming pH: 7.4—blood (balanced synthesizer)	—	—	—
3 Weak Alkaline pH: 6.8 (mixed synthesizer)	Soybean curd (tofu)	4 oz.	80
		3 oz.	60
4 Weak Acid pH: 6.2 (mixed accelerator)	—	—	—
5 Acid Forming pH: 5 (balanced accelerator)	Lentils	1 oz.	85
	Cooked	½ cup	115
	Soybeans		
	Fresh, shelled	1 cup	150
	Dried	½ cup	350
	Cooked	½ cup	150
	Roasted	1 oz.	145
	Soybean milk	¼ cup	40
	Beans, cooked		
	Adzuki	½ cup	115
	Black	½ cup	115
	Kidney	½ cup	115
	Navy	½ cup	115
	Pinto	½ cup	115
	Red	½ cup	115
6 Strong Acid pH: 4.5–4 (accelerator)	Peanuts	1 oz.	160

Fruit: Protein

Combine with slightly starchy and nonstarchy vegetables. *Can* be combined with grains, starches, starchy vegetables, oils, and fats.

FOOD TYPE	FOOD	AMOUNT	CALORIES
1 Strong Alkaline			
pH: 8–7.5 (synthesizer)	Olives	1 oz.	25
2 Alkaline Forming			
pH: 7.4—blood (balanced synthesizer)	—	—	—
3 Weak Alkaline			
pH: 6.8 (mixed synthesizer)	—	—	—
4 Weak Acid			
pH: 6.2 (mixed accelerator)	—	—	—
5 Acid Forming			
pH: 5 (balanced accelerator)	—	—	—
6 Strong Acid			
pH: 4.5–4 (accelerator)	Avocado	½	279

Carbohydrates: High-starch

Grains

Combine with starchy and nonstarchy vegetables, fats, and oils. Do *not* combine with proteins. *Can* be combined with legume proteins, nuts, seeds, and fruit proteins.

FOOD TYPE	FOOD	AMOUNT	CALORIES
1 Strong Alkaline			
pH: 8–7.5 (synthesizer)	Amaranth, cooked	1 cup	100
2 Alkaline Forming			
pH: 7.4—blood (balanced synthesizer)	—	—	—
3 Weak Alkaline			
pH: 6.8 (mixed synthesizer)	—	—	—
4 Weak Acid			
pH: 6.2 (mixed accelerator)	—	—	—
5 Acid Forming			
pH: 5 (balanced accelerator)	Farina		
	Cooked	1 cup	105
	Raw	1 cup	625
	Rice		
	Brown, cooked	½ cup	110
	Brown, raw	½ cup	375
	Wild, cooked	¾ cup	110

FOOD TYPE	FOOD	AMOUNT	CALORIES
	Cakes	2 oz.	225
	Buckwheat		
	Groats, cooked	½ cup	100
	Flour	1 oz.	240
	Bread, wheat or sprouted grain	1 slice	70
	Quinoa, cooked	½ cup	50
6 Strong Acid			
pH: 4.5–4 (accelerator)	Popcorn	1 oz.	110
	Corn grits		
	Cooked	1 cup	125
	Dry	1 cup	580
	Rice bran	1 cup	125
	Wild rice, dry	½ cup	295
	Millet, cooked	½ cup	50
	Barley, cooked	½ cup	200
	Cornmeal, white/yellow	1 oz.	100
	Wheat		
	Whole-grain	1 oz. (1 cup cooked)	100
	Bran	1 oz.	100
	Germ	1 oz.	100
	Bulgur (cracked wheat)	½ cup	120
	Rye	1 oz.	100
	Oats/oat bran, uncooked	1 oz.	110
	Oatmeal, cooked	½ cup	75
	Pastinas (egg)	1 oz.	110

Flour

FOOD TYPE	FOOD	AMOUNT	CALORIES
1 Strong Alkaline pH: 8–7.5 (synthesizer)	Carob	1 oz.	50
2 Alkaline Forming pH: 7.4—blood (balanced synthesizer)	—	—	—
3 Weak Alkaline pH: 6.8 (mixed synthesizer)	—	—	—
4 Weak Acid pH: 6.2 (mixed accelerator)	—	—	—
5 Acid Forming pH: 5 (balanced accelerator)	Chestnut	1 oz.	103

FOOD TYPE	FOOD	AMOUNT	CALORIES
	Sunflower	1 oz.	100
	Soybean	1 cup	230
6 Strong Acid			
pH: 4.5–4 (accelerator)	Corn	1 cup	405
	Rye	1 cup	400
	Wheat	1 cup	456
	Rice	1 cup	550

Legumes: High-starch

Combine with starchy and nonstarchy vegetables, fats, and oils. Do *not* combine with proteins and fruit. *Can* be combined with legume proteins.

FOOD TYPE	FOOD	AMOUNT	CALORIES
1 Strong Alkaline			
pH: 8–7.5 (synthesizer)	—	—	—
2 Alkaline Forming			
pH: 7.4—blood (balanced synthesizer)	—	—	—
3 Weak Alkaline			
pH: 6.8 (mixed synthesizer)	—	—	—
4 Weak Acid			
pH: 6.2 (mixed accelerator)	—	—	—
5 Acid Forming			
pH: 5 (balanced accelerator)	Lima beans		
	Dry	½ cup	265
	Fresh	½ cup	100
	Garbanzo beans, dry	1 cup	755
	Great northern beans, dry	½ cup	300
	Split peas, dry	1 cup	689
	White beans, dry	½ cup	322
6 Strong Acid	Black-eyed peas		
pH: 4.5–4 (accelerator)	(cowpeas), cooked	1 cup	150

Vegetables: High-starch

Combine with starchy and nonstarchy vegetables, fats, and oils. Do *not* combine with proteins and fruit. *Can* be combined with legume proteins.

FOOD TYPE	FOOD	AMOUNT	CALORIES
1 **Strong Alkaline** pH: 8–7.5 (synthesizer)	—	—	—
2 **Alkaline Forming** pH: 7.4—blood (balanced synthesizer)	—	—	—
3 **Weak Alkaline** pH: 6.8 (mixed synthesizer)	Acorn squash	½ cup	50
4 **Weak Acid** pH: 6.2 (mixed accelerator)	Butternut squash	1 cup	35
	Hubbard squash	1 cup	35
	Sweet potatoes	5 oz.	215
	Pumpkin, canned	4 oz.	7
5 **Acid Forming** pH: 5 (balanced accelerator)	Yam	5 oz.	190
	Pumpkin, raw	1 oz.	4
6 **Strong Acid** pH: 4.5–4 (accelerator)	Corn		
	Field	5 oz. (1 ear)	80
	Sweet	5 oz. (1 ear)	100
	Potatoes		
	Raw	1 oz.	25
	Boiled/baked	4 oz.	85

Vegetables: Slightly Starchy

Combine with starchy and nonstarchy vegetables, fats, and oils. Do *not* combine with fruits. *Can* be combined with proteins.

FOOD TYPE	FOOD	AMOUNT	CALORIES
1 **Strong Alkaline** pH: 8–7.5 (synthesizer)	—	—	—
2 **Alkaline Forming** pH: 7.4—blood (balanced synthesizer)	—	—	—

FOOD TYPE	FOOD	AMOUNT	CALORIES
3 Weak Alkaline pH: 6.8 (mixed synthesizer)	Carrots		
	Raw	1 oz.	7
	Steamed	4 oz.	20
	Juice	1 oz.	7
	Rutabagas, cooked	½ cup	30
4 Weak Acid pH: 6.2 (mixed accelerator)	Beets, cooked (steamed)	2 oz.	25
	Parsnip	1 lg.	75
	Jicama, cooked	½ cup	30
5 Acid Forming pH: 5 (balanced accelerator)	Beets, raw	1 oz.	12
		½ cup	35
6 Strong Acid pH: 4.5–4 (accelerator)	—	—	—

Carbohydrates: Nonstarchy—Vegetables

Combine with starchy vegetables, fats, oils, grains, and proteins. Do *not* combine with fruits.

FOOD TYPE	FOOD	AMOUNT	CALORIES
1 Strong Alkaline pH: 8–7.5 (synthesizer)	Kale, cooked	1 cup	45
	Collards	1 cup	75
	Swiss chard, cooked	1 cup	50
	Parsley, fresh	1 tbs.	2
	Mustard greens, cooked	1 cup	30
	Beet greens, cooked	1 cup	40
	Turnip greens, cooked	½ cup	22
	Lamb's-quarters, raw or cooked	1 cup	30
	Mustard spinach, raw or cooked	1 cup	45
	Seaweed		
	Irish moss	2 oz.	12
	Kelp	1 cup cooked	45
	Dulse	4 oz.	23
	Arame	4 oz.	23
2 Alkaline Forming pH: 7.4—blood (balanced synthesizer)	Dock, cooked	1 cup	10

FOOD TYPE	FOOD	AMOUNT	CALORIES
	Chicory greens	30 leaves	20
	Horseradish	1 tsp.	5
	Cabbage, cooked	1 cup	40
	Okra, cooked	1 lb.	150
	Swiss chard, raw	1 cup	50
	Spinach, cooked	1 cup	45
	Kale, raw	4 cups	45
	Lettuce		
	Cos	2 oz.	7
	Romaine	2 oz.	7
	Dark green	2 oz.	7
	White	2 oz.	7
	Watercress	1 cup	10
	Alfalfa sprouts	1 cup	10
	Dandelion greens		
	Steamed	1 cup	75
	Raw	1 cup	100
	Arugula	1 cup	10
	Beet greens, raw	1 cup	10
3 Weak Alkaline pH: 6.8 (mixed synthesizer)	Summer squash, cooked	4 oz.	15
	Leeks	4 oz.	25
	Cress, garden	1 cup	10
	Chinese cabbage	1 cup	15
	Beans		
	Snap	1 cup	25
	Yellow	1 cup	25
	Turnips	½ cup	21
	Scallions	5	25
	Broccoli	1 cup	45
	Lettuce		
	Butter	2 oz.	7
	Boston	2 oz.	7
	Iceberg	2 oz.	7
	Celery, raw	1 cup	18
	Endive/radicchio	1 oz.	3
	Dock, raw	1 cup	10
	Cabbage, raw	¾ cup	20
	Okra, raw	½ cup	40
	Spinach, raw	1 cup	10
	Fennel	1 cup	10
4 Weak Acid pH: 6.2 (mixed accelerator)	Cauliflower, cooked	1 cup	30

FOOD TYPE	FOOD	AMOUNT	CALORIES
	Eggplant, raw	1 oz.	4
	Artichoke	1 lg.	70
	Heart	1	50
	Shallot	1 clove	2
	Gingerroot, fresh	4 oz.	52
	Salsify, cooked	½ cup	55
	Soybean sprouts	1 cup	50
	Kohlrabi		
	Cooked	1 cup	45
	Raw	1 cup	40
	Chicory		
	Boiled	4 oz.	6
	Raw	1 cup	2
	Onions	1 oz.	7
	Cucumber	1 oz.	3
	Radishes	1 oz.	4
	Summer squash		
	Steamed	4 oz.	15
	Raw	4 oz.	15
5 Acid Forming			
pH: 5 (balanced accelerator)	Bamboo shoots, canned	1 oz.	8
	Peas, cooked		
	Green	1 cup	80
	Sugar snap	1 cup	120
	Mung bean sprouts	1 cup	50
	Peppers, chili	1 oz.	4
	Asparagus	4 oz.	10
	Beans, mung	⅓ cup	10
	Celeriac root	1 cup	20
	Peppers, sweet	1 oz.	4
	Brussels sprouts, steamed	4 oz.	20
	Cauliflower, raw	1 cup	25
	Tomatoes	1 oz.	4
6 Strong Acid			
pH: 4.5–4 (accelerator)	Mushrooms	1 oz.	4
	Garlic	1 clove	1

Carbohydrates: Fruits, Sweet Fruits, and Melons

Fruits

Fruits should be eaten by themselves—at least half an hour after meals. The fruits on the following table can be mixed together if they are on your food list.

FOOD TYPE	FOOD	AMOUNT	CALORIES
1 Strong Alkaline pH: 8–7.5 (synthesizer)	Rhubarb, stewed, unsweetened	1 cup	35
2 Alkaline Forming pH: 7.4—blood (balanced synthesizer)	Loganberries	½ cup	45
	Orange	1 med.	75
	Clementine	1 med.	35
	Tangerine	1 med.	35
	Kumquats	6 med.	75
	Kiwifruit	1 med.	60
3 Weak Alkaline pH: 6.8 (mixed synthesizer)	Boysenberries	1 cup	100
	Grapefruit	1 sm.	50
	Raspberries	½ cup	50
	Strawberries	1 cup	50
	Plum	1 med.	20
	Acerola cherries	1 cup	60
	Blueberries	1 cup	100
	Nectarine	1 med.	50
	Gooseberries	1 cup	60
	Pokeberries	½ cup	60
	Papaya	½ cup	35
	Grapes		
	Concord	1 cup	85
	Thompson	1 cup	85
	Elderberries	1 cup	50
	Sapotes	¼ lb.	108
	Cranberries	1 cup	55
	Currants		
	Fresh	1 cup	60
	Dried	½ cup	300
	Lemon	1 med.	25
	Cherries		
	Sour	1 cup	65

FOOD TYPE	FOOD	AMOUNT	CALORIES
	Sweet	15 lg.	85
	Blackberries	1 cup	100
	Lime	1 med.	20
4 Weak Acid			
pH: 6.2 (mixed accelerator)	Guava	1 med.	50
	Loquats	10	60
	Cherimoya	1 cup	80
	Grapes		
	Muscat	1 cup	100
	Tokay	1 cup	100
	Quince	1 med.	20
	Tamarinds	¼ lb.	130
	Apples	6 oz.	50
	Apricot		
	Raw	1	9
	Dried	1	25
	Prickly pears	1 med.	52
	Pear	1 med.	95
	Mango	1 av.	100
5 Acid Forming			
pH: 5 (balanced accelerator)	Litchis	¼ lb.	44
	Passion fruit	4 oz.	15
	Groundberries	1 cup	50
	Pomegranate pulp	1 med. fruit	75
	Crab apples	2 oz.	45
	Peach	1 med.	45
6 Strong Acid			
pH: 4.5–4 (accelerator)	—	—	—

Sweet Fruits

The fruits on the following table *can* be mixed together, as long as you pick your appropriate row.

FOOD TYPE	FOOD	AMOUNT	CALORIES
1 Strong Alkaline			
pH: 8–7.5 (synthesizer)	—	—	—
2 Alkaline Forming			
pH: 7.4—blood (balanced synthesizer)	Pineapple		
	Fresh	1 cup	75
	Crushed, unsweetened	½ cup	100

FOOD TYPE	FOOD	AMOUNT	CALORIES
3 Weak Alkaline			
pH: 6.8 (mixed synthesizer)	Figs	4 oz.	120
	Dried	1 oz.	50
4 Weak Acid			
pH: 6.2 (mixed accelerator)	Apricots, dried	2	50
	Raisins	1 oz.	70
	Prunes	1 oz.	40
	Dates, pitted	1 oz.	70
5 Acid Forming			
pH: 5 (balanced accelerator)	Persimmons, raw	1 oz.	15
	Plantain	1 med.	135
	Banana	1 lg.	100
6 Strong Acid			
pH: 4.5–4 (accelerator)	—	—	—

Melons

It's best to eat melons by themselves—at least half an hour after meals.

FOOD TYPE	FOOD	AMOUNT	CALORIES
1 Strong Alkaline			
pH: 8–7.5 (synthesizer)	—	—	—
2 Alkaline Forming			
pH: 7.4—blood (balanced synthesizer)	—	—	—
3 Weak Alkaline			
pH: 6.8 (mixed synthesizer)	—	—	—
4 Weak Acid			
pH: 6.2 (mixed accelerator)	Watermelon	1 med. slice	100
	Muskmelon	¼	65
	Cantaloupe	½	100
	Honeydew	¼	65
	Casaba	¼	65
	Crenshaw	½	100
5 Acid Forming			
pH: 5 (balanced accelerator)	—	—	—
6 Strong Acid			
pH: 4.5–4 (accelerator)	—	—	—

Fats and Oils

Combine well with grains, legumes, and starchy and nonstarchy vegetables. Do *not* combine with proteins.

FOOD TYPE	FOOD	AMOUNT	CALORIES
1 Strong Alkaline			
pH: 8–7.5 (synthesizer)	—	—	—
2 Alkaline Forming			
pH: 7.4—blood (balanced synthesizer)	—	—	—
3 Weak Alkaline			
pH: 6.8 (mixed synthesizer)	Butter	1 oz.	210
	Margarine	1 oz.	210
4 Weak Acid			
pH: 6.2 (mixed accelerator)	—	—	—
5 Acid Forming			
pH: 5 (balanced accelerator)	Mayonnaise	1 tbs.	100
6 Strong Acid			
pH: 4.5–4 (accelerator)	Oil		
	Avocado	1 tbs.	125
	Corn	1 tbs.	100
	Soybean	1 tbs.	125
	Peanut	1 tbs.	100
	Cottonseed	1 tbs.	125
	Olive	1 tbs.	125
	Safflower	1 tbs.	125
	Sunflower	1 tbs.	125
	Walnut	1 tbs.	125
	Apricot	1 tbs.	125
	Almond	1 tbs.	125

Beverages

FOOD TYPE	FOOD	AMOUNT	CALORIES
1 Strong Alkaline			
pH: 8–7.5 (synthesizer)	—	—	—
2 Alkaline Forming			
pH: 7.4—blood (balanced synthesizer)	Juice		
	Carrot	4 oz.	45
	Fig, unsweetened	6 oz.	60

FOOD TYPE	FOOD	AMOUNT	CALORIES
	Loganberry	6 oz.	80
	Tangerine	4 oz.	50
	Orange	4 oz.	55
	Pineapple	8 oz.	125
3 Weak Alkaline			
pH: 6.8 (mixed synthesizer)	Juice		
	Apple	8 oz.	125
	Apple cider	6 oz.	75
	Apricot	6 oz.	120
	Blackberry	6 oz.	75
	Blueberry	4 oz.	70
	Cranberry	4 oz.	94
	Grape	4 oz.	75
	Lemon	4 oz.	30
	Lime	4 oz.	30
	Nectarine	6 oz.	100
	Papaya	6 oz.	75
	Raspberry	6 oz.	100
4 Weak Acid			
pH: 6.2 (mixed accelerator)	Juice		
	Pear	4 oz.	55
	Quince	4 oz.	45
5 Acid Forming			
pH: 5 (balanced accelerator)	Juice		
	Clam	6 oz.	50
	Passionfruit	4 oz.	75
	Peach	4 oz.	50
	Tomato	8 oz.	50
6 Strong Acid			
pH: 4.5–4 (accelerator)	—	—	—

Miscellaneous

FOOD TYPE	FOOD	AMOUNT	CALORIES
1 Strong Alkaline			
pH: 8–7.5 (synthesizer)	Molasses		
	Light	1 tbs.	50
	Blackstrap	1 tbs.	45
	Brown sugar	1 tbs.	50
	Sorghum syrup	1 tbs.	55

FOOD TYPE	FOOD	AMOUNT	CALORIES
	Maple syrup	1 tbs.	60
2 Alkaline Forming			
pH: 7.4—blood (balanced synthesizer)	Cane syrup	1 tbs.	50
3 Weak Alkaline			
pH: 6.8 (mixed synthesizer)	Pickle, dill	1 lg.	15
	Cane sugar	1 tsp.	18
4 Weak Acid			
pH: 6.2 (mixed accelerator)	Vinegar	1 tbs.	20
	Soy sauce	1 tbs.	7
	Honey	1 tbs.	60
	Mustard	1 tsp.	5
5 Acid Forming			
pH: 5 (balanced accelerator)	—	—	—
6 Strong Acid			
pH: 4.5—4 (accelerator)	Yeast		
	Baker's	1 oz.	24
	Brewer's	1 tbs.	22

Index

About the Author

DR. ELIZABETH DANE is a practitioner of complementary medicine. She has a Ph.D. in Chinese medicine and philosophy and has worked with people from all walks of life for decades. Among her celebrity clients are Ann Reinking, Bebe Neuwirth, James Taylor, Anjelica Huston, and Mercedes Ellington.